Clinical Chemistry in Diagnosis and Treatment

This book is to

The Educational Low-Priced Books Scheme is funded by the Overseas Development Administration as part of the British Government overseas aid programme. It makes available low-priced, unabridged editions of British publishers' textbooks to students in developing countries. Below is a list of some other medical books published under the ELBS imprint.

Baron, Whicher and Lee
A New Short Textbook of Chemical Pathology
Edward Arnold

Govan
Pathology Illustrated
Churchill Livingstone

Kumar and Clark (editors)
Clinical Medicine
Baillière Tindall

MacSween and Whaley (editors)
Muir's Textbook of Pathology
Edward Arnold

Munro and Edwards (editors)
MacLeod's Clinical Examination
Churchill Livingstone

Ogilvie and Evans
Chamberlain's Symptoms and Signs in Clinical Medicine
Butterworth-Heinemann

Swash
Hutchison's Clinical Methods
Baillière Tindall

Weatherall, Ledingham and Warrell (editors)
Oxford Textbook of Medicine Vols 1 and 2
Oxford University Press

Clinical Chemistry in Diagnosis and Treatment

Sixth Edition

Philip D Mayne

MD (Dublin), BA (Mod), MSc (London), FRCPI, FRCPath, FFPath (RCPI)
Consultant in Chemical Pathology, The Children's Hospital, Temple Street
and The Rotunda Hospital, Dublin;
Formerly, Senior Lecturer in Chemical Pathology, Charing Cross and
Westminster Medical School, London

Formerly Zilva . Pannall . Mayne

A member of the Hodder Headline Group
LONDON • SYDNEY • AUCKLAND
Co-published in the USA by
Oxford University Press, Inc., New York

First published in Great Britain 1971 by
Lloyd-Luke (Medical Books) Ltd

Second edition 1975
Third edition 1979
Asian edition published by
PG Publishing Pte Ltd, 1983
Fourth edition 1984
Asian edition published by
PG Publishing Pte Ltd, 1984
Fifth edition 1988
Reprinted with corrections 1989
Sixth edition 1994
Third impression 1998 by Arnold
a member of the Hodder Headline Group plc,
338 Euston Road, London NW1 3BH

(This work has also been translated into Spanish, Serbo-Croat,
Italian, Turkish, Greek, Russian and Bahasa Malaysia)

Co-published in the United States of America by
Oxford University Press, Inc.,
198 Madison Avenue, New York, NY 10016
Oxford is a registered trademark of Oxford University Press

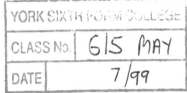
Whilst the advice and information in this book is believed to be true and
accurate at the date of going to press, neither the author nor the publisher
can accept any legal responsibility for any errors or omissions that may be
made. In particular (but without limiting the generality of the preceding
disclaimer) every effort has been made to check drug dosages; however, it
is still possible that errors have been missed. Furthermore, dosage
schedules are constantly being revised and new side effects recognized.
For these reasons the reader is strongly urged to consult the drug
companies' printed instructions before administering any of the drugs
recommended in this book.

British Library Cataloguing in Publication Data
A catalogue record for this book is available from the British Library

Library of Congress Cataloging-in-Publication Data
A catalog record for this book is available from the Library of Congress

ISBN 0 340 57647 2

Composition by Scribe Design, Gillingham, Kent
Printed and bound in Great Britain by Bath Press Colourbooks, Glasgow

Foreword to the first edition

This book aims at giving, within a single cover, all the relevant biochemical and pathological facts and theories necessary to the intelligent interpretation of the analyses usually performed in departments of Clinical Chemistry or Chemical Pathology. The approach is firmly based on general principles and the authors have gone to great trouble to ensure that the development of ideas is logical and easy to follow. A basic knowledge of medicine and of elementary biochemistry is assumed but, given this, the reader should be able to understand even the more involved interrelationships without undue difficulty and should thereafter be in a strong position to apply this knowledge in medical practice.

I have appreciated very much the opportunity of reading this book during its preparation and feel that it represents a distinctly novel approach to the interpretation of biochemical data. In my opinion it could be read with advantage by all categories of reader mentioned in the Preface, and moreover I believe that they will enjoy the experience.

N F Maclagan
January, 1971

Preface to the first edition

This book is intended primarily for medical students and junior hospital staff. It is based on many years' practical experience of undergraduate and postgraduate teaching, and of the problems of a routine chemical pathology department. It is written for those who learn best if they understand what they are learning. Wherever possible, explanations of the facts are given: if the explanation is working a hypothesis (like, for instance, that for the ectopic production of hormones) this is stressed, and where no explanation is known, this is stated. Our experience of teaching and our discussions with students have led us to believe that many of them are willing to read a slightly longer book if it gives them a better understanding than a shorter one. Electrolyte and acid–base balance have been discussed in some detail because, in our experience, these are the most common problems of chemical pathology met with by junior clinicians and ones in which there are often dangerous misunderstandings. Some subjects, such as the porphyrias and conditions of iron overload, are discussed in greater detail than is necessary for undergraduate examinations: however, the incidence of these is high in some ares of the world, and an elementary source of reference seemed to be needed.

We have tried to stress the clinical importance of an understanding of the subject: by including in the chapter appendices some details of treatment, difficult to find together in other books, we hope that this one may appeal to clinicians as well as to students. Two chapters are included on the best use of the laboratory, including precautions that should be taken in collecting specimens and interpreting results. As we have stressed, pathologists and clinicians should work as a team, and full consultation between the two should be the rule. The diagnostic tests suggested are those which we have found, by experience, to be the most valuable. For instance, in the differential diagnosis of hypercalcaemia we find the steroid suppression test very helpful, phosphate excretion indices fallible and tedious to perform and estimation of urinary calcium useless.

Our own junior staff have found the drafts helpful in preparing for the Part I examination for the Royal College of Physicians, as well as for the primary examination for Membership of the Royal College of Pathologists, and our Senior Technicians are using it to study for the Special Examination for Fellowship in Chemical Pathology of the Institute of Medical Laboratory Technology. We feel that those studying for the primary examination for the Fellowship of the Royal College of Surgeons might also make use of it. It could provide the groundwork for study for the final examination for the Membership of the Royal College of Pathologists in Chemical Pathology, and for the Mastership in Clinical Biochemistry.

Initially each chapter should be worked through from beginning to end. For revision purposes there are lists and tables, and summaries of the contents of each chapter. The short subindices in the Table of Contents should facilitate the use of the book for reference.

Appendix A lists some analogous facts that we hope may help understanding and learning. The list must be far from complete, and the student should seek examples for himself.

We wish to thank Professor NF Maclagan for his unfailing encouragement and his helpful advice and criticisms. We are also indebted to a great many other people foremost among whom we should mention Dr JP Nicholson who has read and commented on the whole book, and Professor MD Milne, Professor DM Matthews, Mr KB Cooke and Dr BW Gilliver for helpful advice and criticism on individual chapters. Many registrars and senior house officers in the departments, in particular Dr Krystyna Rowland, Dr Elizabeth Small, Dr Nalini Naik and Dr Noel Walmsley, have been closely involved in the preparation of the book and have provided invaluable suggestions and criticisms. Students, too, have read individual chapters for comprehensibility, and we would particularly like to thank Mr BP Heather, Mr J Muir and Miss HM Merriman for helpful comments. Mr CP Butler of the Westminster Hospital Pharmacy was most helpful during the preparation of the sections on therapy. Mrs Valerie Moorsom and Mrs Marie-Lise Pannall, with the help of Mrs Brenda Sarasin and Miss Barbara Bridges, have borne with us during the typing of the drafts and the final transcript. The illustrations were prepared by Mr David Gibbons of the Department of Medical Photography and Illustration of the Westminster Medical School.

Finally, we would like to thank the publishers for their cooperation and understanding during the preparation of this book.

JFZ
PRP
May, 1971

Preface to the sixth edition

This book was first published in September 1971. Since then five editions have appeared and it has been translated into seven languages. This is surely a testament to its success, which was undoubtedly due to Professor Joan Zilva's and Dr Peter Pannall's experience in both the clinical and laboratory aspects of the subject and in teaching medical and postgraduate students. The book is therefore based on practical experience and on the authors' belief that a clear understanding of normal physiological principles should help to ensure intelligent, selective investigation, so minimizing the risk of dangerous misinterpretation of results.

Both Professor Joan Zilva and Dr Peter Pannall have decided to 'call it a day'. I was a coauthor of the 5th edition and, as the sole author of this one, have continued to stress their philosophy. Although I have not made extensive changes to the text I have revised it where necessary and have again, by seeking comments and discussing difficulties with students and colleagues, tried to clarify some points.

In the first edition neither further reading lists nor reference ranges were included. The authors reluctantly added them from the second edition onward in response to criticisms of their omissions in reviews. I, like Professor Zilva and Dr Pannall, believe that reading lists add little to this type of book, mainly because they are often out-of-date by the time the book is published. Also like the original authors, I feel strongly that students should refer to their own laboratory's reference ranges; students and staff all too often misinterpret data, sometimes with disastrous consequences, because, despite clear warnings in the text and in tables, they failed to take this elementary precaution. I have therefore taken my courage in both hands and reverted to their original practice in this edition.

As always, I would welcome comments and criticism of the text and of the above changes.

I am extremely grateful to both Professor Zilva and Dr Pannall for inviting me to collaborate in the preparation of the 5th edition and to continue what they initiated. I hope that this edition is a worthy successor. I am indebted to them and to Philip Nicholson who has again read and commented on the whole text and on the proofs and to many other colleagues for their helpful comments on the revised chapters. In particular, I wish to thank, in alphabetical order, Drs James Alaghband-Zadeh, Graham Ball, Andrew Day, Margaret Hancock, Michael Feher, Professor Pamela Riches and Ms Joanne Sheldon, and the staff of the Westminster Hospital Pharmacy for checking the details of the pharmaceutical preparations. The electrophoretic strips were prepared by Ms Joanne Sheldon and photographed by the Department of Medical Illustration and Teaching Services of the Charing Cross and Westminster Medical School.

Finally, I would like to thank the publishers, and in particular Mr Nicholas Dunton and Ms Diane Leadbetter-Conway, for their assistance and cooperation during the preparation of this edition.

PDM
September 1993

Contents

The Kidneys and Renal Calculi

1

The kidneys

RENAL PHYSIOLOGY

The kidneys excrete waste products of metabolism and play an essential homeostatic role by controlling the body water and solute balance. Each kidney contains about 10^6 (1 000 000) nephrons and each nephron is made up of five main functional segments (Fig. 1.1).

- *The glomeruli*, in the cortex of the kidney, are invaginated around a capillary network of blood vessels derived from the afferent, and draining into the efferent, arterioles. Water and small molecules are passively filtered during passage of blood through these capillaries, the ultrafiltrate passing through the vessel walls and the glomerular membranes into the glomerular spaces (Bowman's capsules).
- *The proximal convoluted tubules*, also in the cortex, receive filtrate from the glomerular spaces. Convolution increases the tubular length and therefore contact between the luminal fluid and the proximal tubular cells, thus facilitating more solute reclamation than would occur if the loops were shorter.
- *The loops of Henle* are formed as the tubules extend down, for a variable distance, into the medulla. The descending and first part of the ascending limbs are thin but the latter become thicker as they near the cortex.
- *The distal convoluted tubules* in the cortex, important for fine adjustment of luminal fluid, lie near the afferent arterioles with the juxtaglomerular apparatus (p.**28**) between them; the production of renin by the latter is modified by flow in these blood vessels.
- *The collecting ducts* start as the distal tubules turn down into the medulla and end by opening into the renal pelvis. Their anatomical proximity to the loops of Henle is important for final modification of urinary composition (p.**8**). Thus the urine, much modified from the original filtrate, flows from the collecting ducts into the renal tract.

Normal function of the kidneys depends on:

- the integrity of the glomeruli and the tubular cells;
- a normal blood supply – under normal circumstances about 20 per cent of the cardiac output flows through the kidneys;
- normal secretion and feedback control of hormones acting on the kidney

In addition to the excretory function, the kidneys have important endocrine functions producing hormones that act both peripherally and locally. These include:

- *renin*, produced by the juxtaglomerular apparatus;
- *1,25-dihydroxyvitamin D*, the active metabolite of vitamin D, produced following hepatic hydroxylation of 25-hydroxyvitamin D (p.**176**);
- *erythropoietin*, which stimulates erythropoiesis.

Passive filtration

Under normal circumstances, about 200 litres of plasma ultrafiltrate enter the tubular lumina each day, mainly by glomerular filtration into glomerular capsules but also through the spaces between cells lining the

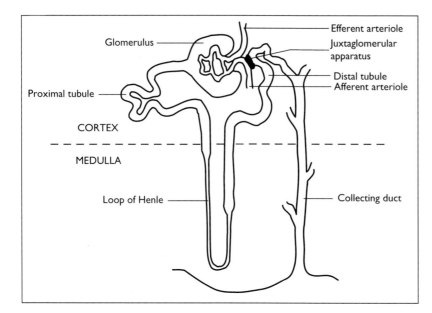

Fig 1.1 Anatomical relation between the individual segments of the nephron and the juxtaglomerular apparatus.

tubules ('tight junctions'). The production of ultrafiltrate depends on the blood flow through normal glomeruli and on the difference between the hydrostatic pressure gradient and the plasma effective colloid osmotic (oncotic) pressure gradient (p.**35**) across the membranes (Fig. 1.2) and tight junctions. The colloid osmotic effect is so weak relative to the hydrostatic gradient that it can usually be ignored. However, it does facilitate some reabsorption of fluid from the proximal renal tubules.

Because filtration is a passive process, the filtrate contains diffusible constituents at almost the same concentrations as in plasma. About 30 000 mmol of sodium, 800 mmol of potassium, 300 mmol of free-ionized calcium, 1000 mmol (180 g) of glucose and 800 mmol (48 g) of urea are filtered in the 200 litres daily. Proteins and protein-bound substances are filtered in only small amounts by normal glomeruli and most are reabsorbed. The very large volume of filtrate allows adequate elimination of waste products such as urea; death from water and electrolyte depletion would occur within a few hours unless the bulk of the water and essential solutes were reclaimed.

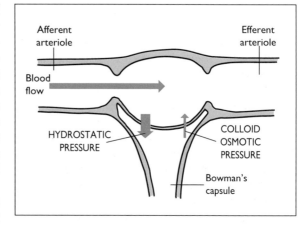

Fig 1.2 Relation between flow of blood through the glomerulus and the factors that effect the rate of filtration across the glomerular basement membrane.

Tubular function

Changes in filtration rate alter the total amount of water and solute filtered, but not the composition of the filtrate. From the 200 litres of plasma filtered a day, only about 2 litres of urine are formed. The composition of urine differs markedly from that of plasma and therefore from the filtrate. The concentrations of individual constituents not only vary independently of each other, but also vary widely as physiological requirements alter. The reabsorption of about 99 per cent of the filtered volume, and adjustment of individual solutes, indicates that tubular cells have carried out active transport, sometimes selectively, against physicochemical gradients. Energy production, mainly in the form of ATP needed for active transport, may be impaired by enzyme poisons, hypoxia and cell death. Transport of charged ions tends to produce an electrochemical gradient that inhibits further transport. This is minimized by two processes:

- **isosmotic transport**. This occurs mainly in the *proximal tubules* and reclaims the bulk of filtered essential constituents. Active transport of one ion leads to passive movement of an ion of the opposite charge in the same direction, along the electrochemical gradient. For instance, isosmotic reabsorption of sodium (Na^+) depends on the availability of diffusible negatively charged ions, such as chloride (Cl^-). The process is 'isosmotic' because the active transport of solute causes equivalent movement of water in the same direction. Isosmotic transport also occurs in the distal part of the nephron, but is quantitatively less at this site.
- **ion exchange**. This occurs mainly in the more *distal parts of the nephrons*, and is important for fine adjustment after bulk reabsorption has taken place. Ions of the same charge, usually cations, are exchanged and neither electrochemical nor osmotic gradients are created. Therefore, during cation exchange there is insignificant net movement of anion or water. For example, Na^+ may be reabsorbed in exchange for potassium (K^+) or hydrogen ions (H^+). Na^+ and H^+ exchange also occurs proximally, but at that site it is more important for bicarbonate reclamation than for fine adjustment of solute reabsorption (see Chapter 4).

All body cells carry out both types of ion transport, but in most cells the pumps are uniformly distributed on the membrane surrounding the cell and solute passes into or out of the cell. In the cells lining the renal tubules, the intestine and many secretory organs, the pumps are located on the membrane on one side of the cell only and therefore solute flows in one direction.

Other substances, such as phosphate and urate, are secreted into, as well as reabsorbed from, the tubular lumen. Waste products, such as urea and creatinine, are not actively handled significantly by tubular cells. Most filtered urea is passed in urine but some diffuses back passively from the collecting ducts with water (p.**7**); by contrast, some creatinine is secreted into the tubular lumen.

Reclamation of solute from the proximal tubule

Over 70 per cent of the filtered sodium, free-ionized calcium and magnesium and almost all the potassium is actively reabsorbed from the proximal tubules.

Some free-ionized calcium is reabsorbed at more distal sites, possibly from the loops of Henle. This reabsorption may be stimulated by parathyroid hormone (PTH) and inhibited by loop diuretics such as frusemide (furosemide). Only about two per cent of filtered calcium appears in the urine.

Many inorganic anions follow an electrochemical gradient; the reabsorption of sodium is limited by the availability of chloride, the most abundant diffusible anion in the filtrate (p.**96**). Bicarbonate is almost completely recovered, following exchange of sodium and hydrogen ions (Fig. 1.3; see Chapter 4 for further details). Specific active transport mechanisms result in almost complete reabsorption of glucose, urate and amino acids. Some urate is secreted into the tubular

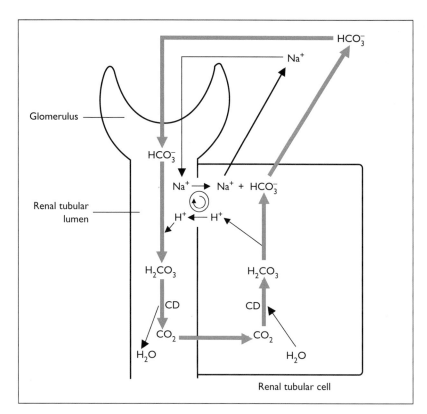

Fig 1.3 'Reclamation' of filtered bicarbonate by the renal tubular cell (see Chapter 4 for explanation).

lumina, mainly in the proximal tubules but most of this is reabsorbed.

There is incomplete phosphate reabsorption; *phosphate in tubular fluid is important for buffering hydrogen ions.* Inhibition of phosphate reabsorption by PTH occurs in both the proximal and distal convoluted tubules and accounts for the hypophosphataemia of PTH excess (p.**174**).

Thus almost all the reusable nutrients and the bulk of electrolytes are reclaimed from the proximal tubules, with fine homeostatic adjustment taking place more distally. Almost all the filtered metabolic waste products, such as urea and creatinine, which cannot be reused by the body, remain in the luminal fluid.

WATER REABSORPTION: URINARY CONCENTRATION AND DILUTION

Water is always reabsorbed passively along an osmotic gradient. However, active solute transport is necessary to produce this gradient. Two main processes are involved in water reabsorption:

- *isosmotic reabsorption of water from the proximal tubules.* The nephrons reabsorbs 99 per cent of the filtered water, about 70 to 80 per cent (140 to 160 litres a day) of which is returned to the body from the proximal tubules. Active solute reabsorption from the filtrate is accompanied by passive reabsorption of an osmotically equivalent amount of water. Therefore, fluid entering the lumina of the loops of Henle, although much reduced in volume, is still almost isosmotic.
- *dissociation of water reabsorption from that of solute in the loops of Henle, distal tubules and collecting ducts.* Normally between 40 and 60 litres of water enter the loops of Henle daily. This volume is reduced to about 2 litres as varying amounts of water are reabsorbed, helping to correct for changes in extracellular

osmolality. At extremes of water intake urinary osmolality can vary from about 40 to 1400 mmol/kg. Because the proximal tubules cannot dissociate water and solute reabsorption, the adjustment must occur between the end of the proximal tubule and the end of the collecting duct. Two mechanisms are involved.

Countercurrent multiplication is an active process occurring in the loops of Henle, whereby a high osmolality is created in the renal medulla and urinary osmolality is reduced. This can occur in the absence of antidiuretic hormone (ADH) and a dilute hypo-osmolal urine is produced.

Countercurrent exchange is a passive process, only occurring in the presence of ADH. Water without solute is reabsorbed from the collecting ducts into the ascending vasa recta along the osmotic gradient created by countercurrent multiplication and by the high osmolality in the medulla. By this means a concentrated urine is produced.

Countercurrent multiplication occurs in the loops of Henle. It depends on the close apposition of the descending and ascending limbs of the loops to the vasa recta. The vasa recta make up a capillary network derived from the efferent arterioles and like the loops of Henle pass deep into the medulla. The descending limbs are permeable to water but the thick ascending limbs are impermeable to water and solute. Chloride is probably actively pumped from the thick ascending to the descending limbs as fluid flows through the lumina of the loops; positively charged Na+ ions follow along the electrochemical gradient. Thus the osmolality progressively increases in the descending limbs and renal medullary interstitium; it decreases in the ascending limbs but as these are impermeable to water, this change is not transmitted to the interstitium.

Fluid entering the descending limbs is almost isosmolal, having the same osmolality as the general circulation, just under 300 mmol/kg. If the fluid in the loops were stationary and no pumping had taken place,

the osmolality throughout the loops and the adjacent medullary tissue would be about 300 mmol/kg.

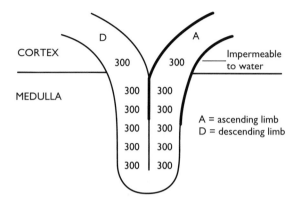

Suppose the fluid column remained stationary and 1 mmol of solute per kg were pumped from the ascending into the descending limb, the result would be:

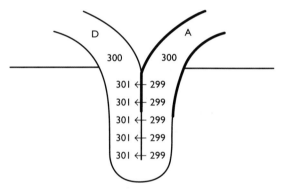

If this pumping continued and there were no flow, the fluid in the descending limb would become hyperosmolal and that in the ascending limb correspondingly hypo-osmolal.

Suppose that the fluid flowed so that each figure 'moved two places':

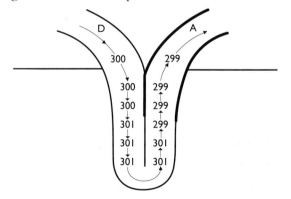

As this happened more solute would be pumped from the ascending to the descending limbs:

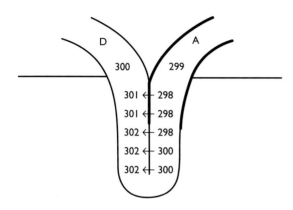

If the fluid again flowed 'two places', then the situation would be:

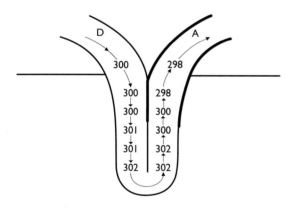

If these steps occurred simultaneously and continuously, the consequences would be:

- increasing osmolality in the tips of the loops of Henle. Because the walls of most of the loops are permeable to water and solute, osmotic equilibrium would be reached with the surrounding tissues in the deeper layers of the medulla, including the plasma within the vasa recta;
- hypo-osmolal fluid leaving the ascending limbs.

The final result might be:

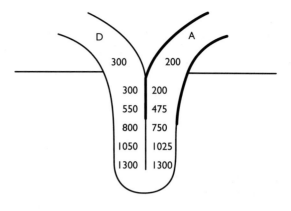

In the absence of ADH the walls of the collecting ducts are impermeable to water, and therefore no further change in osmolality occurs. A hypo-osmolal urine would be passed.

Countercurrent exchange is essential, together with multiplication, for the osmolal concentration of urine. It can only occur in the presence of ADH and depends on the 'random' apposition of the collecting ducts and the ascending vasa recta (Fig. 1.4). ADH increases the permeability of the cell membranes lining the distal parts of the collecting ducts to water which then moves passively along the osmotic gradient created by multiplication. Consequently luminal fluid is concentrated as the collecting ducts pass into the increasingly hyperosmolal medulla.

The increasing concentration of the fluid would reduce the osmotic gradient as it passes down the ducts if it did not meet even more concentrated plasma flowing in the opposite (countercurrent) direction. The gradient is thus maintained, and water continues to be reabsorbed until the fluid reaches the deepest layers, where the osmolality is about four or five times that of plasma. The low capillary hydrostatic pressure at this site and the osmotic effect of plasma proteins ensure that much of the reabsorbed water within the interstitium enters the vascular lumina. The diluted blood is carried towards the cortex and ultimately enters the general circulation and helps to dilute the extracellular fluid.

The osmotic action of urea in the medullary interstitium may potentiate the

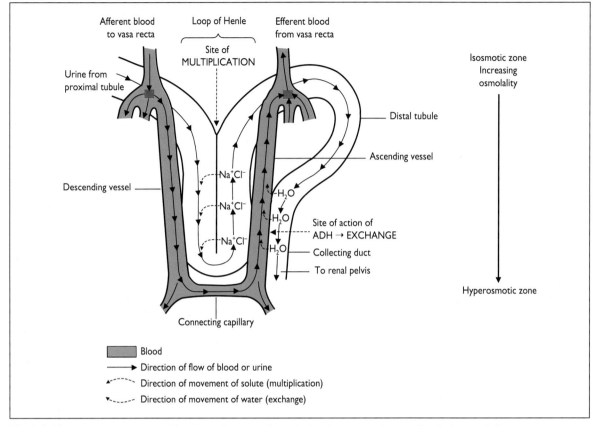

Fig 1.4 The countercurrent mechanism, showing the relation between the renal tubules and the vasa recta.

countercurrent multiplication. As water is reabsorbed from the collecting ducts under the influence of ADH the luminal urea concentration increases. Because the distal collecting ducts are permeable to urea, it enters the deeper layers of the medullary interstitium, increasing the osmolality and drawing water from the lower parts of the descending limbs of the loops. The amount of urea reabsorbed depends on:

- the amount filtered;
- the rate of flow of tubular fluid. As much as 50 per cent of filtered urea may be reabsorbed when flow is significantly reduced.

Thus both concentration and dilution of urine depend on active processes, which may be impaired if tubules are damaged.

HOMEOSTATIC CONTROL OF WATER EXCRETION

The mechanism involved in the normal homeostatic control of urinary water excretion will now be discussed at extremes of water intake.

Water load. A high water intake dilutes the extracellular fluid and the consequent fall in plasma osmolality reduces ADH secretion (p.29). Therefore the walls of the collecting ducts remain impermeable to water and the countercurrent multiplication, acting alone, produces a dilute urine and a high osmolality within the medulla and medullary vessels. Blood from the latter flows into the general circulation, so helping to correct the fall in systemic osmolality.

During a maximal water diuresis the osmolality at the tips of the medullary loops may be 600 mmol/kg or less, rather than the maximum of about 1400 mmol/kg. Increasing the circulating volume increases renal blood flow; the rapid flow in the vasa recta 'washes out' medullary hyperosmolality, returning some of the solute, without extra water, to the circulation. Thus, not only is more water than usual lost in the urine, but more solute is 'reclaimed'. Because medullary hyperosmolality, and therefore the ability to concentrate the urine maximally, is dependent on medullary blood flow, under normal circumstances urinary osmolality will only be fully restored several days after a prolonged water load has stopped. Results of a urine concentration test, performed to differentiate between suspected primary polydipsia and diabetes insipidus, both of which present with a high urine output, must be interpreted with this in mind (water deprivation test, p.**74**).

Water restriction, by increasing the plasma osmolality, increases ADH secretion and allows countercurrent exchange with enhanced water reabsorption. Reduced circulatory volume results in a sluggish blood flow in the vasa recta and increased urea reabsorption, allowing a build-up of the medullary hyperosmolality produced by multiplication. This potientiates water reabsorption in the presence of ADH. The reduced capillary hydrostatic pressure and increased colloid osmotic pressure, due to the haemoconcentration following non-protein fluid loss, ensures that much of the reabsorbed water enters the vascular compartment.

Osmotic diuresis. An excess of filtered solute in the proximal tubular lumina impairs the bulk water reabsorption from this site by its osmotic effect. This excess may be because the cells are not only physically impermeable but also lack an active transport mechanism for the substance, or because the capacity for active or passive reabsorption is exceeded. Unabsorbed solute concentration rises progressively as water is reabsorbed with other solute during passage through the proximal tubules and this opposes further water reabsorption. Thus a larger volume than normal reaches the loops of Henle. Moreover, fluid leaving the proximal tubules, although still isosmotic with plasma, contains a lower sodium concentration than that of plasma, the difference being made up of the unabsorbed solute. The relative lack of the major cation, sodium, to accompany the anion chloride along the electrochemical gradient, inhibits the pump in the loops. The resulting impairment of build-up of medullary osmolality inhibits distal water reabsorption, under the influence of ADH from the collecting ducts, resulting in a diuresis.

The most effective osmotic diuretics are substances that cannot cross cell membranes to any significant degree; therefore they must be infused as they cannot be absorbed from the gut. The most potent tend to be exogenous in origin. The commonest example is mannitol, a sugar alcohol, which is sometimes used therapeutically as a diuretic.

Normally most filtered water leaves the proximal tubular lumina with reabsorbed solute. Enough, for example, glucose (with an active transport system) or urea (which diffuses back passively) may be filtered to exceed the proximal tubular reabsorptive capacity. They too can act as osmotic diuretics and cause water depletion. This is important, for example, in diabetes mellitus or in uraemia (p.**16**).

HOMEOSTATIC SOLUTE ADJUSTMENT IN THE DISTAL TUBULE AND COLLECTING DUCT

Sodium reabsorption in exchange for hydrogen ions occurs throughout the nephrons. In the proximal tubules the main effect of this exchange is on the reclamation of filtered bicarbonate. In the distal tubules and collecting ducts, the exchange process is usually associated with net generation of bicarbonate to replace that lost in extracellular buffering, and so with the fine adjustment of hydrogen ion homeostasis (Fig. 1.3). Potassium and hydrogen ions compete for secretion in exchange for sodium ions. The possible mechanism stimulated by aldosterone is discussed in Chapter 4. The most important stimulus to aldosterone secretion is mediated by the effect of renal blood flow on the release of renin from the juxtaglomerular apparati; this method of reabsorption is part of the homeostatic mechanism controlling sodium and water balance (Chapter 2).

In summary:

- the very large daily volume of filtrate allows waste products, such as urea and creatinine, to be excreted at a rate equal to their production.
- most of the filtered water, electrolytes and reusable metabolites are reclaimed from the proximal tubular lumina.
- fine homeostatic adjustments are made in the more distal segments of the nephron often under hormonal control.

Clinical chemistry of renal disease

PATHOPHYSIOLOGY

Different parts of the nephrons are in close anatomical association and are dependent on a common blood supply. Renal dysfunction of any kind affects all parts of the nephrons to some extent, although sometimes either glomerular or tubular dysfunction is predominant. The net effect of renal disease on plasma and urine depends on the proportion of glomeruli to tubules affected, and the number of nephrons involved. However, it may be easier to understand the consequences of renal disease if we start by considering *hypothetical* individual nephrons, first with a low glomerular filtration rate (GFR) and normal tubular function, and then with tubular damage but a normal GFR. *It must be stressed that these are hypothetical examples.*

REDUCED GFR WITH NORMAL TUBULAR FUNCTION

The total amounts of *urea* and *creatinine* excreted are affected by the GFR. If the rate of filtration fails to balance that of production, plasma concentrations will rise.

Phosphate and *urate* are released during cell breakdown. Plasma concentrations rise because less than normal is filtered. Most of the reduced amount reaching the proximal tubule can be reabsorbed and the capacity for secretion is impaired if the filtered volume is too low to accept the ions; these factors further contribute to high plasma concentrations.

A large proportion of the reduced amount of filtered *sodium* is reabsorbed by isosmotic mechanisms; less than usual is available for exchange with hydrogen and potassium ions distally.

This has two important results:

- *reduction of hydrogen ion secretion* throughout the nephron. Bicarbonate can only be reclaimed if hydrogen ion is secreted (p.**84**); plasma bicarbonate concentrations will fall;
- *reduction of potassium secretion* in the distal tubule, with potassium retention (potassium can still be reabsorbed proximally).

If there is a *low GFR accompanied by a low renal blood flow:*

- *systemic aldosterone secretion will be maximal* (p.**45**); in such cases any sodium reaching the distal tubule will be almost completely reabsorbed in exchange for H⁺ and K⁺, and the urinary sodium concentration will be low;
- *antidiuretic hormone secretion will be increased*; ADH, acting on the collecting ducts, allows water to be reabsorbed in excess of solute, further reducing urinary volume and increasing urinary osmolality well above that of plasma. This high urinary osmolality is mainly due to substances not actively handled by the tubules. For example, the urinary urea concentration will be well above that of plasma. This distal response will only occur in the presence of ADH; in its absence normal nephrons will form a dilute urine.

If the capacity of the proximal tubular cells to reabsorb solute, and therefore water, is normal a larger proportion than usual of the reduced filtered volume will be reclaimed by isosmotic processes. This will further reduce urinary volume.

Thus the findings in venous plasma and urine from the affected nephrons will be:

Plasma:

- high urea and creatinine concentrations;
- low bicarbonate concentration, with low pH;
- hyperkalaemia;
- hyperuricaemia and hyperphosphataemia.

Urine:

- reduced volume;
- a low (appropriate) sodium concentration, *only if renal blood flow is low, stimulating aldosterone secretion*;
- a high (appropriate) urea concentration and therefore a high osmolality, *only if ADH secretion is stimulated.*

REDUCED TUBULAR WITH NORMAL GLOMERULAR FUNCTION

Damage to tubular cells impairs the adjustment of the composition and volume of the urine.

Impaired solute reabsorption from proximal tubules reduces isosmotic water reabsorption. Countercurrent multiplication may also be affected and hence the ability of the collecting ducts to respond to ADH is reduced. *A large volume of inappropriately dilute urine is produced.*

The tubules cannot secrete hydrogen ions and therefore *cannot reabsorb bicarbonate normally nor acidify the urine.*

The response to aldosterone, and therefore the exchange mechanisms involving reabsorption of sodium are impaired; the urine contains an *inappropriately high concentration of sodium for the renal blood flow.*

Potassium reabsorption from the proximal tubule is impaired and *plasma potassium concentrations may be low.*

Reabsorption of glucose, phosphate, magnesium, urate and amino acids is impaired. *Plasma phosphate, magnesium and urate concentrations may be low.*

Thus the findings in venous plasma and urine from the affected nephrons will be

Plasma:

- normal urea and creatinine concentrations (normal glomerular function);
- due to *proximal* or *distal* tubular failure: low bicarbonate concentration with low pH; hypokalaemia.
- due to *proximal* tubular failure: hypophosphataemia, hypomagnesaemia and hypouricaemia.

Urine:

- due to *proximal* and/or *distal* tubular failure: increased volume; pH inappropriately high for that of plasma.
- due to *proximal* tubular failure: generalized aminoaciduria; phosphaturia; glycosuria.
- due to *distal* tubular failure: *even if renal blood flow is low*, an inappropriately high sodium concentration (inability to respond to aldosterone); *even if ADH secretion is stimulated*, an inappropriately low urea concentration, and therefore osmolality (inability of the collecting ducts to respond to ADH).

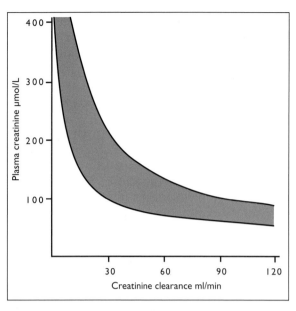

Fig 1.5 The relation between creatinine clearance and plasma creatinine concentration, showing the approximate 95 per cent confidence intervals.

Clinical syndromes of renal disease

There is a spectrum of conditions in which the proportion of glomerular to tubular dysfunction varies. The biochemical findings and urine output depend on the relative contribution of each.

When the GFR falls substances which are little affected by tubular action, such as *urea* and *creatinine*, are retained. Although their plasma concentrations start rising above the baseline for that individual soon after the clearance falls, they seldom rise above the reference range for the population until the GFR is below about 60 per cent of normal (Fig. 1.5) although, in an individual patient, they do rise above baseline.

The degree of *potassium, phosphate* and *urate* retention depends on the balance between the degree of glomerular retention

and the loss due to a reduced proximal tubular reabsorptive capacity. If glomerular dysfunction predominates, so little is filtered that despite failure of reabsorption plasma concentrations rise. If tubular dysfunction predominates glomerular retention is more than balanced by impaired reabsorption of filtered potassium, urate and phosphate, and therefore plasma concentrations may be normal or even low.

A low plasma *bicarbonate* concentration is a constant finding. The associated metabolic acidosis may aggravate the hyperkalaemia of glomerular dysfunction.

The plasma *sodium* concentration is not *primarily* affected by renal disease.

The urinary *volume* depends on the balance between the volume filtered and the proportion reabsorbed by the tubules. At the glomerular end of the spectrum little is filtered and the patient is almost anuric. Since 99 per cent of filtered water is normally reabsorbed, a very small impairment of reabsorption causes a large increase in urine volume. Consequently if tubular dysfunction predominates, impairment of water reabsorption causes polyuria, even though glomerular filtration is reduced.

Plasma concentrations of urea and creatinine depend largely on glomerular function (Fig. 1.6). By contrast, *urinary concentrations* depend almost entirely on tubular function. However, little is filtered at the glomeruli, the concentrations of substances in the initial filtrate are those of a plasma ultrafiltrate. Any difference between these concentrations and those in the urine is due to tubular activity. The more the tubular function is impaired the nearer the plasma concentrations will be to those of urine. Urinary concentrations *inappropriate to the state of hydration* suggest tubular damage, whatever the degree of glomerular dysfunction.

ACUTE OLIGURIA

In adults oliguria is defined as a urine output of less than 400 ml a day, or, in the short term, less than 15 ml an hour; it usually indicates a low GFR. Oliguria may be caused by:

- reduced GFR with minimal renal damage (renal circulatory insufficiency or 'prerenal uraemia');
- intrinsic renal damage;
- intra- or extrarenal obstruction to outflow ('postrenal uraemia').

Acute oliguria, with reduced GFR and with minimal renal damage, is caused by factors that reduce the hydrostatic pressure gradient between the renal capillaries and the tubular lumen. A low intracapillary pressure is the most common cause. It is known as *renal circulatory insufficiency* ('prerenal uraemia') and may be due to:

- intravascular depletion of:
  whole blood (haemorrhage); plasma volume usually due to gastrointestinal loss, or reduced intake.
- reduced pressure due to the vascular dilatation caused by 'shock', causes of which include many severe conditions, such as myocardial infarction, rupture of an ectopic pregnancy, acute pancreatitis or perforation of a peptic ulcer, and intravascular haemolysis including that due to mismatched blood transfusion.

A low GFR due to renal circulatory insufficiency is probably the commonest cause of acute oliguria if tubular function is relatively normal. The patient is usually hypotensive and clinically volume depleted. If renal blood flow is restored within a few hours the condition is reversible, but the longer it persists the greater the danger of intrinsic renal damage.

Since most glomeruli are involved and tubular function is relatively normal, the biochemical findings in plasma and urine are those described on p.**11**. In addition, unless whole blood is lost there may be haemoconcentration. Uraemia due to renal dysfunction may be aggravated if there is increased protein breakdown due to tissue damage, a large haematoma or to the presence of blood in the gastrointestinal lumen; intravenous amino acid infusion may have the same effect because the urea is derived, by hepatic metabolism, from the amino groups of amino acids. Increased tissue breakdown may also aggravate hyperkalaemia, hyperuricaemia and hyperphosphataemia.

Acute oliguria due to renal damage may be due to:

- prolonged renal circulatory insufficiency;
- acute glomerulonephritis, usually in children. The history of a sore throat and the finding of red cells in the urine usually make the diagnosis obvious;
- septicaemia, which should be considered when the cause of oliguria is obscure;
- ingestion of a variety of poisons.

The most difficult problem in the differential diagnosis of acute oliguria is to distinguish between renal circulatory insufficiency, as described above, and intrinsic renal damage that may have followed it. Acute oliguric renal dysfunction often follows a period of reduced GFR and renal circulatory insufficiency. The oliguria is due to reduced cortical blood flow with glomerular damage, aggravated by back pressure on the glomeruli due to obstruction to tubular flow by oedema. At this stage, the concentration of many constituents in plasma, such as urea and creatinine, are raised; tubular damage results in an inappropriately dilute urine for the degree of hypovolaemia.

During recovery oliguria is followed by polyuria. When cortical blood flow increases, and as tubular oedema resolves, glomerular function recovers before that of the tubules. The biochemical findings gradually progress to those of tubular dysfunction until they approximate to those for 'pure' tubular lesions. Urinary output is further increased by the osmotic diuretic effect of the high load of urea. The polyuria may cause water and electrolyte depletion. The initial hyperkalaemia may be followed by hypokalaemia. Mild acidosis, common to both glomerular and tubular disorders, persists until late. Finally, recovery of the tubules restores full renal function.

Acute oliguria due to intrinsic renal damage may be differentiated from that due to renal circulatory insufficiency using laboratory tests, although these are rarely necessary.

In patients with renal circulatory insufficiency urine output increases if normal renal blood flow is restored by correcting blood pressure and circulating volume. If the urine volume fails to rise after rehydration, or if the patient is already normotensive and well hydrated, it is likely that there is renal damage.

Fluid must be given with caution, and only until volume depletion has been corrected; there is a danger of overloading the circulation if the glomerular membranes are unable to filter normally, despite an adequate hydrostatic gradient.

Laboratory tests may be useful but their *limitations must be understood.*

- *Urinary sodium estimation* may be used to differentiate acute oliguria due to renal damage from that due to renal circulatory insufficiency. *Aldosterone secretion will only*

be maximal if renal blood flow is reduced; in such circumstances functioning tubules respond appropriately by selectively reabsorbing sodium by distal tubular exchange mechanisms. A urinary sodium concentration of less than about 30 mmol/L, and certainly less than 20 mmol/L, although not strictly normal if there is a very low renal blood flow, is usually taken to indicate that tubular, and therefore overall renal function, is not significantly impaired. *Measurement of urinary sodium concentration cannot be used to test tubular function once renal blood flow has been restored and the stimulus to aldosterone secretion has therefore been removed.* In the absence of aldosterone the appropriate response of normal tubules is a reduction in differential sodium reabsorption, and the urinary sodium concentration will rise.

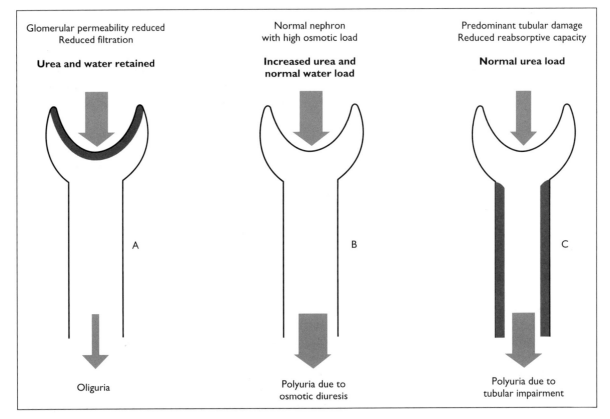

Glomerular permeability reduced Reduced filtration	Normal nephron with high osmotic load	Predominant tubular damage Reduced reabsorptive capacity
Urea and water retained	**Increased urea and normal water load**	**Normal urea load**
A	B	C
Oliguria	Polyuria due to osmotic diuresis	Polyuria due to tubular impairment

Fig 1.6 The effects of glomerular and tubular dysfunction on urinary output and on plasma concentrations of retained 'waste' products of metabolism, the volume depending on the proportion of nephrons involved (see text).

- *Measurement of urinary osmolality* or other indicators of selective water reabsorption, such as urinary urea or creatinine concentrations, are even less valuable than assaying urinary sodium concentration, since ADH secretion is not invariably stimulated.

Acute oliguria caused by intra- or extrarenal obstruction to outflow. A rise in tubular luminal pressure as a primary cause of oliguria is rare. The cause is usually, but not always, clinically obvious and may be due to:

- *intrarenal obstruction*, with blockage of the tubular lumina by haemoglobin, myoglobin, and very rarely urate or calcium. Obstruction caused by casts and oedema of tubular cells is usually the result of true renal damage;
- *extrarenal obstruction*, due to calculi, neoplasms, strictures or prostatic hypertrophy, any of which may cause sudden obstruction. The finding of a palpable bladder indicates urethral obstruction and in the male it is most likely to be due to prostatic hypertrophy, although there are other rarer causes.

Early correction of outflow obstruction rapidly increases the urine output. The longer it remains untreated the greater the danger of ischaemic or pressure damage to renal tissue.

CHRONIC RENAL DYSFUNCTION (CHRONIC RENAL FAILURE – CRF)

Chronic renal dysfunction is usually the end result of a variety of chronic conditions which include glomerulonephritis, obstructive uropathy, polycystic disease, renal artery stenosis, and tubular dysfunction (p.**17**). It may follow an episode of acute oliguric renal failure. Sometimes there is no obvious precipitating factor.

In most cases of acute oliguric renal disease there is diffuse damage involving the majority of nephrons and, if untreated, this results in early nephron damage. A patient who survives long enough to develop chronic renal disease must have

Table 1.1   Some causes of polyuria

Increased fluid intake
   oral or intravenous
Osmotic diuresis
   endogenous substances
      glycosuria
      uraemia (unless due to predominant glomerular
      dysfunction)
   exogenous substances
      mannitol infusion (used therapeutically)
Impaired ADH production
   cranial diabetes insipidus
      congenital or acquired
Impaired renal tubular response to ADH
   nephrogenic diabetes insipidus
      congenital
      acquired
         interstitial nephritis
         medullary cystic disease
         hypercalcaemia or hypokalaemia
         drugs
            lithium carbonate
            demeclocycline
   predominant tubular dysfunction
Other drugs
   diuretics

some functioning nephrons. Histological examination shows that not all nephrons are equally affected. Some may be completely destroyed and others almost normal; some segments of the nephrons may be more affected than others. Some of the effects of chronic renal disease can be explained by this patchy distribution of damage; acute renal disease may show the same picture (Fig. 1.6).

Chronic and sometimes acute renal dysfunction may pass through two main phases:

- an initially polyuric phase;
- subsequent oliguria or anuria, sometimes needing dialysis or renal transplantation.

Polyuric phase. At first glomerular function may be adequate to maintain plasma urea and creatinine concentrations within the reference range. As more glomeruli are involved the rate of urea excretion falls and cannot balance the rate of production; as a consequence the plasma urea, and therefore glomerular filtrate concentrations through the essentially normal glomeruli, rise. This causes an osmotic diuresis in functioning nephrons (Fig. 1.6, B); in other nephrons the tubules may be damaged out of proportion to the glomeruli (Fig. 1.6, C). Both tubular dysfunction in nephrons with functioning glomeruli and the osmotic diuresis through intact nephrons contribute to the polyuria. If the fluid lost is replaced by an equal increase in intake urea excretion can continue through the functioning glomeruli at a higher rate than normal; the increased excretion through normal glomeruli may balance the effects of reduced permeability of others, and a new steady state is reached at a higher concentration of plasma urea. If these subjects are kept well hydrated they may remain in a stable condition, with a moderately raised plasma urea and creatinine concentrations, for years. Other causes of polyuria must be excluded (Table 1.1).

During the polyuric phase, the plasma concentration of many substances, other than urea and creatinine, may be anywhere between the glomerular and tubular ends of the spectrum. Plasma potassium concentrations are very variable but tend to be slightly raised; a metabolic acidosis is always present.

Oliguric phase (Fig. 1.6, A). If nephron destruction continues, the findings approximate more to those of pure glomerular dysfunction. Glomerular filtration decreases significantly and urine output falls; oliguria precipitates a steep rise in plasma urea, creatinine and potassium concentrations. The acidosis becomes more severe. If untreated this stage is often terminal. Before assuming that this is the case, care should be taken to ensure that the sudden rise is not due to obstruction of urine outflow or to electrolyte and water depletion.

The diagnosis of chronic renal failure is usually obvious. Biochemical testing on urine is rarely helpful. In the early phase, before plasma urea or creatinine concentrations have risen significantly, there may be microscopic haematuria or proteinuria. However haematuria may originate from either the kidney or urinary tract and may therefore indicate the presence of other conditions, such as tumours, urinary tract infections or renal calculi.

INCIDENTAL ABNORMAL FINDINGS IN RENAL FAILURE

Other abnormalities, not useful in diagnosis or needing treatment but which may be misinterpreted, may be present.

- *Plasma urate concentrations* rise in parallel with plasma urea. A high plasma concentration does not necessarily indicate primary hyperuricaemia; clinical gout is rarely present (p.**370**).
- *Plasma phosphate concentrations* rise and *plasma total calcium concentrations* fall; the increased hydrogen ion concentration increases the proportion of free-ionized calcium, the plasma concentration of which does not fall in parallel with the total calcium concentration (p.**173**). Impaired renal tubular function and the raised phosphate concentration inhibits the conversion of vitamin D to the active metabolite and this contributes to the fall in the plasma calcium concentration (p.**175**). *Hypocalcaemia should only be treated after correction of hyperphosphataemia* (p.**188**). After several years of chronic renal failure secondary hyperparathyroidism may cause decalcification of bone, with a rise in the *plasma alkaline phosphatase activity* (p.**181**).
- *Normochromic, normocytic anaemia* due to erythropoietin deficiency is common and does not respond to iron therapy.

MILD URAEMIA WITH NORMAL URINARY VOLUME

A slight rise of plasma urea concentration is a common incidental finding especially in elderly subjects. It almost certainly indicates some degree of renal damage which, unless progressive, is unlikely to need treatment. Congestive cardiac failure may impair renal circulation enough to cause mild uraemia.

SYNDROMES REFLECTING PREDOMINANT TUBULAR DAMAGE – RENAL TUBULAR ACIDOSIS

A group of conditions primarily affects tubular function more than that of the glomeruli. However, eventually scarring involving whole nephrons may cause chronic renal dysfunction. Impaired function may involve a single transport system, in particular disorders associated with amino acid (p.**359**) or phosphate transport (p.**184**), or may affect multiple transport systems. Conditions associated with multiple transport defects may cause *renal tubular acidoses* (*RTA*) – renal tubular disorders associated with a systemic metabolic acidosis because of impaired reclamation of bicarbonate or excretion of H$^+$ (see Chapter 4).

Disorders affecting the urine concentrating mechanism and causing nephrogenic diabetes insipidus, but which rarely in themselves cause a metabolic acidosis, are discussed elsewhere (p.**46**).

NEPHROTIC SYNDROME

The nephrotic syndrome is caused by increased glomerular basement membrane permeability, resulting in protein loss, by definition, of more than 5 g a day, with consequent hypoalbuminaemia and oedema. All but the highest molecular weight plasma proteins can pass the glomerulus. The main effects are on *plasma proteins* and the subject is discussed more fully in Chapter 16. Uraemia only occurs in late stages of the disorder, when many glomeruli cease to function.

Low plasma urea concentration

Occasionally the plasma urea concentration may be as low as 1 mmol/L; causes include:

- *those due to increased GFR* (common):
  pregnancy (the commonest cause in young women);
  overenthusiastic intravenous infusion (p.**42**) (the commonest cause in hospitals);
  'inappropriate' ADH secretion (p.**49**).
- *those due to decreased synthesis*:
  use of amino acids for protein anabolism during growth, especially in children;
  low protein intake;
  very severe liver disease; ⎫
  inborn errors of the urea   ⎬ rare
  cycle (infants only).   ⎭

Diagnosis of renal dysfunction

GLOMERULAR FUNCTION TESTS

The biochemical investigation of renal dysfunction can be divided into the following groups:

- to diagnose the presence of renal dysfunction;
- to diagnose the presence of complications (p.**16**);
- to monitor the severity of the disorder and the response to treatment.

As glomerular function deteriorates, substances that are normally cleared by the kidneys accumulate in plasma. Such substances include urea and creatinine.

MEASUREMENT OF PLASMA CONCENTRATIONS

Urea is derived in the liver from amino acids and therefore from protein, whether originating from the diet or tissues. The normal kidney can excrete large amounts of urea. If the rate of production exceeds the rate of clearance plasma concentrations rise. The rate of production is accelerated by:

- a high protein diet;
- increased catabolism due to starvation, tissue damage, sepsis or steroid treatment;
- absorption of amino acids and peptides from digested blood after haemorrhage into the gastrointestinal lumen or soft tissues.

In catabolic states, glomerular function is often impaired due to circulatory factors and this contributes more to the uraemia than does increased production. A significantly elevated plasma urea concentration above about 15 mmol/L (blood urea nitrogen 42 mg/dl), usually indicates impaired glomerular function. Measurement of plasma creatinine may occasionally help to resolve any doubt.

Creatinine is mostly derived from endogenous sources by tissue creatine breakdown. Plasma concentrations in normal individuals are related to muscle mass. The plasma creatinine concentration varies more than that of urea during the day due to protein intake in meals. However, sustained high protein diets and catabolic states probably affect the plasma creatinine concentration less than that of urea. For this reason many laboratories prefer to measure the plasma creatinine concentration to assess renal function. However, this estimation is less precise than that of urea, and is prone to analytical interference by substances such as bilirubin, acetoacetate and many drugs.

Whether plasma urea, creatinine or both are used as the first line investigation of glomerular function remains a matter of local choice. If the plasma concentration of either is significantly raised, and especially if it is rising, impaired glomerular function can safely be diagnosed. Changes reflect changes in the GFR (Fig. 1.5; p.12); progress can best be monitored using plasma concentrations alone.

If renal dysfunction is caused by a reduction in GFR, plasma urea concentrations tend to rise faster than those of creatinine and tend to be disproportionately higher with respect to the upper reference limit. The rate at which urea is reabsorbed from the collecting ducts is dependent on the amount filtered by the glomerulus and by the rate of luminal fluid flow.

CLEARANCE AS AN ASSESSMENT OF GLOMERULAR FILTRATION RATE (GFR)

For a substance (S) that is filtered by the glomerulus, but not reabsorbed from or secreted into the tubules, the amount filtered (GFR $\times$ plasma [S]) must equal the amount excreted in the urine (urinary [S] $\times$ volume per unit time)

$$\text{GFR} \times \text{plasma [S]} = \begin{array}{c} \text{urinary [S]} \\ \times \\ \text{urine volume per unit time} \end{array}$$

$$\text{GFR} = \frac{\text{urinary [S]} \times \text{urine volume per unit time}}{\text{plasma [S]}}$$

The GFR thus measured is referred to as the *clearance* – the volume of plasma that could theoretically be completely cleared of a substance in a minute.

Only substances freely filtered by glomeruli and not acted on by the tubules truly measure GFR. There is no such endogenous substance, but *inulin*, a polysaccharide, fulfils the criteria closely. Because it is not produced by the body, it must be given either by constant infusion, in order to maintain steady plasma concentrations during the period of the test, or by a single injection followed by serial blood sampling to enable the concentration at the midpoint of the collection to be calculated. Similar considerations apply to the use of radiochromium labelled EDTA. Such exogenous clearances are not very practicable for routine use.

Endogenously produced substances are usually present at a fairly steady plasma concentration for the period of the test and blood need only be taken at the midpoint of the urine collection. Creatinine clearances or, more rarely urea clearances, are used but neither fulfils the necessary criteria. There is nothing to choose between the two in practice; neither measures true GFR, both parallel it.

Using the formula already given for GFR where S equals creatinine:

$$\begin{array}{c} \text{Creatinine} \\ \text{clearance} \\ \text{(ml/min)} \end{array} = \frac{\text{urinary [creat]} \times \text{urine volume (ml)}}{\text{plasma [creat]} \times \text{collection period (min)}}$$

Because some creatinine is secreted by the tubules, the creatinine clearance is higher than that of inulin. Urea clearance is lower than that of inulin by about the same amount as that of creatinine is higher as some urea is reabsorbed.

Precision and validity of clearances. Several factors make measurement of clearances more imprecise and inaccurate than those of plasma urea or creatinine concentrations.

- *Every laboratory assay has an inherent imprecision.* The combined imprecision of two assays is greater than that of one. Urine as well as plasma is assayed for clearance measurements.
- *The biggest error of any method depending on a timed urine collection is in the measurement of urine volume.* Even highly motivated patients find accurate collection difficult; collection by patients or staff who do not understand the concept of timing a urine collection (p.**427**) yields very misleading results. The difficulties are increased in infants and young children, and in patients who have difficulty in bladder emptying. Unlike analytical imprecision, the probable magnitude of these errors cannot be estimated; it is likely to be much larger than those of laboratory assays. *This error is decreased by lengthening the collection period.*
- Both creatinine and urea may be partly destroyed by bacterial action in infected or old urine. *This error is increased by lengthening the collection period.*

Interpretation of glomerular function tests. For an individual patient, plasma creatinine concentrations may rise above the baseline level but remain within the population reference range despite a deterioration in glomerular function. The plasma creatinine concentration may not exceed the upper limit of the reference range until the GFR, and therefore the creatinine clearance, has been reduced by approximately 60 per cent (Fig. 1.5; p.12). Consequently, the measurement of creatinine clearance is a more sensitive indicator of early glomerular dysfunction than that of plasma creatinine concentration.

Clearance values will be low whether the reduced GFR is due to renal circulatory insufficiency, intrinsic renal damage, or 'postrenal' causes, and cannot distinguish between them.

Serial creatinine clearance studies are often performed on patients who are receiving potentially nephrotoxic drugs; in view of the imprecision, serial plasma concentrations are probably more reliable for this purpose.

Tubular function tests

Reduced tubular function, with normal glomerular function, impairs the adjustment of the composition and volume of the urine with minimal effect on the plasma urea or creatinine concentration. The investigations used to diagnose tubular disorders can be divided into those that predominantly identify proximal tubular dysfunction and those that predominantly identify distal tubular dysfunction.

Proximal tubular function tests. Impaired solute reabsorption from the proximal tubules reduces isosmotic water reabsorption. Countercurrent multiplication may also be affected and hence the ability to respond to ADH is reduced. A large volume of inappropriately dilute urine is produced.

The tubules cannot secrete hydrogen ions and so *cannot reabsorb bicarbonate normally.* Therefore the urine is inappropriately alkaline for the degree of acidosis in the blood.

The reabsorption of potassium, phosphate, magnesium, urate, glucose and amino acids is impaired. The following findings may be present and measurement may occasionally be useful

Plasma:

- normal urea and creatinine concentrations (normal glomerular function);
- low bicarbonate concentration with low pH;
- hypokalaemia, hypophosphataemia, hypomagnesaemia and hypouricaemia.

Urine:

- increased volume;
- pH inappropriately high for that of plasma;
- phosphaturia, glycosuria;
- generalized aminoaciduria.

If there is detectable glycosuria, phosphaturia and non-selective aminoaciduria the condition is known as the Fanconi syndrome.

Distal tubular function tests. Impaired distal tubular function primarily affects urine acidification, with a failure to excrete hydrogen ions; the urine pH rarely falls below 5.5. There is an impaired response to aldosterone of the exchange mechanism involving reabsorption of sodium, and the urine contains an *inappropriately high concentration of sodium* for the renal blood flow. The associated findings may include:

Plasma:

- low bicarbonate concentration with low pH;
- hypokalaemia.

Urine:

- increased volume;
- pH inappropriately high for that of plasma; impaired response to an ammonium chloride load (p.**103**);
- an inappropriately high sodium concentration, even if renal blood flow is low (inability to respond to aldosterone);
- an inappropriately low urea concentration, and therefore osmolality, even if ADH secretion is stimulated. The *water deprivation test* may be used if tubular damage is suspected. The ability to form a concentrated urine in response to fluid deprivation depends on normal tubular function (countercurrent multiplication) and on the presence of ADH. Failure of this ability is usually due to renal disease, but if there is any suspicion of cranial diabetes insipidus the test can be repeated after giving the synthetic analogue of ADH, DDAVP (p.**75**).

*Proposed schemes for investigating patients with suspected renal disease, polyuria or oliguria are outlined on p.**72**.*

Biochemical principles of treatment of renal dysfunction

Oliguric renal dysfunction. The oliguria of volume depletion, often causing a reduced GFR without significant glomerular membrane damage, should be treated with the appropriate fluid (Table 2.7, p.**54**).

If oliguria is due to parenchymal damage the aims are:

- to restrict fluid and sodium intake, giving only enough fluid to replace losses (p.**30**);
- to provide an adequate non-protein energy source using carbohydrate with or without lipid, to minimize aggravation of uraemia and hyperkalaemia by increased endogenous catabolism;
- to prevent dangerous hyperkalaemia (p.**64**).

Some diuretics increase renal blood flow. Recovery may sometimes be hastened by giving an osmotic diuretic such as mannitol, or other diuretics such as frusemide (furosemide) or ethacrynic acid in large doses.

In chronic renal failure with polyuria the aim is *cautiously* to replace fluid and electrolyte losses. Sodium and water depletion may reduce the GFR further, and so aggravate the uraemia. If there is no response discontinue this replacement.

Dialysis removes urea and other toxic substances from the plasma and corrects electrolyte balance by dialysing the patient's blood against fluid containing no urea and appropriate concentrations of electrolytes, free-ionized calcium and other plasma constituents. The principal forms of dialysis include:

- *haemodialysis* in which blood is passed through an extracorporal circulation and dialysed across an artificial membrane with a solution of low solute concentration before being returned to the body; negative pressure on the dialysate side of the membrane can be varied to adjust the amount of water removed;

- *haemofiltration* is a form of haemodialysis in which large volumes of fluid and solute can be removed through a highly permeable membrane; dialysis is dependent primarily on the blood pressure. Fluid is replaced by intravenous administration;
- *intermittent and continuous ambulatory peritoneal dialysis (CAPD)* in which the folds of the peritoneum are used as the dialysing membrane with capillaries on one side, and an appropriate fluid of higher osmolality infused into the peritoneal cavity on the other. After a suitable time to allow for equilibration of diffusible solutes, depending on the type of peritoneal dialysis, the peritoneal cavity is drained and the cycle is repeated.

The plasma urea concentration should be reduced relatively slowly because of the danger of cellular overhydration if extracellular osmolality falls too fast (p.**34**). The urine output often falls after successful dialysis because the lower plasma urea concentration reduces the osmotic load on functioning nephrons; this does not necessarily indicate deterioration in renal function. Dialysis is used in cases of acute renal failure until renal function improves, or as a regularly repeated procedure in suitable cases of chronic renal failure. It may also be used to prepare patients for transplantation and to maintain them until the transplant functions adequately.

Renal calculi

Renal calculi are usually composed of products of metabolism present in normal glomerular filtrate, often at concentrations near their maximum solubility. Minor changes in urinary composition may cause precipitation of such constituents in the substance of the kidney (see causes of tubular damage, p.**17**), or as crystals or calculi in the renal tract. Although this discussion deals with stone formation, crystalluria or parenchymal damage can occur under the same circumstances, and the treatment of all such conditions is similar.

Conditions favouring calculus formation

- *A high urinary concentration of one or more constituents of the glomerular filtrate*, due to:

  a low urinary volume, with normal renal function, because of restricted fluid intake or excessive fluid loss over a long period of time; this is particularly common in the tropics. It favours formation of most types of calculi, especially if one of the other conditions listed below is also present;
  a high rate of excretion of the metabolic product forming the stone, due either to a high plasma and therefore filtrate levels, or to impairment of normal tubular reabsorption from the filtrate.
- *Changes in pH* of the urine, often due to bacterial infection, which favour precipitation of different salts at different hydrogen ion concentrations.
- *Urinary stagnation* due to obstruction to urinary outflow.
- *Lack of normal inhibitors.* Urine normally contains inhibitors, such as pyrophosphate and glycoproteins, which inhibit the growth of calcium phosphate and calcium oxalate crystals respectively. It has been

suggested that their absence in the urine of some patients may make them more liable to form recurrent calcium stones.

Constituents of urinary calculi

- Calcium-containing salts:

  $\left.\begin{array}{l} \text{calcium oxalate} \\ \text{calcium phosphate} \end{array}\right\}$ with or without magnesium ammonium phosphate;

- Urate;
- Cystine;
- Xanthine.

CALCULI COMPOSED OF CALCIUM SALTS

Between 70 and 90 per cent of all renal stones contain calcium. Precipitation is favoured by hypercalciuria, and the type of salt depends on urinary pH and on the availability of oxalate. Any patient presenting with calcium-containing calculi should have plasma calcium and phosphate estimations performed, and if the results are normal they should be repeated at regular intervals, to exclude primary hyperparathyroidism.

Hypercalcaemia causes hypercalciuria if glomerular function is normal, and estimation of urinary calcium concentration in such cases does not help diagnosis. The causes and differential diagnosis of hypercalcaemia are discussed on p.**178**. In many subjects with calcium-containing renal calculi the plasma calcium concentration is normal. Any *increased release of calcium from bone*, as in actively progressing osteoporosis, in which loss of matrix causes secondary decalcification or in prolonged acidosis in which ionization of calcium is increased, causes hypercalciuria; hypercalcaemia is very rare in such cases. In distal renal tubular acidosis (p.**93**) there is an increased calcium load and, because of the relative alkalinity of the urine, calcium precipitation in the kidney and renal tract may occur; this is a rare cause.

Hyperoxaluria favours the formation of the very poorly soluble calcium oxalate, even if calcium excretion is normal. The source of the oxalate may be dietary. Oxalate absorption is increased by fat malabsorption; calcium in the bowel is bound to fat instead of precipitating with oxalate which is then free to be absorbed. Primary hyperoxaluria, a rare inborn error, should be considered if renal calculi occur in childhood.

Alkaline conditions favouring calcium phosphate precipitation and stone formation are particularly common in patients with *chronic renal infection* due to urease-containing (urea-splitting) organisms, such as *Proteus vulgaris*. These bacteria convert urea to ammonia and bicarbonate.

A significant proportion of cases remain in which there is no apparent cause for calcium precipitation. The commonest cause of *hypercalciuria with normocalcaemia* is so-called *idiopathic hypercalciuria*, a name which reflects our ignorance of the aetiology of the condition. It is in such cases that estimation of urinary excretion may help.

Calcium-containing calculi are usually *hard, white and radiopaque*. Calcium phosphate may form 'staghorn' calculi in the renal pelvis, while calcium oxalate stones tend to be smaller and to lodge in the ureters, where they are compressed into a fusiform shape.

Treatment of calcium-containing calculi depends on the cause. Urinary calcium concentration should be reduced:

- by treating the primary condition, such as urinary infection or hypercalcaemia;
- if this is not possible, by reducing dietary calcium and oxalate intake;
- by reducing the *concentration* by maintaining a high fluid intake day and night, unless there is glomerular failure. Thiazide diuretics reduce urinary calcium excretion. *The concentration rather than the 24 hour output determines the tendency to precipitation.*

URIC ACID STONES

About 10 per cent of renal calculi contain uric acid; these are sometimes associated with *hyperuricaemia*, with or without clinical gout. In most cases no predisposing cause can be found. Precipitation is favoured in an *acid urine*.

Uric acid stones are usually *small, friable and yellowish-brown*, but can occasionally be large enough to form 'staghorn' calculi. They are *radiotranslucent* but may be visualized by ultrasound or by an intravenous pyelogram.

Treatment of hyperuricaemia is discussed on p.**371**. If the plasma urate concentration is normal, fluid intake should be kept high and the urine alkalinized. A low purine diet may help to reduce urate production and excretion.

CYSTINE STONES

Cystine stones are rare. In normal subjects the concentration of cystine in urine is well within its solubility but in homozygous *cystinuria* (p.**360**) this may be exceeded and the patient may present with *radio-opaque* renal calculi. Like urate, cystine is more soluble in alkaline than acid urine; the principles of treatment are the same as for uric acid stones. Penicillamine can also be used to treat the condition.

XANTHINE STONES

Xanthine stones are very uncommon and may be the result of the rare inborn error, xanthinuria (p.**371**). They have *not* been reported during treatment with xanthine oxidase inhibitors such as allopurinol, which impair the conversion of xanthine to urate.

*A proposed scheme for the investigation of a patient with renal calculi is given on p.**77**.*

Summary

The kidneys

1. Normal renal function depends on a normal filtration rate and normal tubular function.
2. A low glomerular filtration rate (GFR) leads to:
   - oliguria;
   - uraemia and retention of other nitrogenous end-products including creatinine and urate, and of phosphate;
   - a low plasma bicarbonate with metabolic acidosis;
   - hyperkalaemia.
3. Tubular damage leads to:
   - polyuria. The urine is inappropriately dilute and contains an inappropriately high sodium concentration in relation to the patient's state of hydration;
   - a low plasma bicarbonate concentration with metabolic acidosis;
   - hypokalaemia;
   - hypophosphataemia and hypouricaemia.
4. In most cases of renal disease impairment of glomerular and tubular function coexist. The clinical findings depend on the proportions of each and on the total number of nephrons involved.
5. A low GFR without significant renal damage may be due to a reduced hydrostatic pressure gradient between the capillary plasma and the tubular lumen. This is most commonly due to renal circulatory insufficiency but may be caused by postglomerular obstruction.
6. In acute oliguric renal damage plasma

findings cannot distinguish the condition from renal circulatory insufficiency.

7. The differentiation between the oliguria of renal circulatory insufficiency with relatively normal tubular function and of acute oliguric renal failure is best made on clinical grounds; if a laboratory test is felt to be necessary the urinary sodium concentration is the best indicator, but can only be interpreted if the renal blood flow was low when the specimen was secreted.

8. In most cases plasma urea or creatinine concentrations reflect changes in renal clearance and assay of one or both is adequate to diagnose and to monitor glomerular dysfunction. Tubular function may be tested by assessing the concentrating capacity of the kidney.

9. Compared with plasma assays clearance tests are relatively imprecise and inaccurate.

Renal calculi

1. The formation of renal calculi is favoured by: *

   - a high concentration of the constituents of the calculi, whether due to oliguria or a high rate of excretion of the relevant substances;
   - a urinary pH which favours precipitation of the constituents of the calculi;
   - urinary stagnation.

2. Seventy to 90 per cent of all renal calculi contain calcium. Calcium-containing stones are most commonly idiopathic in origin, but hypercalcaemia, especially that of primary hyperparathyroidism, should be excluded as a cause.

3. Uric acid stones account for about 10 per cent of renal calculi.

4. Rare causes are cystinuria, xanthinuria and hyperoxaluria.

Sodium and water metabolism

Water is an essential body constituent. Homeostatic processes ensure that:

- the *total water balance* is maintained within narrow limits;
- the *distribution of water* between the vascular, interstitial and intracellular compartments is maintained. This distribution depends on hydrostatic and osmotic forces acting across cell membranes.

Sodium is the most abundant extracellular cation and, with its associated anions, accounts for most of the osmotic activity of the extracellular fluid (ECF); it is important in determining water distribution across cell membranes. *Osmotic activity depends on concentration*, and therefore on the relative amounts of sodium and water in the extracellular fluid compartment, rather than on the absolute quantity of either. An imbalance between the two causes either hypo- or hypernatraemia and therefore changes in osmolality. The clinical pictures that may be associated with these findings are due to the consequent movement of water. *If sodium and water are lost or gained in equivalent amounts, the plasma sodium and therefore osmolal concentration is unchanged*; symptoms are then due to extracellular volume depletion or overloading. Of course, osmotic and volume disturbances often occur together.

The concentrations of associated anions such as chloride and bicarbonate usually alter at the same time as those of sodium. Although the transport of sodium, potassium and hydrogen ions across cell membranes is often interdependent, this chapter is separated from those on potassium and on hydrogen ion homeostasis for ease of discussion.

*T*OTAL WATER AND SODIUM BALANCE

In a 70 kg man, the total body water is about 42 litres and contributes about 60 per cent of the total body weight; there are about 3000 mmol of osmotically active sodium, mainly in the ECF.

Water and sodium intake

Water and electrolyte intake usually balance output in urine, faeces, sweat and expired air. The daily water and sodium intakes are very variable, but in an adult amount to about 1.5 to 2 litres and 60 to 150 mmol respectively.

Loss through the kidneys and gastrointestinal tract

The kidneys and intestine handle water and electrolytes in very similar ways. Net loss through both organs depends on the balance between the volume filtered proximally and that reabsorbed more distally. Any factor affecting either passive filtration or epithelial cellular function may disturb this balance.

Approximately 200 litres of water and 30 000 mmol of sodium are filtered by the kidneys each day; a further 10 litres of water and 1500 mmol of sodium enter the intestinal lumen. The whole of the extracellular water and sodium could be lost by passive filtration in little more than an hour but, under normal circumstances, about 99 per cent is reabsorbed. Consequently the net daily losses amount to about 1.5 to 2 litres of water and 100 mmol of sodium in the urine, and 100 ml and 15 mmol respectively in the faeces.

Fine adjustment of the relative amounts of water and sodium excretion occurs in the distal nephron and the large intestine, often under hormonal control. The effects of *antidiuretic hormone* (ADH) and the mineralocorticoid hormone *aldosterone* on the kidney are the most important physiologically.

Loss in sweat and expired air

About 900 ml of water is lost daily in sweat and in expired air; less than 30 mmol of sodium a day is lost in sweat. Although ADH and aldosterone have some effect on the composition of the latter, its volume is primarily controlled by skin temperature. Respiratory water loss depends on the respiratory rate and bears no relation to the body's need for water. Normally losses in sweat and expired air are rapidly corrected by changes in renal and intestinal loss. However, because neither of the former can be controlled to meet sodium and water requirements they may contribute considerably to abnormal balance when homeostatic mechanisms fail, or if there is gross depletion, either due to poor intake or to excessive losses by other routes.

CONTROL OF SODIUM AND WATER BALANCE

Control of sodium balance

The most important factors controlling sodium balance are renal blood flow and aldosterone. This hormone controls loss from the distal renal tubule and colon. There seems to be little, if any, control of sodium intake.

ALDOSTERONE

Aldosterone is secreted by the zona glomerulosa of the adrenal cortex (p.**118**). It affects sodium-potassium and sodium-hydrogen ion exchange across *all* cell membranes. Its principal effect is on renal tubular cells, but it also affects loss in faeces, sweat and saliva, and the distribution of electrolytes in the body.

Aldosterone stimulates sodium reabsorption from the lumen of the distal renal tubule in exchange for either potassium or hydrogen ion (Fig 2.1). The net result is retention of more sodium than water, and loss of potassium and hydrogen ions. If the circulating aldosterone concentration is high, and *tubular function is normal, the urinary sodium concentration is low.*

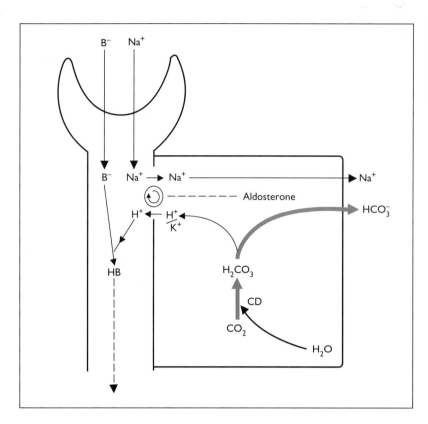

Fig. 2.1 The action of aldosterone on the reabsorption of Na+ in exchange for either K+ or H+ from the distal renal tubules (see Chapter 4 (p.84) for further details).

Many factors have been implicated in the feedback control of aldosterone secretion. These include local electrolyte concentrations, such as potassium in the adrenal gland, but they are almost certainly of less physiological and clinical importance than the effect of the renin–angiotensin system.

THE RENIN–ANGIOTENSIN SYSTEM

Renin is a proteolytic enzyme secreted by the juxtaglomerular apparatus, a cellular complex adjacent to the renal glomeruli lying between the afferent arteriole and the distal convoluted tubule (p.**2**). Secretion increases in response to a reduction in renal artery blood flow, possibly mediated by changes in the mean pressure in the afferent arterioles. Renin splits a decapeptide, *angiotensin I*, from a circulating α_2-globulin known as renin substrate. Another proteolytic enzyme, *angiotensin-converting enzyme*, located

predominantly in the lungs but also within other tissues such as the kidneys, splits off a further two amino acid residues; the remaining octapeptide *angiotensin II*, has a number of important actions:

- it acts directly on capillary walls, causing *vasoconstriction*, and so probably helps to maintain blood pressure and alter the glomerular filtration rate;
- it stimulates the cells of the zona glomerulosa to *synthesize and secrete aldosterone*;
- it *stimulates the thirst centre* and so promotes oral fluid intake.

Poor renal blood flow is often associated with an inadequate systemic blood pressure. The release of renin produces angiotensin II which tends to correct this by causing:

- vasoconstriction which may raise the blood pressure before the circulating volume can be restored;

- aldosterone release, which stimulates sodium and subsequently water retention and hence restores the circulating volume.

Thus aldosterone secretion responds, via renin, to a reduction in renal blood flow. *Sodium excretion is not directly related to total body sodium content nor to plasma sodium concentration.*

ATRIAL NATRIURETIC PEPTIDES

A peptide hormone or hormones, secreted from the right atrial wall in response to stimulation of stretch receptors, may cause a high sodium excretion (natriuresis) by increasing the GFR and by inhibiting renin and aldosterone secretion. However, its importance in the physiological control of sodium excretion and in pathological states has not yet been fully elucidated.

Control of water balance

Both intake and loss of water are controlled by the osmotic gradients across cell membranes in hypothalamic centres. These centres, which are closely related anatomically, control *thirst* and secretion of *antidiuretic hormone.*

ANTIDIURETIC HORMONE (ADH; ARGININE VASOPRESSIN)

ADH is synthesized in the hypothalamus and, after transport down the pituitary stalk, is secreted from the posterior pituitary gland (p.**107**).

Control of ADH secretion. ADH secretion is stimulated by flow of water out of cells caused by a relatively high extracellular osmolality (p.**36**). If the osmolality inside cells is unchanged, an extracellular increase of only two per cent quadruples ADH output; an equivalent fall almost completely inhibits

it. This represents a change in plasma sodium concentration of only about 3 mmol/L. In more chronic changes, when the osmotic gradient has been minimized by solute redistribution (p.**33**), there may be little or no effect. In addition stretch receptors in the left atria, and baroreceptors in the aortic arch and carotid sinus, influence ADH secretion in response to the low intravascular pressure of severe hypovolaemia, stimulating ADH release. This sometimes overrides the inhibition due to low plasma osmolality, which is then not fully corrected.

Actions of ADH. ADH enhances water reabsorption, *in excess of solute*, from the collecting ducts and so dilutes the extracellular osmolality (p.**7**). When ADH secretion is a response to a high extracellular osmolality with the danger of cell dehydration, this is an appropriate response. However, if secretion is in response to a low circulating volume alone, it is inappropriate to the osmolality. The retained water is then distributed throughout the total body water space, entering cells along the osmotic gradient; the correction of extracellular depletion with water alone is thus relatively inefficient in correcting hypovolaemia (p.**44**).

Sometimes the effectiveness of ADH is opposed by other factors. For example during an osmotic diuresis the urine, although hypo-osmolal, contains more water than sodium. Patients being fed intravenously, or who, because of tissue damage, are breaking down more protein than usual, and so are producing more urea from the released amino acids, may become water depleted even if there is adequate ADH; urinary osmolality will be high in these cases.

Assessment of sodium and water balance

Although it is easy to measure the water and sodium intake of patients receiving oral or intravenous liquid feeds, it is less so when a solid diet is being taken. Fortunately, accurate assessment is rarely needed in such cases.

Renal loss should be easy to measure *if the principles of collection are understood* (p.**72**) and if the patient is not incontinent or otherwise unable to cooperate. That lost in formed faeces, sweat and expired air ('insensible loss') is more difficult to assess. These losses may be important when homeostatic mechanisms have failed or there are very high losses by extrarenal routes in, for example, unconscious patients or infants (p.**72**). The aim should be to ensure that, once such subjects are normally hydrated, they are kept 'in balance'. The doctor has the difficult task of imitating normal homeostasis without the help of the sensitive, interlinked mechanisms of the body.

Assessment of the state of hydration

Assessment of the state of hydration of a patient relies on clinical examination and on laboratory evidence of haemoconcentration or haemodilution. Both these methods are crude and quite severe disturbances can occur before there are detectable clinical or laboratory findings.

- *Haemoconcentration.* Extracellular fluid is usually lost from the vascular compartment first and, unless the fluid is whole blood, depletion of water and small molecules results in a rise in concentrations of large molecules, such as proteins and all types of blood cells with a rise in blood haemoglobin concentration and haematocrit.
- *Haemodilution.* Increasing plasma volume with protein-free fluid leads to a fall in the concentrations of proteins and haemoglobin. However, these findings may be affected by pre-existing abnormalities of

protein or red cell concentrations, and although changes are almost always more informative than single readings, both protein and haemoglobin concentrations may alter following, for example, blood transfusion or because of the primary disease.

It may be very difficult to assess hydration, but it is usually possible if the history and clinical and laboratory findings are all taken into account. Occasionally measurement of the urinary sodium concentration may help (p.**46**).

Monitoring total fluid balance

By far the most important measurements in assessing changes in day-to-day fluid balance are accurate records of fluid intake and output. 'Insensible loss' is usually assumed to be about 900 ml/day, but there is endogenous water production of about 500 ml/day by metabolic processes. Therefore the *net* daily 'insensible loss' is about 400 ml. The required daily intake may be calculated from the output during the previous day plus 400 ml to allow for 'insensible loss'; this method is satisfactory if the patient is normally hydrated before day-to-day monitoring is started.

A pyrexial patient may lose a litre or more of fluid in sweat, and, if he is also hyperventilating, respiratory water loss may be considerable. In such cases an allowance of 400 ml for insensible loss may be totally inadequate. In addition, many very ill patients may be incontinent of urine, thus making accurate assessments of fluid losses very difficult.

In most circumstances carefully recorded fluid balance charts are of more importance than frequent electrolyte estimations. *Inaccurate measurement and charting is useless and may be dangerous.*

DISTRIBUTION OF WATER AND SODIUM IN THE BODY

In mild disturbances of water and electrolyte balance their total amounts in the body may be of less importance than their distribution between body compartments.

Water is distributed between the main body fluid compartments in which different electrolytes contribute to the osmolality. These compartments are:

- **intracellular**, in which *potassium* is the predominant cation;
- **extracellular**, in which *sodium* is the predominant cation and which can be subdivided into:

  interstitial of very low protein concentration;

  intravascular (plasma) containing protein in relatively high concentration.

Distribution of electrolytes between cells and interstitial fluid

Sodium is the predominant extracellular cation, the intracellular concentration being less than a tenth of that within the ECF; the intracellular potassium concentration is about 30 times that of the ECF. About 95 per cent of the osmotically active sodium is outside cells and about the same proportion of potassium is intracellular. These differential concentrations are maintained by cell-surface energy-dependent sodium/potassium ATPase pumps.

Other ions tend to move across cell membranes in association with sodium and potassium. The movement of hydrogen ions has already been mentioned. Magnesium and phosphate ions are predominantly intracellular and those of chloride extracellular. The distribution of these and of

bicarbonate is often affected by the same factors that influence sodium and potassium distribution.

Distribution of electrolytes between plasma and interstitial fluid

The cell membranes of the capillary endothelium are more permeable to small ions than those of tissue cells. The plasma protein concentration is relatively high, but that of interstitial fluid very low. The osmotic effect of the intravascular proteins is balanced by very slightly higher interstitial electrolyte concentrations ('Gibbs Donnan effect'); this difference is small and, for practical purposes, plasma electrolyte concentrations can be assumed to be representative of those in the extracellular fluid as a whole.

Distribution of water

Over half the body water is inside cells (Table 2.1). About 15 to 20 per cent of the extracellular water is intravascular; the remainder constitutes the interstitial fluid.

The distribution of water across biological membranes depends on the balance between the hydrostatic pressure and the *in vivo* effective osmotic pressure differences on each side of the membrane. Correct interpretation of plasma electrolyte results depends on a clear understanding of these factors.

Table 2.1 The approximate volumes in different body compartments through which water is distributed, in a 70 kg adult

	Volume (litres)
Total body water	42
Intracellular compartment	24
Extracellular compartment	18
interstitial space	13
intravascular space (blood volume)	5

OSMOTIC PRESSURE

Net movement of water across a membrane permeable only to water depends on the concentration gradient of particles, either ions or molecules, across that membrane; this is known as the *osmotic gradient*. However, *for any weight to volume ratio*, the larger the particles the fewer there are per unit volume, and therefore the less osmotic effect they exert. If the membranes were freely permeable to ions and smaller particles as well as to water, these diffusible particles would exert no osmotic effect across membranes and therefore the larger ones would become more important in affecting water movement. This phenomenon gives rise to the *effective colloid osmotic (oncotic) gradient*. To explain water distribution in the body it is essential to understand the importance of these three factors:

- number of particles per unit volume;
- concentration gradient across the membrane;
- particle size relative to membrane permeability.

UNITS OF MEASUREMENT OF OSMOTIC PRESSURE

Osmolar concentration can be expressed as:

- *the osmolarity* in mmol/L of *solution*;
- *the osmolality* in mmol/kg of *solvent*.

If solute is dissolved in pure water at concentrations such as those in body fluids, osmolarity and osmolality will hardly differ.

However, as plasma is a complex solution containing large molecules such as proteins, the total volume of solution (water + protein) is greater than the volume of solvent only (water) in which the small molecules are dissolved. At a protein concentration of 70 g/L the volume of water is about six per cent less than the total volume of the solution (that is, the molarity should theoretically be about six per cent less that the molality). Most methods for measuring individual ions assess them in molarity (mmol/L). If the concentration of proteins in plasma is grossly increased, the volume of solvent is significantly reduced but the volume of solution remains unchanged. Therefore the molarity of certain ions, such as sodium, in mmol/L will be reduced but the molality will be unaltered (Fig. 2.2). This apparently low sodium concentration is known as pseudo-hyponatraemia (p.**38**).

Measured plasma osmolality. Osmometers measure changes in properties of a solution, such as freezing-point depression or vapour pressure which depend on the total osmolality of the solution – the osmotic effect that would be exerted by the sum of all the dissolved molecules and ions across a membrane permeable only to water. These properties are known as *colligative properties*. Sodium and its associated anions, mainly chloride, contribute 90 per cent or more to this measured plasma osmolality, the effect of protein being negligible (Table 2.2). As the only major difference in composition between plasma and interstitial fluid is in protein content, the plasma osmolality is almost identical with that of the interstitial fluid surrounding cells.

Calculated plasma osmolarity. It is the osmol*al*, rather than the osmol*ar*, concentration that exerts an effect across cell membranes and which is controlled by homeostatic mechanisms. However, as discussed below, the calculated plasma osmolarity is usually as informative as the measured plasma osmolality.

Although, because of the space occupying effect of protein, the measured osmolality of

Table 2.2 Approximate contributions of solutes to plasma osmolality

	Osmolality (mmol/kg)	Per cent total
Sodium and anions	270	92
Potassium and anions	7	
Calcium (ionized) and anions	3+	
Magnesium and anions	1+	8
Urea	5	
Glucose	5	
Protein	1 (approx)	
Total	292 (approx)	

plasma should be higher than the osmolarity, calculated from the sum of the molar concentrations of all the ions, there is usually little difference between the two figures. This is because there is incomplete ionization of, for example NaCl to Na^+ and Cl^-; this reduces the osmotic effect by almost the same amount as the volume occupied by protein raises it. Consequently the calculated plasma osmolarity is a valid approximation to the true measured osmolality. However, if there is gross *hyperproteinaemia* or *hyperlipidaemia* such that either protein or lipid contributes much more than six per cent to the measured plasma volume, the calculated osmolarity may then be significantly lower that the true osmolality in the plasma water. A hypothetical example is shown in Fig. 2.2.

Many formulae of varying complexity have been proposed to calculate plasma osmolarity. None of them can predict the osmotic effect, but the following formula gives a close approximation to plasma osmolality.

Plasma osmolarity = 2([Na$^+$] + [K$^+$]) + [urea] + [glucose] in mmol/L

The factor of 2, which is applied to the sodium and potassium concentrations, allows for the associated anions and assumes complete ionization. This calculation is not valid if:

- an unmeasured osmotically active solute, such as mannitol or alcohol, is circulating in plasma. A significant difference between measured and calculated osmotic pressures, in the absence of hyperproteinaemia or hyperlipidaemia, may suggest alcohol or other poisoning. For example, a plasma alcohol concentration of 100 mg/dl contributes about 20 mmol/kg to the osmolality. This osmotic difference is known as the *osmolar gap* and can be used to assess the presence in plasma of *unmeasured* osmotically active particles;
- gross hyperproteinaemia or hyperlipidaemia is present.

In such cases the plasma sodium concentration may be misleading as a measure of the osmotic effect and plasma osmolality should be measured.

Calculation of urinary osmolarity is not feasible because of the considerable variation in the concentrations of different, sometimes unmeasured, solutes; the osmotic pressure of urine can only be determined by measuring the osmolality.

DISTRIBUTION OF WATER ACROSS CELL MEMBRANES

Osmotic pressure gradient. Because the hydrostatic pressure difference across the cell membrane is negligible cell hydration depends on the effective osmotic difference between intra- and extracellular fluids. The cell membranes are freely permeable to water and to some solutes but different solutes diffuse, or are actively transported, across cell membranes at different rates, but always much more slowly than water. In a stable state the total intracellular osmolality, due mostly to potassium and associated anions, equals that of the interstitial fluid, due mostly to sodium and associated anions; consequently there is no *net* movement of water into or out of cells. In some pathological states rapid changes of extracellular solute concentration affect cell hydration; slower changes may allow time for redistribution of solute and have little or no effect.

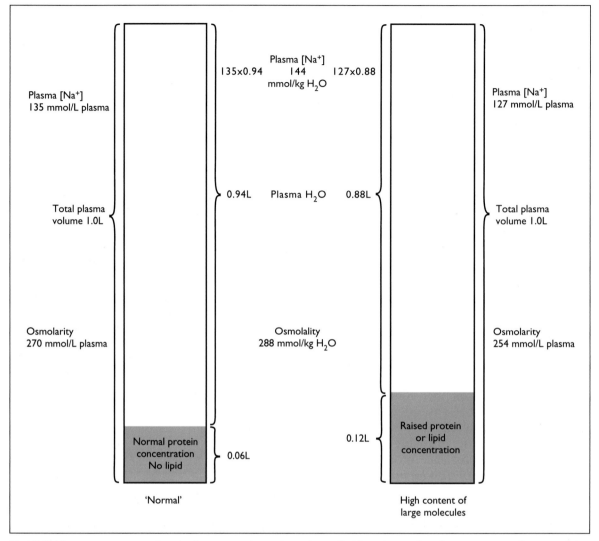

Plasma [Na⁺]
135x0.94   144   127x0.88
mmol/kg H₂O

Plasma [Na⁺]
135 mmol/L plasma

Plasma [Na⁺]
127 mmol/L plasma

0.94L   Plasma H₂O   0.88L

Total plasma
volume 1.0L

Total plasma
volume 1.0L

Osmolarity
270 mmol/L plasma

Osmolality
288 mmol/kg H₂O

Osmolarity
254 mmol/L plasma

Normal protein
concentration
No lipid

0.06L

0.12L

Raised protein
or lipid
concentration

'Normal'

High content of
large molecules

Fig. 2.2 The consequence of gross hyperproteinaemia or hyperlipidaemia on the plasma water volume and its effect on the calculated plasma osmolarity and the true plasma osmolality.

- **Sodium**. Rapid changes in the concentration of extracellular sodium and its associated anions, because they account for at least 90 per cent of the extracellular osmolality in normal subjects, affect cell hydration; if there is no significant change in the other solutes, a rise causes cellular dehydration and a fall causes cellular overhydration.
- **Urea**. Normal extracellular concentrations are so low as to contribute very little to the measured plasma osmolality. However, concentrations 15-fold or more above normal can occur in severe uraemia and can then make a significant contribution. However, urea does diffuse into cells very much more slowly than water. Consequently in acute uraemia the increased osmotic gradient alters cell hydration, but in chronic uraemia, although the measured plasma osmolality is frequently increased, the *osmotic effect of urea is*

reduced as the concentrations gradually equalize on the two sides of the membrane.

- **Glucose**. Like urea, the normally low extracellular concentration does not contribute significantly to the osmolality. However, unlike urea, glucose is actively transported into many cells, but once there it is rapidly metabolized, even at high extracellular concentrations and the intracellular concentration remains low. Severe hyperglycaemia, whether acute or chronic, causes a marked osmotic effect across cell membranes, with movement of water from cells into the extracellular compartment causing cellular dehydration.

Although uraemia and hyperglycaemia can both cause cellular dehydration, the contribution of normal urea and glucose concentrations to plasma osmolality is so small that reduced levels of these solutes, unlike those of sodium, do not cause cellular overhydration.

Increases in concentrations of other endogenous solutes, such as calcium, potassium or magnesium, enough significantly to affect the osmotic gradient across cell membranes are incompatible with life for other reasons.

Exogenous substances such as mannitol, not transported into cells, remain within the extracellular compartment and contribute to the osmolality, can be infused into the circulation to reduce cerebral oedema. Like urea and glucose, mannitol can cause an osmotic diuresis (p.**16**). Alcohol may have a similar effect.

Large rises in the osmotic gradient across cell membranes may result in the movement of enough water from the intracellular compartment to dilute extracellular constituents. Consequently, if the change in osmolality has not been caused by sodium and its associated anions, a fall in plasma sodium concentration is appropriate to the state of osmolality. If, under such circumstances the plasma sodium concentration is not low this indicates hyperosmolality (p.**32**).

In almost all circumstances plasma osmolarity, calculated from sodium, potassium, urea and glucose concentrations, is at least as clinically valuable as measurement of plasma osmolality. It has the advantage that the solute responsible, and therefore its likely osmotic effect, is often identified.

DISTRIBUTION OF WATER ACROSS CAPILLARY MEMBRANES

Maintenance of blood pressure depends on the retention of fluid within the intravascular compartment at a higher hydrostatic pressure than that of the interstitial space. Hydrostatic pressure in capillary lumina tends to force fluid into the extravascular space. In the absence of any effective opposing force fluid would be lost rapidly from the vascular compartment. Unlike other cell membranes, those of the capillaries are permeable to small ions. *Therefore sodium alone exerts almost no osmotic effect and the distribution of water across capillary membranes is little affected by changes in electrolyte concentration.*

Colloid osmotic pressure. The very small osmotic effect of plasma protein molecules produces an effective osmotic gradient across capillary membranes; this is known as the *colloid osmotic*, or *oncotic pressure*. It is the most important factor opposing the net outward hydrostatic pressure (Fig. 2.3). Albumin (molecular weight 65 000), present intravascularly at significant concentration and extravascularly at very low concentration because it cannot pass freely across the capillary wall, is the most important protein contributing to the colloid osmotic pressure. The measurement of plasma albumin concentration is a crude guide to the plasma colloid osmotic pressure. Larger molecular weight proteins, although present at much the same weight per volume as albumin, contribute much less to this effect because of their larger sizes. Because proteins contribute negligibly to total plasma osmotic pressure (Table 2.2; p.**33**), *measurement of plasma osmolality cannot be used to assess colloid osmotic effects across capillary walls.*

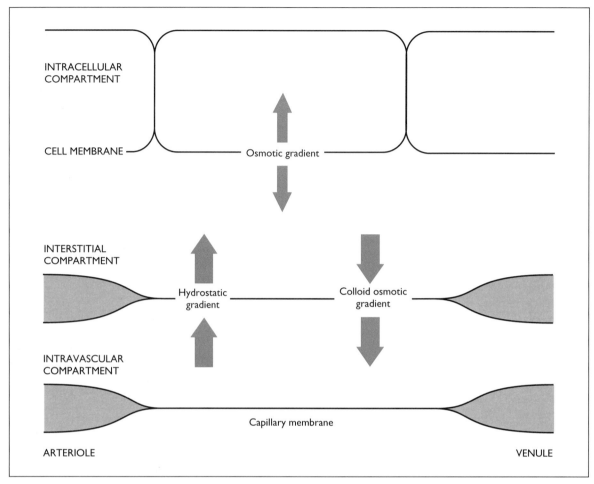

Fig. 2.3 Osmotic factors which control the distribution of water between the fluid compartments of the body.

Relation between sodium and water homeostasis

In normal subjects the concentrations of sodium and its associated anions are the most important osmotic factors affecting ADH secretion. Plasma volume, by its effect on renal blood flow, controls aldosterone secretion and therefore sodium balance. The homeostatic mechanisms controlling sodium and water excretion are interdependent. A simplified scheme is shown in Fig. 2.4.

Thirst depends on a rise in extracellular osmolality, whether due to water depletion or sodium excess, and also by a very large increase in the activity of the renin–angiotensin.

A rise in extracellular osmolality reduces water loss by stimulating ADH release and increases intake by stimulating thirst; both these actions dilute the extracellular osmolality. Osmotic balance, and therefore cellular hydration, is rapidly corrected. If the primary abnormality is in sodium rather than in water balance, cellular hydration is sometimes protected at the expense of aggravating abnormalities in total body volume.

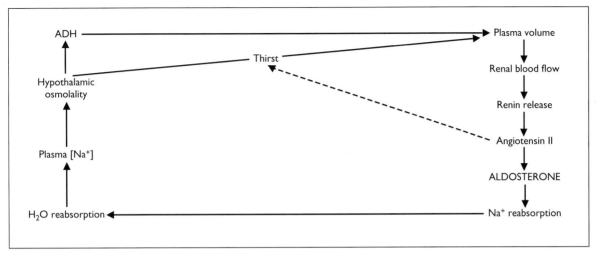

Fig. 2.4 Control of water and sodium homeostasis.

Assessment of sodium status

As discussed, the plasma sodium concentration is important because of its osmotic effect on fluid distribution. Plasma sodium concentrations should be monitored while volume is being corrected to ensure that the distribution of fluid between the intra- and the extracellular compartments is optimal. The presence of other osmotically active solutes should be taken into account. Measurement of total body sodium is not a useful investigation

Clinical Features of Sodium and Water Disturbances

The initial clinical consequences of:
- primary sodium disturbances depend on changes of extracellular osmolality and hence of cellular hydration;
- primary water disturbances depend on changes in extracellular volume.

Clinical features of disturbances of sodium concentration

Measuring the plasma sodium concentration is usually a substitute for measuring plasma osmolality. Plasma sodium concentrations *per se* are not important, but their effect on the osmotic gradient across cell membranes is. It is important to understand that the one does not always reflect the other.

If the concentration of plasma sodium alters rapidly, and those of other extracellular solutes remain the same, most of the clinical features are due to the consequence of the osmotic difference across cell membranes, with redistribution of fluid between cells and the extracellular fluid. However, gradual changes, which allow time for redistribution of diffusible solute, such as urea, and so for equalization of osmolality without major shifts of water, may produce little effect on fluid distribution.

Hyponatraemia is usually caused by excess water relative to sodium within the extracellular compartment and may reflect extracellular hypo-osmolality (Table 2.3). If this is so it may cause cellular overhydration. However, hyponatraemia, *associated with a normal plasma osmolality* may occur in the following situations:

- *artefactual hyponatraemia* may be due to taking blood from the limb into which fluid of low sodium concentration is being infused, and may not reflect the sodium concentration in the general circulation (p.**425**);
- *appropriate hyponatraemia* may be due, for example, to acute uraemia, hyperglycaemia, infusion of amino acids or mannitol, a high plasma alcohol or other solute concentrations. All these may increase extracellular osmolality; the consequent homeostatic dilution of total extracellular solute concentration towards normal causes hyponatraemia which reflects partial or complete compensation of hyperosmolality, rather than hypo-osmolality;
- *'pseudohyponatraemia'* may be due to gross hyperlipidaemia or to hyperproteinaemia. The sodium concentration in plasma water, and therefore the osmolality at cell membranes, may then be normal (Fig. 2.2; p.**34**).

Infusion of isosmolal sodium-containing fluids, with the aim of 'correcting' artefactual, appropriate or pseudohyponatraemia, is dangerous.

When hyponatraemia reflects true hypo-osmolality cerebral cellular overhydration may cause headache, confusion, fits and even death.

Hypernatraemia *always reflects hyperosmolality*, with the danger of cellular dehydration *providing artefactual causes, such as the use of excess sodium heparin as an anticoagulant, have been excluded* (p.**426**). Severe hypernatraemia can never be appropriate to the osmolal state; the plasma concentrations of solutes other than sodium are very low and do not contribute significantly to the plasma osmolality (Table 2.2; p.33). For example, although hyperglycaemia can increase the plasma osmolality by as much as 50 mmol/kg in 290 mmol/kg (about 18 per cent), complete absence of glucose would only reduce it by about 5 mmol/kg (about two per cent). Some causes of hypernatraemia are shown in Table 2.4.

The clinical effects of cerebral cellular dehydration are *thirst, mental confusion* and later *coma*.

Table 2.3 Some causes of hyponatraemia

Plasma osmolality normal or increased
  artefactual
  appropriate hyponatraemia
    acute uraemia
    diabetes mellitus
    infusion of amino acids or mannitol
    alcohol
  pseudohyponatraemia
    hyperlipidaemia or hyperproteinaemia

Plasma osmolality low
  intravascular volume depletion
    diuretic treatment
    adrenal insufficiency (Addison's disease)
  increased extracellular fluid volume
    inappropriate composition of fluid replacement
    inappropriate ADH secretion
  increased extracellular fluid volume with oedema
    congestive cardiac failure
    nephrotic syndrome

Table 2.4 Some causes of hypernatraemia, once artefactual causes have been excluded

Inadequate water intake
   unavailability of water
   failure to drink
      unconsciousness or confusion
      infants
      damage to thirst centre

Impaired water retention
   osmotic diuresis such as
      glycosuria
      increased urea load
   diabetes insipidus

Excessive sodium intake
   drugs
      some antibiotics
         carbenicillin
         metronidazole
   diet (very rare)

Excessive sodium retention
   excess mineralocorticoid
      Conn's syndrome
      Cushing's syndrome

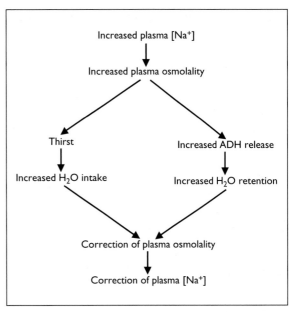

Fig. 2.5 Homeostatic mechanisms involved in the correction of hypernatraemia.

Hyponatraemia is a much commoner finding than hypernatraemia and is often appropriate to the osmolal state. If artefactual causes are excluded, the incidence of true hypo-osmolality is probably not much higher than that of hypernatraemia, which always reflects hyperosmolality. Figure 2.5 outlines the physiological mechanisms that prevent significant hypernatraemia developing in the conscious individual who has access to water.

Disturbances of sodium and water metabolism

Disturbances of sodium and water balance are most commonly due to excessive losses from the body, usually of gastrointestinal fluid. These losses may be inappropriately increased if the volume or composition of infused fluid is incorrect; repletion will then be relatively ineffective and the increased gastrointestinal excretion may aggravate the clinical abnormalities.

More rarely the primary defects are excessive or deficient secretion of aldosterone or ADH.

WATER AND SODIUM DEFICIENCY

Apart from loss of solute-free water in expired air, water and sodium are always lost together from the body. An imbalance between the degree of their deficiencies is relatively common and may be due to the composition of the fluid lost or to that of the fluid given to replace it.

The initial effects depend on the composition of the fluid lost compared with that of plasma.

- *Isosmolar volume depletion* results if the sodium concentration of the fluid lost is similar to that of plasma; *changes in plasma sodium concentration are then rare.*
- *Predominant sodium depletion is usually the result of inappropriate treatment,* since no body fluid has a significantly higher

sodium concentration than that of plasma, apart from concentrated bile. *Hyponatraemia results.*

- *Predominant water depletion* results if the *sodium concentration of the fluid lost is much lower than that of plasma.* *Hypernatraemia* indicates loss of relatively more water than sodium, even if there is little evidence of volume depletion.

Subsequent effects depend on the efficiency of homeostatic mechanisms and on the availability and composition of fluid replacement.

We believe that the term 'dehydration' should be abandoned. It is often used to describe all the conditions listed above, although the clinical and biochemical findings are very different. The consequent confusion may lead to inappropriate and possibly dangerous treatment. An attempt should be made to assess the approximate composition of fluid lost by identifying its origin.

Isosmolar volume depletion

CAUSES OF ISOSMOLAR FLUID LOSS

The sodium concentrations of all small intestinal secretions and of the urine passed, when tubular function is grossly impaired, are between 120 and 140 mmol/L. Clinical conditions causing approximately isosmolar loss are therefore:

- small intestinal fistulae, including new ileostomies;
- small intestinal obstruction and paralytic ileus, in which the fluid accumulating in the gut lumen has, like urine in the bladder, been lost from the ECF;
- severe renal tubular damage with minimal glomerular dysfunction; for example, the recovery phase of acute oliguric renal dysfunction, or polyuric chronic renal dysfunction.

Intestinal losses are much more likely to produce severe volume depletion than renal tubular disease.

RESULTS OF ISOSMOLAR FLUID LOSS

Hypovolaemia reduces renal blood flow and causes renal circulatory insufficiency with *oliguria, uraemia* and the other changes described on p.**10**. Sodium and water are lost in almost equivalent amounts and the plasma sodium concentration is usually normal; for this reason the patient may not complain of thirst despite some volume depletion.

Haemoconcentration confirms considerable loss of fluid other than blood, although its absence does not exclude such loss. Apart from the possibility of pre-existing abnormalities of haemoglobin and plasma protein concentrations, increased capillary permeability, which frequently accompanies conditions associated with the 'shock' syndrome, may enable albumin to diffuse more freely than usual into the interstitial fluid resulting in hypoalbuminaemia.

Postural hypotension, a fall in blood pressure on standing, is a relatively early sign of volume depletion. Severe hypovolaemia causes *hypotension* even in the supine position.

CHANGES PRODUCED BY HOMEOSTATIC MECHANISMS

The ability to respond to hormonal homeostatic changes depends mainly on renal tubular function and does not occur if the isosmolar volume depletion is due to tubular damage.

The reduced intravascular volume impairs renal blood flow and stimulates renin and therefore aldosterone secretion. There is selective sodium reabsorption from the distal tubules and a *low urinary sodium concentration* (Fig. 2.6).

The tendency of the retained sodium to increase plasma osmolality stimulates ADH secretion and water is reabsorbed; this tends to correct the circulating volume and keep the plasma sodium concentration normal. *Severe* intravascular volume depletion may also stimulate ADH secretion and therefore water retention, causing mild hyponatraemia. This additional water is distributed throughout the total body water space and moves from the depleted, and now slightly hypo-osmolar, ECF into the relatively well-hydrated intracellular compartment.

Even maximal renal water and sodium retention cannot correct extrarenal losses that exceed those of a normal urine output. Water and sodium must be replaced in adequate amounts to provide 'substrate' for the kidneys. However, it is important to understand that excessive replacement, especially with fluid of an inappropriate concentration, has undesirable side effects. Replacement of isosmolar fluid loss with fluid of low sodium concentration is the commonest cause of predominant sodium depletion; this is discussed below.

EFFECTS OF INTRAVENOUS VOLUME REPLACEMENT

Patients unable to absorb adequate amounts of oral fluid because of gastrointestinal loss usually need intravenous replacement. The following discussion applies to such cases and assumes normal renal function.

Fluid replacement in a patient who presents with hypovolaemia can be monitored by clinical observation and by the measurement of urine output. There is always the danger that overcorrection will increase intestinal loss of fluid and result in the accumulation of more fluid in an already distended bowel caused by an intestinal obstruction or paralytic ileus.

Infusion of protein-free fluid increases the hydrostatic gradient and reduces the opposing colloid osmotic gradient by diluting plasma proteins. The desirable increase in glomerular filtration, caused by the overcorrection of hypovolaemia, results in an increase in urine output and is a common cause of a low plasma urea concentration. This is inevitably accompanied by a less desirable increase in intestinal and renal loss. The reduction in the intravascular colloid osmotic pressure could be minimized if the infused fluid contained molecules of about the size of albumin. This would also minimize fluid loss from the vascular compartment into the interstitial space. Unfortunately infused albumin

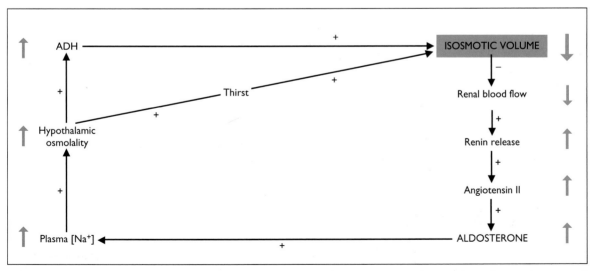

Fig. 2.6 Homeostatic correction of isosmotic volume depletion. The reduced intravascular volume impairs renal blood flow and stimulates renin and therefore aldosterone secretion. There is selective sodium reabsorption from the distal tubules and a low urinary sodium concentration (shaded area indicates primary change).

has a very short intravascular half-life; most other colloid preparations have some disadvantages and, unless salt has been extracted during preparation, contain relatively high sodium concentrations.

It is difficult to assess clinically when volume repletion is adequate but not excessive. Measurement of urinary sodium concentration may sometimes help. If tubular function is adequate, a urinary sodium concentration of less than about 20 mmol/L suggests that renal blood flow is still low enough to stimulate maximal renin and aldosterone secretion, and infusion should be increased. A urinary sodium concentration much higher than 30 mmol/L *in a patient with adequate tubular function* suggests overcorrection and the need to slow the rate of infusion. Urinary sodium levels may sometimes need to be monitored in this way until intestinal obstruction is relieved. In cases in which all losses can be measured, further maintenance of normal balance should be based on *accurate* fluid balance charts.

Predominant sodium depletion

EFFECTS OF THE COMPOSITION OF INFUSED FLUID

No body secretion has a sodium concentration significantly higher than that of plasma. Predominant sodium depletion is almost always due to infusion of fluid of inappropriate composition. The composition of the fluid is even more important than the volume. The effect of the absence of colloid in electrolyte solutions has already been discussed.

Patients with isosmolar fluid depletion, or recovering from major surgery, are often infused with fluid such as 'dextrose saline' which contains about 30 mmol/L of sodium.

Glucose in the infused fluid renders it isosmolar despite the low sodium concentration, but the glucose is metabolized and both plasma sodium and osmolality are diluted by the remaining hypo-osmolar fluid. Homeostatic mechanisms tend to correct this hypo-osmolality but may to be overwhelmed if the infusion rate is high (Fig. 2.7).

The excess hypo-osmolar infused fluid dilutes the plasma sodium causing a dilutional hyponatraemia with hypo-osmolality. The homeostatic mechanisms that tend to correct this hypo-osmolality involve the inhibition of ADH secretion. The excess water is lost in the urine until restoration of normal plasma osmolality again stimulates normal ADH secretion. Correction of osmolality may occur at the expense of intravascular volume. This would stimulate renin and aldosterone secretion and sodium would be retained with the consequent restoration of osmolality and normal ADH secretion.

However, if intravascular volume is maintained by replacing the urinary volume with effectively hypotonic fluid, hypo-osmolality with hyponatraemia persists and sodium depletion is aggravated. As shown in Fig. 2.7, restoration of the plasma volume inhibits renin and aldosterone secretion and sodium is lost in the urine despite hypo-osmolality. The net effect of this procedure is restoration of circulating volume at the expense of sodium depletion and cellular overhydration.

The clinical findings include:

- those due to hypo-osmolality;
- a large volume of dilute urine due to inhibition of ADH secretion (p.**29**).

The laboratory findings include:

- hyponatraemia.

If fluid intake is excessive, the following also occur:

- haemodilution;
- a low plasma urea concentration due to the high GFR. Excessive intravenous infusion is one of the commonest causes of a low plasma urea concentration;

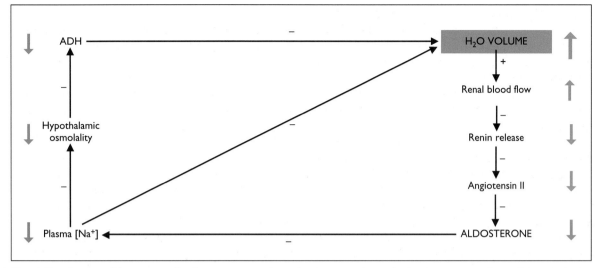

Fig. 2.7 Infusion of hypotonic fluid as a cause of predominant sodium depletion. Increased circulating volume with reduction in plasma osmolality inhibits aldosterone and ADH secretion (shaded area indicates primary change).

- *high urinary sodium concentration, due to inhibition of aldosterone secretion.*

During the immediate postoperative period, pain and stress also stimulate ADH secretion and therefore water retention; this effect is short lived. Hyponatraemia is rarely a problem unless hypo-osmolar saline is being infused. Taking all these factors into account, it is not surprising that postoperative hyponatraemia is so common.

In subjects with normal renal function the mechanisms described above rapidly correct both sodium and water balance when the infusion is stopped, and no serious harm is done. However, by alternating 'dextrose saline' and isotonic saline, we find that most patients can maintain relatively normal plasma sodium and urea concentrations, while passing an adequate volume of urine; the danger of overloading the circulation is minimal if renal and cardiac function are normal. Infusion should be stopped as soon as the patient can take oral fluids. Infusion of 'dextrose saline' without any other fluid into seriously ill patients whose homeostatic mechanisms may be impaired is even more likely to cause dangerous hyponatraemia.

FAILURE OF HOMEOSTATIC MECHANISMS CONTROLLING SODIUM

Aldosterone deficiency, such as occurs in *Addison's disease* (p.**126**), the least rare cause, is a much more uncommon cause of sodium depletion than that described above. *Initial* homeostatic reactions tend to maintain osmolality at the expense of volume.

Although less than 1.5 per cent of the filtered sodium is reabsorbed in the renal distal convoluted tubules, this is where the fine adjustment is made in the ratio of sodium to water and therefore to plasma osmolality and hence normal cell hydration is safeguarded. If aldosterone cannot be secreted normally in response to an increase in those of renin and angiotensin, this adjustment cannot be made (Fig. 2.8). Under such circumstances, although a greater proportion of sodium may be reabsorbed from the proximal tubules, there may still be relative sodium deficiency and hypovolaemia. *Initially*, plasma osmolality, and therefore plasma sodium concentration, are maintained by excess water loss; loss of sodium in excess of water reduces plasma osmolality and cuts off ADH secretion.

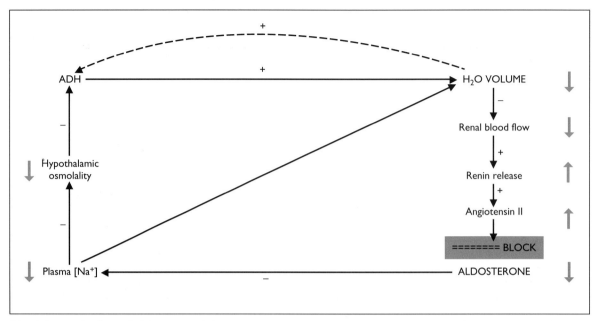

Fig. 2.8 Initial effect of aldosterone deficiency results in impaired sodium retention and hypovolaemia; later, severe hypovolaemia stimulates increased ADH secretion with water retention sometimes causing a dilutional hyponatraemia (shaded area indicates the primary change).

Later, hypovolaemia stimulates ADH secretion, with water retention in excess of sodium; dilutional hyponatraemia may occur despite intravascular volume depletion.

The clinical features include circulatory insufficiency with postural hypotension.

The laboratory findings include:

- haemoconcentration due to fluid depletion;
- renal circulatory insufficiency with mild uraemia, due to volume depletion;
- an inappropriately high urinary sodium concentration in the presence of volume depletion;
- *later* dilutional hyponatraemia and hyper-kalaemia.

Predominant water depletion

Predominant water depletion is caused by loss of water in excess of sodium. It is usually due either to loss of fluid which has a sodium concentration less than that of plasma, or to deficient water intake. The rise in extracellular osmolality stimulates both ADH secretion, which minimizes water loss, and thirst. Because of the latter effect, laboratory abnormalities are most marked if the patient is unable to respond to thirst. Causes of predominant water depletion can be divided into the following groups.

Predominant water depletion with normal homeostatic mechanisms.

- Excessive loss of fluid that has a sodium concentration less than that of plasma. These include:
  loss of large amounts of sweat, such as in pyrexial patients;
  loss of gastric fluid;
  loss of fluid stools of low sodium con-centration, usually in infantile gastro-enteritis;
  excessive respiratory loss;
  loss of fluid from extensive burns.

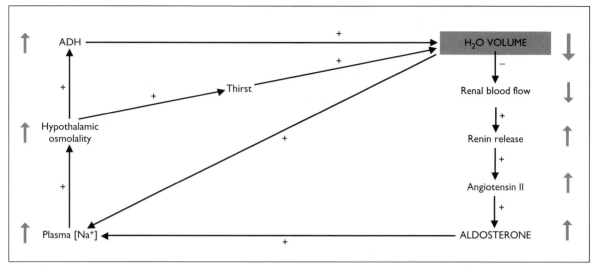

Fig. 2.9 Homeostatic correction of predominant water depletion. Reduced circulating water volume and hypernatraemia, due to water depletion, stimulate aldosterone and ADH secretion (shaded area indicates the primary change).

- Deficiency of water intake:
  inadequate water supply, or mechanical obstruction to its intake.

Failure of homeostatic mechanisms controlling water retention

- Inadequate response to thirst:
  comatose or confused patients;
  infants;
  damage to the thirst centre. Significant water depletion is very rare if the response to thirst is normal and water is available.
- Impaired water retention, with passage of urine of low sodium concentration:
  cranial diabetes insipidus due to ADH deficiency;
  overriding of ADH action by osmotic diuresis;
  nephrogenic diabetes insipidus due to failure of tubular cells to respond normally to ADH.

In most clinical conditions associated with predominant water depletion more than one of these factors is contributory.

Predominant water depletion with normal homeostatic mechanisms. *Immediate effects*

of water depletion are shown in Fig 2.9 and result in:

- *loss of water in excess of sodium*. The plasma sodium concentration and hence osmolality increase;
- *reduction of circulating volume*, which reduces renal blood flow and stimulates aldosterone secretion. Sodium is retained and hypernatraemia is aggravated.

Compensatory effects occur because the increase in the plasma osmolality stimulates:

- *thirst*, increasing water intake, if water is available and if the patient can respond to it;
- *ADH secretion*. Urinary volume falls and water loss through the kidney is reduced.

If an adequate amount of water is available, depletion is rapidly corrected. If there is an inadequate intake to replace the loss *hypernatraemia may occur before clinical signs of volume depletion are detectable*. The clinical features of predominant water depletion include:

- thirst;
- oliguria due to ADH secretion;
- *later*, signs of volume depletion (p.**40**).

The laboratory findings are:

- hypernatraemia;
- haemoconcentration due to fluid depletion;
- mild uraemia, due to volume depletion and hence low GFR;
- a high urinary osmolality and urea concentration due to the action of ADH;
- a low urinary sodium concentration in response to high aldosterone levels, stimulated by the low renal blood flow.

Deficiency of water intake; the unconscious patient. The syndrome of water depletion with hypernatraemia is found most commonly in unconscious or confused patients or in infants with gastroenteritis or pneumonia. In such subjects there is usually more than one cause of water depletion. These include:

- *pyrexia*, with an increase in the loss of hypotonic sweat;
- *hyperventilation* due to pneumonia, acidosis or brain stem damage with an increase in water loss in expired air;
- *osmotic diuresis*, which overrides the effect of ADH, causing further water loss. Some causes are:
  hypertonic intravenous infusions, for example to provide nutrients (glucose or amino acids);
  tissue damage and hence increased production of urea from protein;
  glycosuria in diabetic coma.
- *cranial diabetes insipidus*, which may be caused by head injury;
- *inability to respond to hyperosmolality by drinking*.

A high urinary volume, which may be caused by an osmotic diuresis or diabetes insipidus, contributes to water depletion and does *not* indicate 'good' hydration. The extent of the fluid loss may not be appreciated if the patient is incontinent. In such situations homeostatic responses may not be able to respond to hyperosmolality. *Hypernatraemia may be present before the more usual signs of volume depletion are detectable.* Monitoring cumulative fluid balance of patients at risk of developing hypernatraemia helps to detect water depletion early enough to allow preventive measures to be taken (p.**72**).

Patients with extensive *burns*, especially those unable to drink because they are unconscious or confused, are even more at risk of developing hyperosmolality as the water in exuded ECF evaporates, and some of the electrolyte is reabsorbed into the circulation.

Hyperosmolar saline should never be used as an emetic in cases of poisoning. Movement of water into the gut along the osmotic gradient and absorption of some of the sodium can cause marked hypernatraemia. Death has occurred as a consequence of this practice particularly if the patient could not respond to hyperosmolality by drinking because of vomiting or because he was unconscious.

Failure of homeostatic mechanisms controlling water retention. These syndromes are relatively rare and include:

- *cranial diabetes insipidus (DI)*, a syndrome associated with impairment of ADH secretion. It may be idiopathic in origin or due to either pituitary or hypothalamic damage, caused by head injury or by invasion of the region by tumour. DI following a head injury, after presenting with polyuria, may sometimes pass through a temporary 'recovery' phase following transient release of ADH from the remaining granules in the pituitary stalk, resulting in water retention and occasionally causing a dilutional hyponatraemia. The polyuric phase of established DI ensues. Some patients with DI due to trauma recover partially or completely as cerebral oedema resolves;
- *nephrogenic diabetes insipidus* is caused by the impaired action of ADH on the renal collecting ducts. Although intrinsic renal disorders, such as interstitial nephritis caused by infection or polycystic renal disease, impair the renal concentrating ability, they are not usually included in the classification of nephrogenic DI. The disorder may be either familial or acquired and be due to:

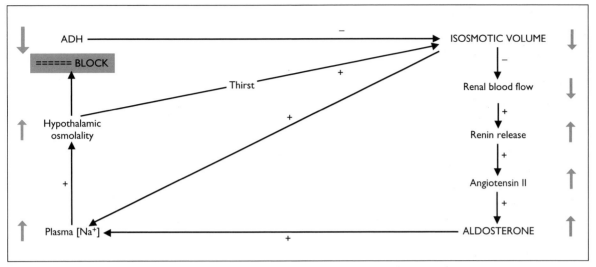

Fig. 2.10 Consequences of ADH deficiency (diabetes insipidus). Impaired water retention results in an increased plasma osmolality with stimulation of thirst and hypovolaemia with increased aldosterone secretion (shaded area indicates the primary change).

a rare inborn error involving renal collecting duct function, inherited as a sex-linked recessive disorder, in which plasma ADH concentrations are high but the tubules cannot respond to it; the newborn infant passes a large volume of urine and rapidly becomes hyperosmolar and volume depleted. Urinary loss is difficult to asses at this age and the cries of thirst may be misinterpreted;

drugs, such as lithium carbonate or demeclocycline, which interfere with the action of ADH causing the clinical picture of nephrogenic DI;

hypercalcaemia or *hypokalaemia*, both of which impair the urine concentrating mechanism and may present with polyuria;

damage to the thirst centre, by invasion by the tumour or granulomatous tissue causing impaired secretion of ADH.

The first phase of ADH deficiency is identical with that described for predominant water depletion (Fig. 2.10). As increased ADH secretion cannot occur in response to water depletion and hyperosmolality, compensation cannot occur except by increasing oral water intake in response to thirst. In some cases the thirst centre may also be involved in the same underlying pathological process.

Clinical features that differ from those described in the previous section are due to ADH deficiency. They are:

- *polyuria*, not oliguria;
- *a dilute*, not concentrated, urine.

The diagnostic procedure is described on p.**73**.

Water and sodium excess

An excess of water and sodium is usually rapidly corrected. Syndromes of excess are usually associated with impaired homeostatic mechanisms.

Volume excess not primarily due to an osmotic difference across cell membranes may cause *hypertension* and *cardiac failure*. Oedema only occurs if:

- the capillary hydrostatic pressure is increased, as in congestive cardiac failure;

- the capillary colloid osmotic pressure is reduced due to hypoalbuminaemia.

Laboratory findings are characteristic of *haemodilution* and, unless there is glomerular dysfunction, *plasma urea concentrations tend to be low.*

Secondary aldosteronism; oedema. By convention the term secondary aldosteronism usually refers to the clinical condition in which long-standing aldosterone secretion is stimulated by the renin–angiotensin system following a low renal blood flow. This may be due to local abnormalities in renal vessels or to a reduced circulating volume.

Secondary aldosteronism may be due to:

- *redistribution of extracellular fluid*, leading to a reduced plasma volume despite a normal or even high total extracellular fluid volume. Such conditions may be caused by a reduction in plasma colloid osmotic pressure and are therefore associated with low plasma albumin concentrations. *Oedema is present.* Persistent hypoalbuminaemia may be due to:

chronic liver disease;
nephrotic syndrome;
protein malnutrition.

- *damage to renal vessels, reducing renal blood flow*. These conditions are *rarely associated with oedema*:
  essential hypertension;
  malignant hypertension;
  renal hypertension, such as that due to renal artery stenosis.

- *cardiac failure*, in which two factors may reduce renal blood flow and a third one aggravates the hyperaldosteronism:
  a low cardiac output results in poor renal perfusion;
  an increased capillary hydrostatic pressure in cardiac failure may cause redistribution of fluid into the interstitial space, with *oedema*;
  impaired aldosteronism catabolism may aggravate the condition.

The mechanisms are outlined in Fig. 2.11. The reduced renal blood flow stimulates aldosterone secretion with enhanced sodium reabsorption from the distal convoluted

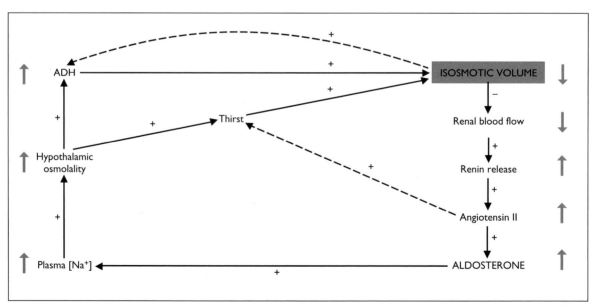

Fig. 2.11 Effect of secondary aldosterone secretion. Decreased effective intravascular volume increases renin and aldosterone secretion; if pronounced, ADH secretion may be increased and thirst stimulated, resulting in hyponatraemia despite an increase in total body sodium (shaded area indicates the primary change).

tubules and subsequent water retention. These processes tend to restore the intravascular volume.

However, if there is hypoalbuminaemia or heart failure, more fluid passes into the interstitial fluid as the retained water dilutes the plasma albumin concentration and therefore lowers the colloid osmotic pressure and raises the capillary hydrostatic pressure. The circulating volume can only be maintained by further fluid retention. A vicious cycle leads to the accumulation of excess fluid in the interstitial compartment (oedema). Some factors that increase fluid accumulation in the interstitial space are summarized in Table 2.5. If the reduced renal blood flow is caused by a narrowing of blood vessels, hypertension rather than oedema results.

Initially, this cycle stimulates a parallel increase in water and sodium retention, with normonatraemia. However, stimulation of ADH secretion by hypovolaemia, if long-standing, may cause enough sodium-free water retention to produce mild hyponatraemia, despite the excess of total body sodium. Angiotensin II also stimulates thirst and therefore increases water intake (p.**28**). It is important to recognize this (Table 2.6) because administration of sodium with the aim of correcting hyponatraemia may be dangerous.

Hypokalaemia is less common in secondary than in primary hyperaldosteronism, perhaps because the low GFR reduces the amount of sodium reaching the distal tubules and therefore the amount available

for exchange for either potassium or hydrogen ions (p.**28**). However, if reabsorption of sodium without water is inhibited by so-called loop diuretics (p.**68**), potassium depletion occurs more readily than in subjects without hyperaldosteronism.

The clinical features found in these patients are those of the underlying primary condition. Laboratory findings include:

- normonatraemia or mild hyponatraemia;
- a low urinary sodium concentration;
- those due to the primary abnormality, such as hypoalbuminaemia.

PREDOMINANT EXCESS OF WATER

Predominant water overload may occur in circumstances in which normal homeostasis has failed, for example:

- *in glomerular dysfunction*, if fluid of low sodium concentration has been infused in excess of that lost. Fluid balance must be carefully controlled in such cases;
- *if there is 'inappropriate' ADH secretion.* Hormone secretion is defined as inappropriate if it continues when it should be cut off by negative feedback control, in this case by a low plasma osmolality. ADH, like many other peptide hormones, can be synthesized by malignant cells in non-endocrine tissues 'ectopic' secretion; (Chapter 21). Inappropriate secretion of ADH, probably from the pituitary or hypothalamus, and therefore not 'ectopic', is very common in many illnesses, in particular disorders of the pulmonary and central nervous systems. The finding of a urine of higher osmolality than plasma, despite plasma hypo-osmolality, is evidence of such inappropriate secretion;
- *during the intravenous administration of the posterior pituitary hormone oxytocin* ('Syntocinon') to induce labour. Oxytocin has an antidiuretic effect similar to that of the chemically closely related ADH (p.**107**). If five per cent glucose or dextrose saline is used as a carrier, the glucose is metabolized and the net effect is retention of solute-free water. Death

Table 2.5 Some factors which increase the accumulation of fluid within the interstitial space, resulting in oedema

Increase in hydrostatic pressure gradient
  heart failure with sodium retention.

Decrease in colloid osmotic pressure gradient
  decrease in plasma colloid osmotic pressure:
    decrease in plasma albumin concentration.
  increase in capillary permeability to albumin:
    'shock' and any severe illness;
    infection with inflammation and therefore increased permeability of the capillary endothelium.

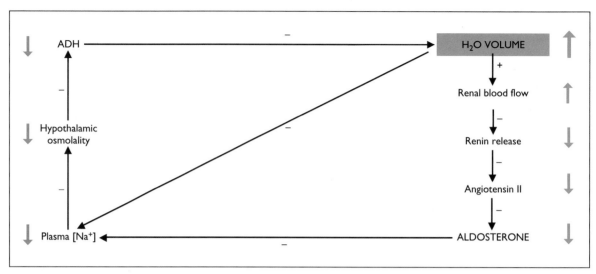

Fig. 2.12 Homeostatic correction of water excess. Increased intravascular water volume, with decreased plasma osmolality, inhibits aldosterone and ADH secretion (shaded area indicates the primary change).

from acute hypo-osmolality has resulted after prolonged infusion; oxytocin should be given in the least possible volume of isotonic saline and the fluid balance and plasma sodium concentrations monitored carefully.

In the presence of normal homeostatic mechanisms (Fig. 2.12), excessive water intake:

- tends to lower plasma sodium concentration and therefore osmolality;
- increases renal blood flow and cuts off aldosterone secretion, increasing urinary sodium loss and therefore further decreasing its plasma concentration;
- lowers plasma osmolality and therefore cuts off ADH secretion; a large volume of dilute urine is then passed.

When glomerular function is impaired, excretion of excess water may be limited. If there is appropriate ADH secretion, or if oxytocin is being infused, for example during labour, water retention continues despite the low plasma osmolality and compensation cannot occur.

The clinical consequences are those of:

- volume excess;
- hypo-osmolality if overhydration is rapid.

The onset of symptoms is related to the rate of fall of rather than to the absolute osmolality. If the onset of hypo-osmolality is gradual, as in patients with inappropriate ADH secretion, and if there has been redistribution of other diffusible solutes across cell membranes, clinical symptoms may be absent despite very severe hyponatraemia. The biochemical findings include:

- haemodilution;
- hyponatraemia.

If there is glomerular dysfunction, there will be uraemia. In the syndrome of inappropriate ADH secretion the GFR is high and plasma urea concentration tends to be low.

PREDOMINANT EXCESS OF SODIUM

Predominant sodium excess is rare. It is usually caused by inappropriate secretion of aldosterone, such as in *primary hyperaldosteronism (Conn's syndrome)* or by other corticosteroids as in *Cushing's syndrome* (p.**122**). In these syndromes sodium retention stimulates that of water, minimizing changes in plasma sodium concentration.

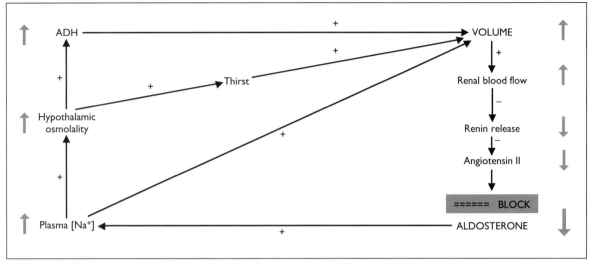

Fig. 2.13 Effect of primary aldosteronism (Conn's syndrome). Aldosterone secretion is relatively autonomous causing sodium retention and increasing the plasma osmolality. This stimulates ADH secretion. The increase in intravascular volume inhibits renin secretion (shaded area indicates the primary change).

Primary hyperaldosteronism (Conn's syndrome). About half the cases of the syndrome are due to a single benign adenoma of the glomerulosa cells of the adrenal cortex, about 10 per cent are multiple, and most of the remaining cases are associated with bilateral nodular hyperplasia of the adrenal cortex. Aldosterone secretion is relatively autonomous (Fig. 2.13).

- Aldosterone excess causes urinary sodium retention.
- The rise in plasma sodium concentration stimulates ADH secretion and water retention.
- Water retention tends to restore plasma sodium concentrations to normal.
- Aldosterone secretion is not subject to normal feedback suppression. Its continued action causes sodium and water retention at the expense of potassium loss; hypokalaemic alkalosis is common.

Typical clinical features are:

- those of hypervolaemia. Patients have mild to moderate hypertension but are rarely oedematous;
- those associated with hypokalaemia (p.**66**).

Laboratory findings include:

- hypokalaemic alkalosis due to excess aldosterone secretion (for explanation of the high plasma bicarbonate concentration see p.**60**);
- a plasma sodium concentration, which may be within the reference range, but is usually greater than 140 mmol/L;
- a low urinary sodium concentration in the early stages. Later sodium excretion may rise, possibly because of hypokalaemic tubular damage (p.**66**).

Hypokalaemic alkalosis is a common finding in potassium depletion from other causes; primary hyperaldosteronism is a very rare condition. However, the association of these findings in a patient without an obvious reason for potassium loss and with mild to moderate hypertension suggests the diagnosis of primary hyperaldosteronism. The investigative procedure described on p.**76** should be followed. If the cause does not become obvious from the results of simple tests the finding of high plasma aldosterone with a low renin activity confirms the diagnosis (Fig. 2.13); in secondary aldosteronism both the plasma aldosterone concentration and renin activity are high (Fig. 2.11).

URINARY SODIUM ESTIMATION

Estimation of daily sodium losses in urine and other biological fluids with a view to quantitative replacement is not only unnecessary but may also be dangerous. *Urinary sodium excretion is not related to body content but to renal blood flow.* Replacement of the small amount of urinary sodium lost in hypovolaemic patients will be inadequate, and of the large amount in volume-expanded patients excessive. Cell hydration must be protected by giving fluid containing the proportion of sodium to water that will maintain plasma sodium concentrations normal; the total volume of this fluid must be determined by the state of volume repletion.

Estimation of the urinary sodium concentration in a random specimen may sometimes be of value to monitor volume requirements (p.**42**). More rarely it may help to differentiate renal circulatory insufficiency from intrinsic renal damage (p.**14**)

*The student should read 'Indications for electrolyte estimation' on p.**75**.*

BIOCHEMICAL BASIS OF TREATMENT OF SODIUM AND WATER DISTURBANCES

It cannot be stressed too strongly that treatment should not be based on plasma sodium concentrations alone. Hyponatraemia *per se* only rarely needs to be treated. Assessment of the history, clinical findings indicating haemoconcentration or haemodilution, and the plasma urea concentration help to unravel the cause of a low plasma sodium concentration and to determine whether its correction is indicated. Rarely it may be useful to know the urinary sodium concentration or osmolality. Hypernatraemia, on the other hand, should always be treated by *slow* infusion of hypotonic fluid.

Table 2.6 uses hypothetical values to illustrate the various combinations of disturbances of sodium and water metabolism and their treatment. Solutions available for intravenous use are listed on p.**54** and p.**55**. These rules can only be a guide to treatment in often complicated clinical situations. They may, however, help to avoid some of the more dangerous and common errors of electrolyte therapy.

If homeostatic mechanisms are impaired, and especially if there is glomerular damage, normal hydration should be maintained according to the principles outlined on p.**72**.

Table 2.6 Hypothetical numerical examples to illustrate conditions associated with normal and abnormal plasma sodium concentrations

	ECF (litre)	ECNa$^+$ (mmol)	Plasma [Na$^+$] (mmol/L)	Features (see text)	Principles of treatment
Normal subject	*20*	*2800*	*140*		
Normonatraemia due to isosmotic changes in volume					
Na$^+$ and H$_2$O loss e.g. diarrhoea	15↓	2100↓	*140*	Volume depletion	Treat cause Isosmolar saline
Na$^+$ and water gain e.g. non-oedematous 2° aldosteronism	30↑	4200↑	*140*	Volume excess	Treat cause Restrict Na$^+$ and H$_2$O
Hyponatraemia due to relative H$_2$O excess					
H$_2$O excess e.g. inapprop. ADH	25↑	*2800*	112↓	Volume excess Hypo-osmolality	Restrict H$_2$O
Na$^+$ depletion e.g. postop. infusion of low [Na$^+$] fluid	*20*	2240↓	112↓	Hypo-osmolality	Give at least isosmolar saline
Na$^+$ and H$_2$O excess e.g. oedematous 2° aldosteronism	30↑	3360↑	112↓	Volume excess Hypo-osmolality	Restrict Na$^+$ and H$_2$O
Na$^+$ and H$_2$O loss plus ADH secretion e.g. late Addison's disease	15↓	1680↓	112↓	Volume depletion Hypo-osmolality	Treat cause Give at least isosmolar saline
Hypernatraemia due to relative Na$^+$ excess					
H$_2$O depletion e.g. unconscious patient	18↓	*2800*	155↑	Hyperosmolality	Give hypo-osmolar saline slowly
Na$^+$ excess (very rare) excessive intake, usually in infants	*20*	3100↑	155↑	Hyperosmolality	Remove Na$^+$ by dialysis

Values are related to those of a hypothetical 'normal subject' (line 1). 'Normal' values are in italics throughout. Shifts of fluid across cell membranes, along the osmotic gradient, would slightly reduce changes in plasma sodium concentrations. Note especially the relatively slight water depletion associated with hypernatraemia.

Table 2.7   Some electrolyte-containing fluids for intravenous infusion

	Na+	K+	Cl-	HCO₃-	Glucose	Ca²⁺	Approximate osmolarity × plasma
	←		(mmol/L)	→	(g/dl)	(mmol/L)	
Saline							
'Normal' (physiological 0.9%)	154	–	154	–	–	–	×1
Twice 'normal' (1.8%)	308	–	308	–	–	–	×2
Half 'normal' (0.45%)	77	–	77	–	–	–	×0.5
Fifth 'normal' (0.18%)	31	–	31	–	–	–	×0.2
'Dextrose' saline							
2.5% 0.45%	77	–	77	–	140 (2.5)	–	×1
4% 0.18%	31	–	31	–	222 (4.0)	–	×1
5% 0.45%	77	–	77	–	278 (5.0)	–	×1.5
Sodium bicarbonate							
1.4%	167	–	–	167	–		×1
2.74%	327	–	–	327	–	–	×2
8.4%*	1000	–	–	1000	–	–	×6
Complex solutions							
Ringer's	147	4.2	156	–	–	2.2	×1
Hartmann's	131	5.4	112	29†	–	1.8	×1
Na+ lactate	167	–	–	167†	–	–	×1

*Most commonly used bicarbonate solution. Note marked hyperosmolarity. Only use if strongly indicated.
†As lactate.

Table 2.8   Composition of some amino acid solutions (all hyperosmolar)

	Na+	K+	Cl⁻	Ca²⁺	PO₄²⁻	Mg²⁺	Nitrogen (g/L)
	←			(mmol/L)		→	
Synthamin 9	73	60	70	–	30	5	9.1
Synthamin 4*	73	60	70	–	30	5	14.0
Synthamin 17	73	60	70	–	30	5	16.5
Vamin 9	50	20	55	2.5	–	1.5	9.4
Vamin 9 glucose**	50	20	55	2.5	–	1.5	9.4
Vamin 14*	100	50	100	5	–	8	13.5
Vamin 18	–	–	–	–	–	–	18.0

*available electrolyte-free.
**provides 1700 kJ (406 kcal)/L, from glucose.

Table 2.9 Electrolyte-free glucose (dextrose) solutions for intravenous administration (mostly used as an energy source)

Dextrose per cent	Glucose mmol/L	Osmolarity	Approximate kJ/L	Approximate kcal/L
5	277	Isosmolar	860	(205)
10	555	Hyperosmolar	1720	(410)
20	1110	Hyperosmolar	3440	(820)
50	2770	Hyperosmolar	8600	(2050)

Table 2.10 Other hyperosmolar solutions (for inducing an osmotic diuresis or for reducing cerebral oedema)

	per cent	mmol/L	Approximate osmolarity × plasma
Mannitol	10	550	× 2
	20	1100	× 4

Summary

1. Homeostatic mechanisms for sodium and water are interlinked. Potassium and hydrogen ions often take part in exchange mechanisms with sodium.
2. Aldosterone secretion is the most important factor affecting body sodium content.
3. Aldosterone secretion is controlled by the renin–angiotensin mechanism, which responds to changes in renal blood flow.
4. Antidiuretic hormone (ADH) secretion is the most important factor affecting body water excretion.
5. ADH secretion is controlled by changes in plasma osmolality, which normally depend on the plasma sodium concentration. A contraction in plasma volume in pathological states may also stimulate its secretion.
6. Distribution of fluid between intra- and extracellular fluid compartments depends on the osmotic difference across the cell membrane. Changes in gradient are usually due to changes in extracellular sodium concentrations.
7. Distribution of fluid between the vascular and interstitial compartments depends on the balance between the capillary hydrostatic pressure and the plasma colloid osmotic pressure; the latter depends mainly on the plasma albumin concentration.
8. Clinical effects of disturbances of water and sodium metabolism are due to:

   - changes in extracellular osmolality, dependent mainly on sodium concentration. In pathological states plasma urea and glucose concentrations and ingested solutes can be important;
   - changes in circulating volume.

Potassium metabolism

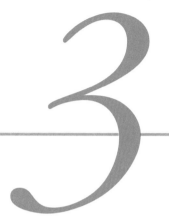

The total amount of potassium in the body is about 3000 mmol, of which about *98 per cent* is *intracellular*. Hence although the plasma potassium concentration is a poor indicator of the total body content it is the changes in the *extracellular (plasma)* concentration of potassium, like those of calcium and magnesium, that affect neuromuscular activity and cardiac action. These changes may be of immediate importance in therapy, irrespective of the amount of intracellular potassium. Both severe hypokalaemia and hyperkalaemia are dangerous and must be treated. However, an attempt should be made to predict, from the history and other findings, if there is a total body deficit so that therapeutic requirements may be anticipated. Measurement of total body potassium is *not* indicated.

FACTORS AFFECTING THE PLASMA POTASSIUM CONCENTRATION

The large amount of intracellular potassium ion (K^+) provides a reservoir for the extracellular compartment. Changes in water balance have little direct effect on the plasma potassium concentration, unlike those on sodium (Na^+). The hyperkalaemia often found when there is volume depletion is the result of renal retention rather than of haemoconcentration (p.**65**).

The normal potassium intake is about 60 to 100 mmol a day. Potassium enters and leaves the extracellular compartment by three main routes:

- the intestine;
- the kidneys:
    the glomeruli;
    the tubular cells;
- through the membranes of all other cells.

THE KIDNEYS

Glomerular filtrate. Potassium is filtered by glomeruli at almost the same concentration as in plasma. Because of the very large volume of the filtrate, about 800 mmol (about a quarter of the total body content) would be lost daily if there were no tubular regulation. The net loss, although very variable, is only about 10 per cent of that filtered.

The tubules. Potassium is normally almost completely reabsorbed in the proximal tubules. Renal tubular dysfunction may cause potassium depletion. Potassium is secreted in the distal tubules and collecting ducts in exchange for sodium; hydrogen ions compete with potassium. *Aldosterone stimulates both exchange mechanisms*. If the proximal tubules are functioning normally, potassium loss in the urine depends on three factors:

- the amount of *sodium available* for exchange. This depends on the filtration rate, filtered sodium load, and sodium reabsorption from the proximal tubules and loops of Henle. Reabsorption in the loops is inhibited by many diuretics (p.**68**).
- the relative *amounts of hydrogen and potassium ions* in the cells of the distal tubules and collecting ducts, and on the *ability to secrete hydrogen ions (H^+) in exchange for Na^+*. This may be impaired during treatment with carbonate dehydratase inhibitors and in some types of renal tubular acidosis.
- the circulating *aldosterone* concentration. This is increased following fluid loss with volume contraction (p.**45**), which usually accompanies intestinal loss of potassium, and in most conditions requiring diuretic therapy.

THE INTESTINE

Potassium is absorbed through the small intestine. Dietary intake replaces net urinary and faecal loss, and amounts to 100 mmol a day or less.

Potassium leaves the extracellular compartment in all intestinal secretions, usually at concentrations near to or a little above that in plasma. A total of about 60 mmol a day is lost into the intestinal lumen, most of which is reabsorbed. Less than 10 mmol a day is present in formed faeces. As in the case of sodium, excessive intestinal potassium loss in diarrhoea stools, in ileostomy fluid or through other fistulae is derived more from the fluid entering the intestinal lumen from the body than from dietary intake. However, prolonged starvation can cause or aggravate potassium depletion with hypokalaemia.

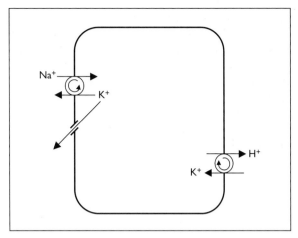

Fig. 3.1 Movement of potassium across cell membranes.

THE CELL MEMBRANES

The high intracellular potassium concentration is maintained by the Na^+/K^+-ATPase 'pump' on cell surfaces. This exchanges three sodium ions out from cells in exchange for two potassium ions in the extracellular fluid (ECF), thus establishing an electrochemical gradient across the cell membrane, with a net positive charge in the ECF. The loss of potassium from cells down the concentration gradient is opposed by this electrochemical gradient. Potassium is also exchanged for hydrogen ions (Fig. 3.1).

A small shift of potassium out of cells may cause a significant rise in plasma concentrations, whether *in vivo* or *in vitro*. In the latter situation, the artefactual hyperkalaemia due to haemolysed or old specimens may be misinterpreted (p.**426**). Usually the shift of potassium across cell membranes is accompanied by a shift of sodium in the opposite direction, but the *percentage* change in extracellular sodium concentrations is much less than that of potassium. For example, if there is a one-to-one exchange of 4 mmol/L of sodium for potassium across the cell membranes, there would be a doubling of the plasma potassium concentration, clinically a very significant change, but the plasma sodium concentration would only fall from about 140 mmol/L to 136 mmol/L.

Increased uptake and *net gain* of potassium by cells may occur:

- if the activity of the pump is increased.
  Insulin enhances the cellular uptake of glucose and potassium. This effect may be used to treat hyperkalaemia. It is the main cause of the change from hyperkalaemia to hypokalaemia during treatment of diabetic ketoacidosis.
  Catecholamines may have a similar effect and it has been suggested that this may contribute to the hypokalaemia sometimes found after the stress of myocardial infarction. However, in patients with phaeochromocytomas, in whom plasma catecholamine concentrations are very high, hypokalaemia is not a common finding.
- in alkalosis due to increased uptake by cells and increased urinary loss. Induction of alkalosis can also be used to treat hyperkalaemia.

There is *net loss* of potassium from cells:

- if potassium is lost from the ECF and replenished from cells;
- if the pump is inefficient, as it is in hypoxia, or if glucose metabolism is impaired as in severe diabetes mellitus;
- in acidosis, when potassium is displaced from cells by hydrogen ions.

RELATION BETWEEN HYDROGEN AND POTASSIUM IONS

The extracellular hydrogen ion concentration affects the entry of potassium into all cells. Changes in the relative proportions of K+ and H+ in distal renal tubular cells affect the urinary loss of potassium.

- *In acidosis* increased loss of potassium from cells into the ECF, coupled with reduced urinary secretion of potassium, causes *hyperkalaemia*.
- *In alkalosis* net increased uptake of potassium into cells and the increased urinary potassium loss causes *hypokalaemia*.

Because the relation between K+ and H+ is reciprocal, changes in K+ balance affect that of hydrogen ions.

In absorptive cells, including those in the renal tubules, the pump is probably situated on the nonluminal surface. In the kidney, sodium derived from the luminal fluid is pumped through the cell in exchange for either K+ or H+. If K+ is lost from the ECF it flows down the increased concentration gradient, so reducing its intracellular content. Unless there is renal tubular cell damage sodium is reabsorbed in exchange for less K+ and more H+ than usual. For each H+ ion formed within the tubular cell by the carbonate dehydratase (CD) mechanism (p.**83**) one bicarbonate ion (HCO_3^-) is produced.

$$H_2O + CO_2 \xrightarrow[CD]{} H^+ + HCO_3^-$$

As more H+ is secreted into the urine the reaction is accelerated and more HCO_3^- is generated, passing into the ECF accompanied by the reabsorbed sodium ion (Fig 3.2 p.**63**). The result is an extracellular alkalosis and an acid urine. Therefore, chronic potassium depletion is usually accompanied by a *high plasma bicarbonate concentration*. If other causes for a raised plasma bicarbonate concentration are excluded, such as severe chronic obstructive airways disease, and especially if factors known to cause potassium depletion are present, such as diuretic therapy, this finding is a sensitive indicator of potassium depletion, even if the plasma potassium concentration is within the reference range. These are the changes of *chronic* potassium depletion.

Table 3.1 The relation between plasma potassium and bicarbonate concentrations

Plasma [K+]	Plasma bicarbonate	Most likely cause	Clinical examples
Low N or ↓	↑	Chronic K+ loss	Diuretic treatment chronic diarrhoea (eg. purgative abusers)
↓ or ↓↓	N or ↓	Acute K+ loss	Severe acute diarrhoea, fistulae etc Hyperchloraemic acidosis Renal tubular acidosis
↓	↓	Respiratory alkalosis	Overtreatment on respirator Hysterical overbreathing
↑	↓	Metabolic acidosis	Renal dysfunction Diabetic ketoacidosis
↑	↑	Respiratory acidosis	Bronchopneumonia
↑	N	Acute K+ load	Excess K+ treatment

N = normal.

The combination of hypokalaemia and a high plasma bicarbonate concentration is more likely to be due to K⁺ depletion, which is common, than to a metabolic alkalosis, which is rare.

After *acute* potassium loss there is a slight lag in potassium release from cells. This may result in more severe hypokalaemia for the same degree of depletion than in the chronic state; plasma bicarbonate concentrations are less likely to be raised, because it takes several days before enough bicarbonate is retained to be detectable.

Theoretically, potassium excess could cause intracellular alkalosis and extracellular acidosis. *The combination of hyperkalaemia and a low plasma bicarbonate concentration is more likely to be caused by a metabolic acidosis, which is common, than by potassium excess, which is extremely rare.*

In a respiratory acidosis the plasma bicarbonate concentration is often high (p.**94**) and the plasma potassium concentration high normal. The relation between the plasma potassium and bicarbonate concentrations are summarized in Table 3.1.

Abnormalities of Plasma Potassium Concentrations

In any clinical situation no single factor accounts for all the changes in plasma potassium concentration. For example, in conditions associated with intestinal potassium loss concomitant fluid loss causes secondary hyperaldosteronism; similarly many conditions requiring diuretic therapy are associated with, or result in, secondary hyperaldosteronism. This aggravates urinary potassium loss and increases entry of potassium into cells. However, if volume and sodium depletion are severe the reduced total amount of sodium filtered through the glomeruli makes less available for exchange with potassium in the distal tubules; consequently aldosterone cannot produce maximal effects: hypokalaemia may then become evident only when the patient is rehydrated.

Hypokalaemia

Hypokalaemia is often the result of potassium depletion, but if the rate of loss of potassium from cells equals or exceeds the loss from the ECF potassium depletion may not cause hypokalaemia. By contrast, hypokalaemia can occur without depletion if there is a shift into cells, as in alkalosis, after taking a large amount of glucose and in the rare condition, familial periodic paralysis.

Misleading transient hypokalaemia may occur for a few hours after ingestion of oral diuretics that enhance potassium loss.

Causes of hypokalaemia, summarized in Table 3.2, may be classified according to the predominant cause.

NONRENAL CAUSES OF HYPOKALAEMIA

Redistribution within the body, by entry into cells:

- *glucose and insulin therapy.* This may be used to treat severe hyperkalaemia;
- *increased secretion of catecholamines,* such as may occur due to the stress of myocardial infarction (p.**59**);

Table 3.2 Some causes of hypokalaemia classified into predominantly nonrenal and renal causes

Nonrenal causes	Renal causes	Nonrenal and renal causes
Redistribution	*Enhanced Na^+/K^+ exchange*	alkalosis
glucose and insulin	secondary hyperaldosteronism	pyloric stenosis
catecholamines	Cushing's syndrome	
familial hypokalaemic periodic paralysis	steroid therapy	
	'ectopic' ACTH secretion	
	primary hyperaldosteronism (Conn's syndrome)	
Intestinal loss	Bartter's syndrome	
prolonged vomiting	carbenoxolone therapy	
diarrhoea	liquorice	
loss through intestinal fistula		
purgative abuse	*Excess Na^+ available for exchange*	
	infusion of saline	
Reduced intake	diuretics ('loop' diuretics)	
poor diet		
reduced intake	*Decreased Na^+/H^+ exchange*	
	carbonate dehydratase inhibitors	
	renal tubular acidosis	
	Impaired proximal tubular reabsorption	
	renal tubular dysfunction	
	Fanconi syndrome	

- *familial hypokalaemic periodic paralysis* (very rare). In this condition episodic paralysis is associated with entry of potassium into cells.

Loss from the ECF into intestinal secretions:

- prolonged vomiting;
- diarrhoea;
- loss through intestinal fistulae;
- *habitual purgative users* may present with hypokalaemia and are often reluctant to admit to the habit.

Intestinal loss is usually aggravated by secondary hyperaldosteronism consequent on fluid depletion. The resultant inappropriately high urinary potassium may sometimes contribute more to depletion than to the original pathology. It must be remembered that:

- the concentration of potassium in fluid from a *recent ileostomy* and in *diarrhoea stools* be may five to 10 times that of plasma, but a prolonged drain of any intestinal secretion, even if its potassium concentration is not very high, causes depletion, especially if urinary loss is increased by secondary hyperaldosteronism;
- *mucus-secreting villous adenomas of the intestine* are very rare but may cause considerable potassium loss.

Reduced potassium intake:

- *chronic starvation.* If water and salt intake is also reduced, secondary hyperaldosteronism may aggravate the hypokalaemia.

RENAL CAUSES OF HYPOKALAEMIA

Enhanced renal secretion of potassium. Increased activity of the pump in distal renal tubules. This is associated with a hypokalaemic alkalosis (Fig 3.2):

- *secondary hyperaldosteronism* often aggravates other causes of potassium depletion;
- *Cushing's syndrome and steroid therapy.* Patients secreting excess of, or on prolonged therapy with, glucocorticoids tend to become hypokalaemic due to the mineralocorticoid effect on the distal renal tubules;
- *'ectopic' ACTH secretion*, which stimulates cortisol secretion (p.**124**);

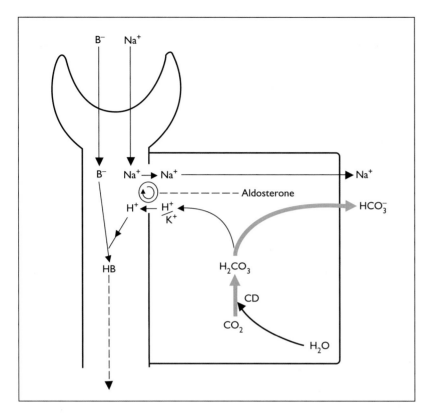

Fig. 3.2 Exchange of Na^+ for either K^+ or H^+ in the renal tubules (for explanation see Chapter 4, p.84).

- *primary hyperaldosteronism* (Conn's syndrome) (p.**51**);
- *Bartter's syndrome* is a very rare condition in which there is hyperplasia of the renal juxtaglomerular apparatus with increased renin and therefore aldosterone secretion. Because angiotensin II activity is impaired, there is no vasoconstriction and consequently the patient is normotensive. This latter finding helps to distinguish the syndrome from that of primary hyperaldosteronism;
- *carbenoxolone therapy* is occasionally used to accelerate the healing of peptic ulcers. It potentiates the action of aldosterone and can cause hypokalaemia;
- *liquorice and tobacco* contain glycyrrhizinic acid which has a mineralocorticoid-like effect. Overindulgence in liquorice-containing sweets or habitual tobacco chewing can cause hypokalaemia.

Excess sodium available for exchange in the distal renal tubules:

- *prolonged infusion of saline;*
- *diuretics inhibiting the pump in the loops of Henle* (p.**68**). The activity of the distal pump is enhanced by secondary hyperaldosteronism.

Reduced proximal tubular potassium reabsorption:

- *renal tubular dysfunction* (for example, the recovery phase of acute oliguric renal failure);
- *Fanconi syndrome* (p.**356**);
- *hypercalcaemia* which may impair the reabsorption of potassium even if there is no renal damage.

Decreased renal Na^+/H^+ exchange because of impaired generation of H^+ within the renal tubular cells, thus favouring Na^+/K^+ exchange associated with a hypokalaemic acidosis. Causes include:

- *carbonate dehydratase inhibitors* (p.**94**);
- *renal tubular acidosis* (p.**93**).

COMBINED NONRENAL AND RENAL CAUSES OF HYPOKALAEMIA

Loss of potassium from ECF by more than one route, may occur from:

- cells and urine:
  alkalosis.
- cells, urine and intestine:
  pyloric stenosis with alkalosis. The losses into urine and cells are probably more important causes of the hypokalaemia than the loss in gastrointestinal secretion.

Hyperkalaemia

Plasma potassium results should not be reported if the specimen is haemolysed or if plasma was not separated from cells within a few hours after the blood was taken (p.**426**). *Pseudohyperkalaemia,* due to *in vitro* leakage of potassium from cells into plasma, is often misinterpreted, sometimes with dangerous consequences. This may occur if there has been a delay in separating the plasma from the cells, *particularly if the blood sample has been placed in a refrigerator,* when activity of the pump is slowed by the low temperature.

The commonest cause of true hyperkalaemia is when the rate of potassium entering the ECF is greater than the rate of excretion from the body.

Causes, summarized in Table 3.3, can be classified into nonrenal and renal causes.

NONRENAL CAUSES OF HYPERKALAEMIA

Gain of potassium by the body either from the intestine or by the intravenous route.

- *Overenthusiastic potassium therapy,* especially in patients with impaired glomerular function.
- *Failure to stop potassium therapy* when depletion has been corrected and the cause removed.

Redistribution within the body, loss from cells.

- *Severe tissue damage.*
- *Familial hyperkalaemic periodic paralysis* is exceedingly rare and is associated with release of potassium from cells.

Table 3.3 Some causes of hyperkalaemia classified into predominantly nonrenal and renal causes

Nonrenal causes	Renal causes
In vitro effects	*Insufficient Na+ available for exchange*
haemolysis	renal glomerular dysfunction
leukocytosis	sodium depletion
thrombocytosis	
delayed separation of plasma	*Decreased Na+/K+ exchange*
	mineralocorticoid deficiency
Increased input	hypoaldosteronism (Addison's disease)
exogenous source	congenital adrenal hyperplasia
endogenous source	hyporeninaemic hypoaldosteronism (Type IV RTA)
severe tissue damage	drugs
haemolysis	Angiotensin converting enzyme inhibitors
familial hyperkalaemic periodic paralysis	diuretics
	spironolactone
	amiloride
Redistribution	
acidosis	
hypoxia	

RENAL CAUSES OF HYPERKALAEMIA

Too little sodium available for exchange in the distal tubules.

- *Renal glomerular dysfunction.* Hyperkalaemia is usually aggravated by the concomitant acidosis and release of potassium from cells.
- *Sodium depletion.*

Impaired renal secretion of potassium. Decreased activity of Na^+/K^+-ATPase pump in the distal renal tubules.

- Mineralocorticoid deficiency:
  hypoaldosteronism as in Addison's disease;
  congenital adrenal hyperplasia in C_{21}-hydroxylase deficiency (p.**128**);
  hyporeninaemic hypoaldosteronism, an uncommon disorder presenting in the elderly, often with renal impairment and glucose intolerance.
- Drugs:
  angiotensin-converting enzyme (ACE) inhibitors, such as captopril and enalapril, which are used to treat hypertension, inhibit the conversion of angiotensin I to angiotensin II and therefore aldosterone secretion (p.**28**). They may cause hyperkalaemia, especially if glomerular function is impaired.
  diuretics acting on the distal tubules and either antagonizing aldosterone activity (spironolactone) or inhibiting the pump (amiloride) (p.**68**).

Gain by ECF by more than one route. Reduced renal excretion despite gain by ECF from cells.

- *Acidosis.*
- *Hypoxia* causes impairment of the pump in all cells, with a net gain of potassium within the extracellular fluid. Such impairment in the distal tubules causes potassium retention. If hypoxia is severe, lactic acidosis aggravates hyperkalaemia.

Diabetic ketoacidosis. In patients with poorly controlled diabetes mellitus, potassium enters the ECF from cells, because normal action of the pump depends on the energy supplied by glucose metabolism. If glomerular function is relatively normal, urinary potassium loss is increased, resulting in total body potassium depletion. Despite this, loss from the plasma into the urine rarely keeps pace with the gain from cells and mild hyperkalaemia is common. As the condition progresses two other factors contribute to hyperkalaemia:

- volume depletion causing a reduced GFR;
- keto-, and sometimes lactic, acidosis

All these factors are reversed during insulin and fluid therapy. As potassium re-enters cells extracellular potassium concentrations fall and the depletion is revealed. *Plasma potassium concentrations must be monitored regularly during therapy* and potassium given as soon as the concentration begins to fall.

MEASUREMENT OF URINARY AND INTESTINAL LOSSES

Pure urinary or intestinal potassium losses as causes of hypokalaemia are very rare. Measurement of such losses, with a view to quantitative replacement, may lead to even more dangerous errors of treatment than in the case of sodium.

- If gain of potassium by the ECF from cells is faster than loss from it into urine and the intestinal lumen, replacement of measured loss could endanger the patient's life by aggravating hyperkalaemia.

• If loss from the ECF into cells is predominant therapy based on urinary excretion may be inadequate.

High urinary potassium excretion may be appropriate when, for instance, trauma has damaged many cells. It would be as rational to replace urinary glucose quantitatively in an uncontrolled diabetic patient as to use urinary potassum measurements in the same way. *It is the plasma potassium concentrations that are important.* In rapidly changing clinical states frequent estimations of these are the only safe way of assessing therapy. In chronic potassium depletion measurement of the plasma bicarbonate concentration may help to indicate the state of cellular repletion.

The diagnostic use of urinary potassium estimations to determine the primary cause of potassium depletion may also be misleading. Most extrarenal causes of potassium loss are associated with volume depletion and therefore with secondary hyperaldosteronism. A high urinary potassium excretion is not proof of a primary renal cause. Excretion of less than about 20 mmol a day can only be expected in the *well-hydrated* hypokalaemic patient with extrarenal losses in whom aldosterone secretion is inhibited. Therefore a low potassium excretion confirms extrarenal loss, but a high one does not prove that it is the primary cause.

CLINICAL FEATURES OF DISTURBANCES OF POTASSIUM METABOLISM

The clinical features of disturbances of potassium metabolism are due to changes in the extracellular concentration of the ion.

Hypokalaemia, by interfering with neuromuscular transmission, causes *muscular weakness*, *hypotonia* and *cardiac arrhythmias*, and may precipitate digoxin toxicity. It may also aggravate paralytic ileus and hepatic encephalopathy.

Intracellular potassium depletion causes extracellular alkalosis (p.**60**). This reduces the plasma free-ionized calcium concentration and, in long-standing depletion of gradual onset, the presenting symptoms may be *muscle cramps* and even *tetany* (p.**173**). This syndrome is accompanied by high plasma bicarbonate concentrations.

Prolonged potassium depletion impairs the renal concentrating mechanism and may cause *polyuria* with potassium depletion.

Hyperkalaemia, particularly if severe, carries the danger of cardiac arrest.

Both hypo- and hyperkalaemia cause characteristic changes in the electrocardiogram. These changes are only obvious if plasma concentrations are grossly abnormal.

• *Hypokalaemia* causes prolongation of the P–R interval, flattening of the T waves and prominent U waves.
• *Hyperkalaemia* causes widening of the QRS complex and tall, 'tented' T waves.

TREATMENT OF POTASSIUM DISTURBANCES

Abnormalities of plasma potassium should be corrected irrespective of total body potassium. However, an attempt should be made to assess the latter so that changes in plasma potassium concentration, for instance, during treatment of diabetic ketoacidosis, can be anticipated. Treatment must be monitored by frequent plasma potassium estimations.

Hypokalaemia. *Mild* hypokalaemia can be treated with *oral* potassium supplements which must be continued until plasma potassium and *bicarbonate* concentrations have returned to normal. Undertreatment is more common than overtreatment. The normal subject loses about 60 mmol of potassium daily in the urine, much larger amounts being excreted during diuretic therapy. By the time hypokalaemic alkalosis is present the total deficit is probably several hundred mmol. A patient with hypokalaemia should be given *at least* 80 mmol a day; much more may be needed if plasma potassium concentrations fail to rise.

It is sometimes suggested that hypokalaemia could be treated by a high intake of fruit or fruit juice. Table 3.4 shows that if it were possible to ingest the quantities required, the consequent diarrhoea might well be self-defeating. The relatively high cost is only a minor disadvantage.

In *severe* hypokalaemia, particularly if the patient is unable to take oral supplements, *intravenous potassium* should be given cautiously (p.**70**). Diarrhoea not only reduces absorption of oral potassium supplements, but may itself be aggravated by them; this too may be an indication for intravenous therapy.

Hyperkalaemia. Treatment of hyperkalaemia is based on three principles. The first two apply in severe hyperkalaemia:

- *reducing the risk of cardiac arrhythmias.* Very severe hyperkalaemia can cause cardiac arrest. Calcium and potassium ions have opposing actions on cardiac muscle; the immediate danger can be minimized by infusing calcium, usually as gluconate (p.**70**). This has no effect on the plasma potassium concentration, but, because it has a rapid effect on cardiac sensitivity, allows time to institute measures to reduce hyperkalaemia.
- *reducing the plasma potassium concentration by stimulating entry into cells.* Plasma potassium can be reduced within an hour by increasing the rate of entry into cells. Insulin enhances the activity of the pump and *must* be given with glucose to prevent hypoglycaemia. It then stimulates entry of potassium into the intracellular compartment. Induction of an alkalosis by infusing bicarbonate also increases the rate of entry into cells (p.**59**). For practical reasons,

Table 3.4 Potassium content of fruit and fruit juice (UK, March 1993)

	Approximate K+ content	Approximate amount containing 50 mmol	Price for 50 mmol relative to 'Slow K'
Tomato juice	82 mmol/L	610 ml	12
Orange juice	30 mmol/L	1700 ml	25
Grapefruit juice	30 mmol/L	1700 ml	27
Orange cordial (*undiluted*)	16 mmol/L	3100 ml	25
Bananas	8 per banana	6 bananas	23
'Slow K'	8 per tablet	6 tablets	1

these treatments, which involve intra-venous infusion, cannot be continued indefinitely, but they allow long-term treatment to be instituted.

- *reducing the total body potassium.* In moderate hyperkalaemia potassium can be removed from the body at a rate higher than, or equal to, that at which it is entering the extracellular fluid by giving ion-exchange resins either by the oral or rectal route. These resins are not absorbed and exchange potassium for either sodium or calcium ions. The plasma potassium concentration is lowered at the expense of body depletion. The potassium may have to be replaced when the primary cause of the hyperkalaemia has been removed. In severe, intractable hyperkalaemia haemodialysis may very occasionally be needed.

Diuretic Therapy

In oedematous states fluid accumulation within the interstitial space is associated with an excess of total body sodium, *even if there is hyponatraemia* (p.48). Diuretics act by inhibiting sodium reabsorption in the renal tubules and thus the isosmotic reabsorption of water. They may be used to treat hypertension as well as oedema. All diuretics tend to affect potassium balance and this effect should be anticipated, especially in patients with secondary hyperaldosteronism or renal dysfunction. Diuretics can be divided into two principal groups, based on their site of action:

- those inhibiting the pump in the loops of Henle and therefore water reabsorption in the distal tubules and collecting ducts. The increased sodium load on the distal tubules and collecting ducts associated with secondary hyperaldosteronism caused by volume depletion increases pump activity with enhanced sodium/potassium exchange. In our experience long-term diuretic therapy almost invariably causes significant potassium depletion and sometimes symptomatic hypokalaemia, even if potassium supplements are given. *A high plasma bicarbonate concentration* is common in such patients and is a more sensitive indicator of cellular K+ depletion than that of plasma potassium. Such diuretics include:

  '*loop diuretics*', frusemide (furosemide), bumetanide and ethacrynic acid which inhibit sodium reabsorption from the ascending limb of the loops of Henle.
  thiazides which act at the junction of the loops and the distal tubules, sometimes called the 'cortical diluting segments'.

- *diuretics that inhibit either aldosterone directly or the exchange mechanisms in the distal tubules and collecting ducts.* These cause *potassium retention* and may lead to hyperkalaemia, especially if glomerular function is impaired. Potassium supplements *should not be* used. Potassium-retaining diuretics include:

  spironolactone, a competitive aldosterone antagonist.
  amiloride and *triamterene*, direct inhibitors of the Na+/K+ exchange mechanism in the distal tubules. These diuretics are often used together with those causing potassium loss when hypokalaemia cannot be controlled by potassium supplementation, or to potentiate sodium loss by inhibiting reabsorption at more than one site. Used alone they have only a weak diuretic action.

Carbonate dehydratase inhibitors, such as acetazolamide, are rarely used as diuretics but are still used to treat glaucoma. They tend to cause a hypokalaemic acidosis (p.94).

Summary

1. Changes in plasma potassium concentrations are the net result of exchanges between ECF and cells, kidney and intestine.
2. In any clinical situation many factors are involved, and monitoring of plasma potassium concentration is the only safe guide to treatment.
3. Because hydrogen and potassium compete for exchange with sodium ions in renal tubules and other cell membranes, disturbances of hydrogen ion homeostasis and potassium balance often coexist. A raised plasma bicarbonate concentration may indicate intracellular potassium depletion.
4. Clinical manifestations of disturbances of potassium balance are due to its action on neuromuscular transmission and on the heart.
5. Commonly used diuretics fall into two main groups:

   • those inhibiting sodium reabsorption from the loops of Henle and distal tubules, causing potassium depletion;
   • those antagonizing aldosterone, either directly or indirectly, by affecting Na^+/K^+ transport mechanisms, causing potassium retention.

TREATMENT OF HYPOKALAEMIA

Potassium-containing Preparations

One gram of potassium chloride contains 13 mmol of potassium.

FOR ORAL USE

1. Potassium effervescent tablets BP; 6.5 mmol K+ per tablet (as bicarbonate and acid tartrate).
2. Slow K (Ciba); 8 mmol K+ per tablet (as bicarbonate and chloride).
3. Sando K (Sandoz); 12 mmol K+ per tablet (as bicarbonate and chloride).

FOR INTRAVENOUS USE

These preparations should only be used if there is significant depletion, or if oral potassium cannot be taken or retained. In most cases oral potassium treatment is preferable. Intravenous potassium should be given with care, especially in the presence of poor glomerular function. The following rules should be observed:

- unless the deficit is unequivocal and severe, intravenous potassium should not be given if there is oliguria;
- potassium in intravenous fluid should not usually exceed a concentration of *40 mmol/L*;
- intravenous potassium should not usually be given at a rate of more than *20 mmol per hour*. In very severe depletion this dose may have to be exceeded; in such cases frequent plasma potassium estimations must be performed.

Strong potassium chloride solution BP; 20 mmol of potassium chloride in 10 ml. It should be added to a full bag of intravenous fluid and mixed well. 10 mL added to 500 ml of fluid, such as five per cent glucose (dextrose), gives a final concentration of 40 mmol/L.

Warning. This solution should *never* be given undiluted.

TREATMENT OF HYPERKALAEMIA

Emergency Treatment

Calcium chloride (or gluconate) 10 ml of a 10 per cent solution is given intravenously with ECG monitoring. This treatment antagonizes the effect of hyperkalaemia on heart muscle, but does not alter potassium concentrations.

Warning. Calcium should never be added to bicarbonate solutions because calcium carbonate is poorly soluble in water. If too much calcium is given, hypercalcaemia may cause cardiac arrest.

Glucose 50 g with 20 units of soluble insulin by intravenous injection starts to lower plasma potassium concentrations within about 30 minutes by increasing potassium entry into cells. If the situation is less urgent 10 units of soluble insulin may be added to a litre of 10 per cent glucose.

40 ml of 8.4 per cent sodium bicarbonate (40 mmol of bicarbonate) may be injected over five minutes as an alternative to glucose and insulin *if a metabolic acidosis is present.* This solution is hyperosmolar.

Long-term Treatment

Sodium or calcium polystyrene sulphonate (Resonium-A or Calcium Resonium; 'Sanofi-Winthrop') 45 to 60 g a day *by mouth* in 15 g doses, or 30 g in methyl cellulose solution as *a retention enema* retained for nine hours. These remove potassium from the body.

*B*IOCHEMICAL INVESTIGATION OF RENAL, WATER AND ELECTROLYTE DISORDERS

Monitoring Fluid Balance

Maintenance and inspection of *accurate* fluid balance charts in the wards is as important as measurement of daily plasma electrolyte concentrations.

Fluid imbalance may develop so gradually in those patients who are unconscious and who have abnormal losses that it may pass unnoticed if individual *daily* charts are relied upon, especially if insensible losses are ignored. Maintenance of a *cumulative* fluid balance record is a more sensitive way of detecting a trend; this may then be corrected before serious abnormalities develop. It is especially important in patients at risk of predominant water depletion, which is less clinically obvious than the more common isosmolal volume depletion (p.**44**) and which may not be noticed until dangerous hypernatraemia has developed.

In the example shown in Table 3.5, *400 ml* has been allowed for as *insensible daily loss*; calculated losses are therefore more likely to be under- than overestimated. The danger of fluid overload by replacement of the stated volume is minimal.

This shows how insidiously a serious deficit can develop over a few days.

The volume of fluid infused should be based on the calculated cumulative balance and on clinical evidence of the state of hydration, and its composition adjusted to maintain the plasma electrolyte concentrations normal. If the cumulative balance figures are plotted on the same graph as plasma sodium and urea concentrations, potential hypernatraemia and renal circulatory insufficiency can often be detected and treated before they become serious and clinically obvious.

If the ambient temperature is high, or if the patient is pyrexial, hyperventilating, or has large unmeasured intestinal losses, as in intestinal obstruction or ileus, more than 400 ml should be allowed for as insensible loss.

Investigation of Acute Oliguria

Correct management of acute oliguria depends on distinguishing between renal and extrarenal causes.

1. Estimate plasma electrolytes (especially potassium) at once. Knowledge of the urea and/or creatinine concentrations is of less immediate therapeutic importance. Treat dangerous hyperkalaemia (p.**70**).
2. Exclude postrenal causes. Urinary obstruction due to prostatic hypertrophy is the commonest cause of oliguria in the adult male with a palpable bladder.
3. Examine the urine for protein and casts: their presence suggests significant renal damage. Microbiological investigation may reveal urinary tract infection.
4. *If the patient is oedematous, perhaps due to congestive cardiac failure, do not continue with steps 5 and 6.* Fluid administration is contraindicated, whether or not there is renal damage.
5. Rehydrate the patient, watching for signs of incipient overhydration, and measure the urine output accurately. If this increases rapidly, and the plasma urea/creatinine concentrations start to level off or fall within 24 hours, the cause is likely to be prerenal. If, after rehydration, the oliguria persists and the plasma urea concentration continues to rise, renal

Table 3.5 Hypothetical cumulative fluid balance chart assuming an insensible daily loss of 400 ml.

	Intake (ml)	Measured output (ml)	Total output (minimum ml)	Daily balance (ml)	Cumulative balance (ml)
Day 1	2000	1900	2300	−300	−300
Day 2	2000	2000	2400	−400	−700
Day 3	2100	1900	2300	−200	−900
Day 4	2200	2000	2400	−200	−1100

damage is likely and fluid balance should be maintained as described on p.**30**.

6. If the cause is still in doubt, estimate the urinary sodium concentration. *This is only useful if the specimen is collected when the patient is still volume depleted*, since only under these conditions is aldosterone secretion likely to be maximal (p.**14**). If the concentration is below about 20 mmol/L, significant renal damage is unlikely and rehydration can safely be continued.

7. Plasma potassium concentrations must be measured at least daily and treatment adjusted appropriately.

Investigation of Polyuria *(Table 1.1; p. 15)*

CONFIRM POLYURIA AND EXCLUDE OBVIOUS CAUSES

1. Take a history.

   - Distinguish between true polyuria (a high 24 hour urinary volume) and frequency (a normal 24 hour volume but abnormally frequent micturition).
   - Is the patient taking diuretics? This cause may easily be forgotten.
   - If there is a recent history of oliguric renal dysfunction the patient has probably entered the polyuric phase, and should be treated accordingly (p.15).

2. Is there a cause for an osmotic diuresis such as:

   - gross glycosuria due to diabetes mellitus or infusion of glucose (dextrose)?
   - severe tissue damage, leading to a high urea load?
   - infusion of amino acids?

If so, investigate and treat, or change the composition of the infusion.

3. If fluid, especially of low sodium concentration, is being infused, adjust accordingly.

4. Is there a possible obvious cause for diabetes insipidus, such as a head injury?

DISTINGUISH BETWEEN POLYURIA APPROPRIATE TO A HIGH INTAKE AND THAT DUE TO FAILURE OF HOMEOSTATIC MECHANISMS

1. Volume depletion suggests failure of homeostasis.

2. Accurately monitor fluid intake and output.

   - *A negative balance* suggests *failure of homeostasis.*
   - *A positive balance* suggests that *polydipsia is primary.*

The patient should be carefully watched for secret fluid ingestion ('hysterical polydipsia') or even addition of fluid to the urine.

3. Estimate plasma urea/creatinine and electrolyte concentrations.

   - *Very high plasma urea/creatinine concentrations suggests renal damage.* Treat and monitor accordingly (p.**20**).
   - *Low or low normal plasma urea/creatinine concentrations, especially if there is*

mild hyponatraemia, suggest that polydipsia is the primary cause and that the polyuria is appropriate. Question the patient about his intake in relation to true thirst. Patients with true 'hysterical polydipsia' may give misleading answers; they rarely complain of nocturia.

- *High normal or high urea/creatinine concentrations*, urea up to about 15 mmol/L (90 mg/dl; urea nitrogen 42 mg/dl), *especially if the plasma sodium concentration is high normal or high, suggest impairment of the tubular ability to concentrate.* Severe hypokalaemia may suggest that this is a cause of tubular dysfunction.

4. If the plasma urea/creatinine concentration is slightly high, cautiously increase fluid intake. A fall in the plasma urea concentration in response to rehydration suggests that glomerular damage is minimal. Seek a cause for tubular damage.

   - Take a drug history.
   - Send urine for microbiological examination to detect pyelonephritis.
   - Estimate plasma calcium and urate concentrations.
   - Exclude the other causes listed on p.**17**.
   - In infants, consider inborn errors of metabolism (Chapter 18).

5. If it is still not possible to distinguish between polydipsia, tubular impairment and diabetes insipidus, *contact the laboratory* to arrange a water deprivation test, if necessary with DDAVP.
6. Treat mild tubular impairment with a high fluid intake.
7. In cases of diabetes insipidus, seek a neurological opinion.

WATER DEPRIVATION TEST

Restriction of water intake for some hours should stimulate ADH secretion (p.**29**). Solute-free water is reabsorbed from the collecting ducts and a concentrated urine is passed. Maximal water reabsorption is impaired if:

- the countercurrent multiplication mechanism is impaired;
- ADH activity is low.

If the feedback mechanism is intact, plasma ADH levels are already high and administration of exogenous hormone will not improve the renal concentrating power; if diabetes insipidus is the cause, tubular function is normal and therefore the administration of ADH will increase the renal concentrating ability and increase the urine osmolality.

Warning *The test should not be performed if the patient is volume depleted or has even mild hypernatraemia.* In such cases the finding of a low urine to plasma osmolality ratio (see below) is diagnostic and further fluid restriction may be dangerous. If the test is necessary, it must be stopped if:

- *the patient becomes distressed.* If the apparent 'distress' does not coincide with a high normal or high plasma osmolality it is likely to be psychological in origin;
- *the plasma osmolality (or sodium concentration) rises to high or high normal concentrations.* Urine and blood specimens should be collected at once;
- *the patient loses more than three per cent of his body weight.*

Procedure. Always contact the laboratory *before* starting the test, both to ensure efficient and speedy analysis, and to check local variations in the protocol.

The patient is allowed no food or water after about 20.00 hours on the night before the test. *He must be in hospital, and kept under observation* during the period of fluid restriction (see above). The duration of water deprivation depends on the clinical presentation and the degree of polyuria.

On the day of the test:

08.00 hours. The bladder is emptied. Blood and urine are collected and plasma and urine osmolalities measured. If the plasma osmolality is low normal or low, water depletion is unlikely and polyuria is probably due to an appropriate response to a high intake. *If the plasma osmolality is high normal or high and the urine osmolality greater than 850 mmol/kg the test should be stopped.* **09.00 hours.** Blood and urine are again collected and the plasma and urine osmolality measured.

Interpretation. The duration of the test depends on changes in the urinary osmolalities:

- If the urinary osmolality exceeds 850 mmol/kg neither significant tubular disease nor diabetes insipidus are present and the test may be stopped.
- If the urinary osmolality is below 850 mmol/kg, and that of plasma is normal, fluid restriction should be continued and the estimations repeated at hourly intervals. The test should be stopped as soon as the urine osmolality exceeds 850 mmol/kg.
- Failure to concentrate three consecutive urine specimens indicates either tubular disease or diabetes insipidus; the differential diagnosis is usually clear on clinical grounds and the test may then be stopped. If the diagnosis of diabetes insipidus is considered, continue with the DDAVP test.

DDAVP TEST

DDAVP (1-**D**eamino-8-**D-A**rginine **V**aso**p**ressin; desmopressin acetate) is a potent synthetic analogue of vasopressin.

Procedure. 4 µg DDAVP is injected intramuscularly; continue to collect urine and plasma samples.

Interpretation. If there is tubular dysfunction or nephrogenic diabetes insipidus there will be no change in the urinary osmolality but the plasma osmolality may increase due to water loss during the test. In cranial diabetes insipidus the urinary osmolality increases usually to a value greater than 850 mmol/L.

Note. After prolonged overhydration, usually due to hysterical polydipsia, concentrating power, even after administration of exogenous hormone, may be impaired. This is due to washing out of medullary hyperosmolality (p.**9**). Unless the patient is volume depleted or there is plasma hyperosmolality, the test should be repeated after several days of relative water restriction. The patient should be kept under careful observation, on the one hand for signs of genuine distress associated with a rise in plasma osmolality, and on the other for surreptitious drinking.

The measurement of urinary specific gravity is too inaccurate to be useful, and should no longer be carried out. If an osmometer is unavailable estimation of the urinary urea concentration may help. Values of about 90 to 100 times that of plasma indicate good concentrating ability.

Investigation of Electrolyte Disturbances

Electrolyte estimations provide the numerical bulk of the workload and are responsible for a large part of the expenditure of most chemical pathology departments. Conditions in which plasma sodium or potassium concentrations may be abnormal have been discussed; abnormal concentrations, especially of sodium, may not be of clinical significance but may indicate a change in plasma osmolality, which, if rapid, may cause redistribution of water across cell membranes; normal levels do not guarantee normal balance.

Before requesting any test it is worth considering whether a high, normal or low result will aid diagnosis or treatment. For technical reasons sodium and potassium are estimated simultaneously by the laboratory, but their clinical value should be considered separately: potassium results are more often useful than those of sodium. This mental discipline may help to avoid some common and dangerous therapeutic errors that arise from a misunderstanding of the underlying pathophysiological processes.

Plasma sodium concentrations should be estimated regularly:

- in unconscious or confused patients and infants losing fluid, because of the danger of hyperosmolality due to hypernatraemia;
- in the patient in diabetic coma or precoma, because of the danger of sustained hyperosmolality due to hypernatraemia despite successful control of plasma glucose concentrations;
- in the patient with intravascular volume depletion, to help diagnosis and to indicate the type of replacement fluid.

Plasma potassium and bicarbonate concentrations should be estimated regularly in any patient in whom there is a possible cause for abnormal concentrations because potassium, unlike sodium, abnormalities must always be treated. Such patients include those:

- with abnormal losses from the gastrointestinal tract or kidneys, especially due to diuretic, steroid or ACTH therapy;
- on potassium supplementation;
- with renal dysfunction;
- in diabetic ketoacidosis or hyperosmolar coma or precoma;
- in whom digoxin toxicity is considered.

The indications for electrolyte estimation are few compared with the numbers usually requested. In the fully conscious, normally hydrated patient with no abnormal losses plasma sodium estimation rarely helps. Mild hyponatraemia is common (p.**38**), but treatment in such subjects is usually contraindicated. In the absence of renal dysfunction potassium estimation is also unhelpful.

Investigation of Hypokalaemia

HYPOKALAEMIC ALKALOSIS

Diuretic therapy is by far the commonest cause of hypokalaemic alkalosis in hypertensive patients. Primary hyperaldosteronism and ectopic ACTH production are very rare.

The following procedure will almost always elucidate the cause without the need for expensive and time-consuming hormone assays.

1. Exclude obvious causes of potassium loss, such as diarrhoea. Prolonged fasting may occasionally cause hypokalaemia.
2. Take a careful drug history, with special reference to potassium-losing diuretics, purgatives, steroid, ACTH or tetracosactrin (for example 'Synacthen') therapy; rare causes of a steroid-like effect are ingestion of carbenoxolone or liquorice.
3. Look at the plasma sodium concentration. If it is above about 140 mmol/L, the hypokalaemia is likely to be due to steroids or a steroid-like effect. If it is low normal or low, another cause, such as potassium-losing diuretics, is probable.
4. If not clinically contraindicated, stop all therapy known to affect potassium loss. This is, in any case, necessary if hormone assays are later indicated, because their results are affected by such treatment.
5. Give adequate oral potassium supplements until both the plasma potassium *and bicarbonate* concentrations are normal.
6. Stop supplements and continue to monitor plasma potassium concentrations for several days. Most cases remain normokalaemic and need no further investigation.

If the plasma potassium concentrations fall again without an obvious cause, or if adequate supplementation fails to correct the hypokalaemia and there is no evidence of renal tubular damage, blood specimens should be taken under carefully controlled conditions for hormone assays. If the patient has mild to moderate hypertension and primary hyperaldosteronism is suspected, *contact the laboratory before taking blood for both renin and aldosterone assays.*

If 'ectopic' ACTH secretion is suspected, measure plasma cortisol, and if the concentration is high, ACTH. ACTH and therefore cortisol secretion are stimulated by stress, and moderately high plasma concentrations of ACTH are not necessarily due to ectopic hormone secretion.

Investigation of a Patient with Suspected Conn's Syndrome

Procedure. The patient should be in hospital for the test and should not be taking diuretics or antihypertensive drugs. He should be normovolaemic and have a daily sodium intake of about 100 mmol. After he has been kept recumbent for at least eight hours blood is taken for plasma electrolyte, renin and aldosterone assays. After the patient has then walked around for 30 minutes a further blood sample is taken for repeat plasma renin activity and aldosterone assays.

Interpretion. The diagnosis can only be made if the plasma aldosterone concentration is high and renin activity inappropriately low for the aldosterone concentration; the latter does not increase significantly after 30 minutes walking around.

HYPOKALAEMIC ACIDOSIS

Hypokalaemic acidosis is relatively rare and the cause is usually obvious.

1. Loss of potassium through fistulae in the proximal small intestine may be accompanied by significant bicarbonate loss.
2. Hypokalaemic acidosis is a complication of transplantation of the ureters into the ileum or colon (p.**93**).
3. If neither of these causes is present, the diagnosis of renal tubular acidosis should be considered (p.**93**).

Investigation of Hyperkalaemia

1. Exclude artefactual causes of hyperkalaemia such as haemolysis or delayed separation of plasma from blood cells (p.**426**).

2. Is there a cause for cell damage, such as hypoxia or severe trauma?
3. What are the plasma urea/creatinine and bicarbonate concentrations? Severe renal glomerular dysfunction is a common cause of hyperkalaemia. Acidosis, whether metabolic (with a low plasma bicarbonate concentration) or respiratory (with a normal or high plasma bicarbonate concentration), may cause mild hyperkalaemia even if glomerular function is normal. A cause for respiratory acidosis is usually obvious clinically.
4. Is the patient taking drugs, such as:

   - potassium supplements? It is surprisingly common for such supplementation to be continued once the need for it has passed and for this cause of hyperkalaemia to be forgotten.
   - potassium-retaining diuretics?
   - an angiotensin-converting enzyme (ACE) inhibitor?

5. The combination of hypotension, skin pigmentation, hyponatraemia with hyperkalaemia and mild uraemia is common in many serious illnesses, and is only rarely due to Addison's disease. However, this diagnosis should not be forgotten. Look for pigmentation of the mucous membranes. If there is any doubt, estimate the plasma cortisol concentration. It should be very high at any time of day in an ill patient: if it is low, or even normal, proceed as on p.**151**. If steroid treatment is required immediately, consider performing a short Synacthen test (p.**152**) which will only delay the onset of treatment by about an hour.

Investigation of a Patient with Renal Calculi

1. If the stone is available, send it to the laboratory for analysis.

2. Exclude *hypercalcaemia* and *hyperuri-caemia*.

3. If the *plasma calcium concentration is normal*, collect a 24-hour specimen of urine for calcium and oxalate estimations; acid must be added to the specimen before analysis to keep calcium in solution.

4. *If all these tests are negative*, and especially if there is a family history of calculi, screen the urine for cystine. If the qualitative test is positive the 24-hour excretion of cystine should be estimated (p.**360**).

5. *If fresh uninfected urine is alkaline despite a systemic metabolic acidosis* the diagnosis of renal tubular acidosis is likely (p.**93**). A pH above 8 is suggestive of a urinary infection with a urea splitting organism, such as *Proteus vulgaris.*

6. In children a low plasma urate and high urinary xanthine suggest xanthinuria. If these values are normal the 24-hour excretion of oxalate should be determined to exclude primary hyperoxaluria.

Hydrogen ion homeostasis

About 50 to 100 *milli*moles of hydrogen ions are released from cells into extracellular fluid each day. Despite fluctuations in the rate of release throughout the day, due to varying loads, the extracellular hydrogen ion concentration ([H$^+$]) is maintained between about 35 and 45 *nano*mol/L (40 nmol/L = pH 7.40). Control of hydrogen ion balance depends ultimately on the secretion of H$^+$ from the body, mainly into the urine. *Renal impairment causes acidosis.*

Aerobic metabolism of the carbon skeletons of organic compounds converts hydrogen, carbon and oxygen to water and carbon dioxide (CO_2). Although CO_2 does not directly affect the hydrogen ion balance, it is an essential component of the extracellular buffering system. *Control of CO_2 depends on normal lung function.*

The principal sources of hydrogen ions are:

- *the metabolism of amino acids.* Conversion of amino nitrogen to urea in the liver, or of the sulphydryl groups of some amino acids to sulphate, releases equimolar amounts of hydrogen ions. Although a high protein diet may increase the H$^+$ load and aggravate a pre-existing acidosis, it is rarely of clinical importance.
- *the incomplete metabolism of carbon skeletons of organic compounds.* Anaerobic carbohydrate metabolism produces lactate (p.**203**) and anaerobic metabolism of fatty acids and of ketogenic amino acids produces acetoacetate (p.**200**); these processes release equimolar amounts of H$^+$, either directly or indirectly. In pathological lactic acidosis or ketoacidosis the rate of these reactions is so rapid that the capacity of the compensatory mechanisms is exceeded and the H$^+$ concentration in blood rises significantly (pH falls).

Many anabolic processes, including gluconeogenesis, use hydrogen ions. Acidosis is commoner than alkalosis because metabolism produces hydrogen and not hydroxyl ions.

DEFINITIONS

An acid can dissociate to produce hydrogen ions (protons: H$^+$) which can be accepted by a *base*. Examples of acids and bases important in hydrogen ion balance are shown in Table 4.1.

An alkali dissociates to produce hydroxyl ions (OH$^-$). Alkalis are of little importance in the present discussion because hydroxyl ions are not primary products of metabolism.

A strong acid is almost completely dissociated in aqueous solution, and so produces many H$^+$. For example, hydrochloric acid is a strong acid and is almost entirely dissociated in water to form H$^+$ and Cl$^-$ ions. The examples given in Table 4.1 are *weak acids*, yielding relatively few hydrogen ions. However very small changes in the hydrogen ion concentration may have important biological consequences.

Buffering is a process by which a strong acid (or base) is replaced by a weaker one, with a consequent reduction in the number of free hydrogen ions and therefore the change in pH, after addition of acid, is less than it would be in the absence of the buffer. For example:

$$H^+Cl^- + NaHCO_3 \longleftrightarrow H_2CO_3 + NaCl$$

| Strong acid | **buffer** | weak acid | neutral salt |

pH is a measure of hydrogen ion activity. It is $\log_{10}$ of the reciprocal of the hydrogen ion concentration ([H$^+$]) in mol/L. The $\log_{10}$ of a number is the power to which 10 must be raised to produce that number:

$\log 100 = \log 10^2 = 2$, and $\log 10^7 = 7$.

If [H$^+$] is 10^{-7} (0.000 000 1) mol/L, then $\log$ [H$^+$] = -7.

Table 4.1   Some weak acids and their conjugate bases, present in biological fluids

	Acid			**Conjugate base**	
Carbonic acid	H_2CO_3	$\leftrightarrow$ H^+ +		HCO_3^-	Bicarbonate ion
Dihydrogen phosphate	$H_2PO_4^-$	$\leftrightarrow$ H^+ +		HPO_4^{2-}	Monohydrogen phosphate ion
Ammonium ion	NH_4^+	$\leftrightarrow$ H^+ +		NH_3	Ammonia
Lactic acid	$CH_3CHOHCOOH$	$\leftrightarrow$ H^+ +		$CH_3CHOHCOO^-$	Lactate ion
Acetoacetic acid	CH_3COCH_2COOH	$\leftrightarrow$ H^+ +		$CH_3COCH_2COO^-$	Acetoacetate ion
3-hydroxy-butyric acid	$CH_3CHOHCH_2COOH$	$\leftrightarrow$ H^+ +		$CH_3CHOHCH_2COO^-$	3-hydroxy-butyrate ion

But

$$pH = \log \frac{1}{[H^+]} = -\log [H^+]$$

Therefore   pH = 7

At pH 6, $[H^+] = 10^{-6}$ (0.000 001) mol/L (1000 nmol/L) and at pH 7, $[H^+] = 10^{-7}$ (0.000 000 1) mol/L (100 nmol/L); *a change of one pH unit represents a 10-fold change in [H⁺]*. Changes of this magnitude do not occur in cells or in extracellular fluid. However, in pathological conditions the blood pH can change by more than 0.3 of a unit; a decrease of pH by 0.3, from 7.4 to 7.1, represents a doubling of [H⁺] from 40 to 80 nmol/L. The use of the pH notation makes a very significant change in [H⁺] appear deceptively small.

Urinary pH is much more variable than that of blood. [H⁺] can vary 1000-fold (a change of 3 pH units).

The Henderson–Hasselbalch equation expresses the relation between pH and a buffer pair, that is a weak acid and its conjugate base (Table 4.1). The equation is valid for any buffer pair, the pH being dependent on the *ratio* of the concentration of base to acid.

$$pH = pK + \log \frac{[base]}{[acid]}$$

The bicarbonate pair is an important biological example. The base is bicarbonate (HCO_3^-) and the acid carbonic acid (H_2CO_3). It is not possible to measure the latter directly; however, it is in equilibrium with dissolved CO_2, of which the partial pressure (P_{CO_2}) *can* be estimated. The concentration of H_2CO_3 is derived by multiplying this measured value by the solubility constant (s) for CO_2. Therefore:

$$pH = pK + \log \frac{[HCO_3^-]}{P_{CO_2} \times s}$$

If the P_{CO_2} is expressed in:

- kilopascals (kPa) s = 0.23;
- mmHg, s = 0.03.

The overall pK of the bicarbonate system is 6.1. Therefore if P_{CO_2} is in kPa:

$$pH = 6.1 + \log \frac{[HCO_3^-]}{P_{CO_2} \times 0.23}$$

This form of the equation for the bicarbonate pair will be used in the rest of the chapter.

*H*YDROGEN ION HOMEOSTASIS

Despite considerable fluctuations in the rate of release of H⁺ into the extracellular fluid, the hydrogen ion concentration, and therefore pH, is relatively tightly controlled in blood by the following mechanisms.

- *Hydrogen ions can be incorporated into water.*

$$H^+ + HCO_3^- \longleftrightarrow H_2CO_3 \longleftrightarrow CO_2 + H_2O$$

This is the normal mechanism during oxidative phosphorylation. As this reaction is reversible, H^+ is inactivated by combining with HCO_3^- only if the reaction is driven to the right by the removal of CO_2. By itself this would cause bicarbonate depletion.

- *Buffering of hydrogen ions is a temporary measure* as the H^+ has not been excreted from the body. The production of the weak acid of the buffer pair causes only a small change in pH (see Henderson–Hasselbalch equation). If hydrogen ions are not completely neutralized or eliminated from the body and if production continues, buffering power will eventually be so depleted that the pH will change significantly.

- *Hydrogen ions can be lost from the body only through the kidneys and the intestine.* This mechanism is coupled with the generation of bicarbonate ion (HCO_3^-). In the kidney this is the method by which secretion of excess H^+ ensures regeneration of buffering capacity.

Control Systems

Carbon dioxide and hydrogen ions are potentially toxic products of aerobic and anaerobic metabolism respectively. Most CO_2 is lost through the lungs but some is converted to bicarbonate, thus contributing important extracellular buffering capacity; inactivating one toxic product provides a means of minimizing the effects of the other.

A buffer pair is most effective at maintaining a pH near its pK, when the ratio of the concentrations of base to acid is close to one. However, the optimum pH of the extracellular fluid is about 7.4 and the pK of the bicarbonate system is 6.1. Although this may appear to be a disadvantage the *bicarbonate*

system is the most important buffer* in the body because:

- it accounts for over 60 per cent of the blood buffering capacity;
- it is necessary for efficient buffering by haemoglobin, which provides most of the rest of the blood buffering capacity;
- H^+ secretion by the kidney depends on it.

THE CONTROL OF CO_2 (P_{CO_2}) BY THE RESPIRATORY CENTRE AND LUNGS

The partial pressure of CO_2 in plasma is normally about 5.3 kPa (40 mmHg) and depends on the balance between the rate of production by metabolism and the loss through the pulmonary alveoli. The sequence of events is as follows:

- inspired oxygen is carried from the lungs to the tissues by haemoglobin (p.**98**);
- the tissue cells use the oxygen for aerobic metabolism; some of the carbon in organic compounds is oxidized to CO_2;
- CO_2 diffuses along a concentration gradient from the cells into the extracellular fluid and is returned by the blood to the lungs, where it is eliminated in expired air;
- the rate of respiration, and therefore the rate of CO_2 elimination, is controlled by chemoreceptors in the respiratory centre in the medulla of the brainstem and by those in the carotid and aortic bodies. The receptors respond to changes in the $[CO_2]$ or $[H^+]$ of plasma or of the cerebrospinal fluid. If the P_{CO_2} rises much above 5.3 kPa or, if the pH falls, the rate of respiration increases. Normal lungs have a very large reserve capacity for CO_2 elimination.

Not only is there a plentiful supply of CO_2, the denominator in the Henderson–Hasselbalch equation, but the normal respiratory centre and lungs can control its concentration within narrow limits by responding to changes in the $[H^+]$ and therefore compensate for changes in acid-base disturbances.

Some diseases of the lungs, or abnormalities of respiratory control, primarily affect the P_{CO_2}.

THE CONTROL OF BICARBONATE BY THE KIDNEYS AND ERYTHROCYTES

The renal tubular cells and erythrocytes generate bicarbonate, the buffer base in the bicarbonate system, from CO_2. Under physiological conditions:

- *the erythrocyte mechanism makes fine adjustments* to the plasma bicarbonate concentration in response to changes in P_{CO_2} in the lungs and tissues;
- *the kidneys play the major role in maintaining the circulating bicarbonate concentration* and in eliminating H+ from the body.

THE CARBONATE DEHYDRATASE SYSTEM

Bicarbonate is produced following the dissociation of carbonic acid formed from CO_2 and H_2O. This is catalysed by carbonate dehydratase (CD; carbonic anhydrase), present in high concentrations in erythrocytes and renal tubular cells.

$$CO_2 + H_2O \underset{CD}{\longleftrightarrow} H_2CO_3 \longleftrightarrow H^+ + HCO_3^-$$

Not only do erythrocytes and renal tubular cells have a high concentration of CD, but they also have means of removing one of the products, H+; thus both reactions continue to the right and HCO_3^- is formed. One of the reactants, water, is freely available and one of the products, H+, is removed. HCO_3^- generation is therefore accelerated if the concentration of:

- CO_2 rises;
- HCO_3^- falls;
- H+ falls because it is either buffered by erythrocytes or excreted from the body by renal tubular cells.

Therefore an increase of intracellular P_{CO_2}, or a decrease in intracellular $[HCO_3^-]$ in the erythrocytes and renal tubular cells maintain the extracellular bicarbonate concentration by accelerating the production of HCO_3^-. This minimizes changes in the ratio of $[HCO_2^-]$ to P_{CO_2} and therefore changes in pH.

In the normal subject, at a plasma P_{CO_2} of 5.3 kPa, (a CO_2 of about 1.2 mmol/L (p.**101**)), erythrocytes and renal tubular cells keep the extracellular bicarbonate at about 25 mmol/L. The extracellular ratio of $[HCO_3^-]$ to $[CO_2]$ (both in mmol/L) is just over 20:1. It can be calculated from the Henderson–Hasselbalch equation that, with a pK of 6.1, this represents a pH very near 7.4. An increase of intracellular P_{CO_2}, or a decrease in intracellular $[HCO_3^-]$, accelerates HCO_3^- production and minimizes changes in the ratio and therefore in pH.

BICARBONATE GENERATION BY THE ERYTHROCYTES (FIG. 4.1)

Haemoglobin is an important blood buffer. However it only works effectively in cooperation with the bicarbonate system.

$$pH = pK + \log \frac{[Hb^-]}{[HHb]}$$

Erythrocytes produce little CO_2 as they lack aerobic pathways. Plasma CO_2 diffuses along a concentration gradient into erythrocytes, where carbonate dehydratase catalyses its reaction with water to form carbonic acid (H_2CO_3) which then dissociates. Much of the H+ is buffered by haemoglobin and the HCO_3^- diffuses out into the extracellular fluid along a concentration gradient. Electrochemical neutrality is maintained by diffusion

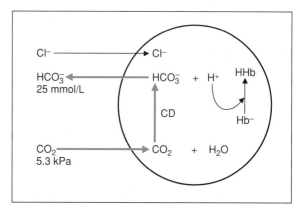

Fig. 4.1 Generation of bicarbonate by erythrocytes, showing the 'chloride shift'.

of chloride in the opposite direction into cells. This movement of ions is known as the 'chloride shift' (Fig. 4.1).

Under normal circumstances the higher Pco_2 in blood leaving tissues stimulates erythrocyte HCO_3^- production; consequently the arteriovenous difference in the ratio $[HCO_3^-] : [CO_2]$, and therefore the pH, is kept relatively constant.

Extra- and intracellular buffers other than bicarbonate and haemoglobin do not contribute significantly to blood buffering. They include:

- *phosphate*, which has a plasma concentration of about 1 mmol/L, but a higher concentration in bone and inside cells where buffering capacity is of more importance;
- *proteins* which, because of their low concentrations in plasma, also have little blood buffering capacity but are more important at the high intracellular concentrations in plasma.

THE KIDNEYS

Carbonate dehydratase is also of central importance in the mechanisms involved in H^+ secretion and in maintaining the bicarbonate buffering capacity in the blood. Hydrogen ions are secreted from renal tubular cells into the lumina where they are buffered by constituents of the glomerular filtrate. Unlike haemoglobin in erythrocytes, urinary buffers are constantly being replenished by continuing glomerular filtration. *For this reason, and because most of the excess H^+ can only be eliminated from the body by the renal route, the kidneys are of major importance in compensating for chronic acidosis.* Without them the haemoglobin buffering capacity would soon become saturated.

Two renal mechanisms control $[HCO_3^-]$ in the extracellular fluid:

- *bicarbonate reclamation ('reabsorption')*, the predominant mechanism in maintaining the steady state. The CO_2 driving the carbonate dehydratase mechanism in renal tubular cells is derived from filtered bicarbonate. *There is no net loss of hydrogen ions;*
- *bicarbonate generation*, a very important mechanism for correcting acidosis, in which the levels of CO_2 or $[HCO_3^-]$ affecting the carbonate dehydratase reaction in renal tubular cells reflect those in the extracellular fluid. *There is a net loss of hydrogen ions.*

Bicarbonate reclamation (Fig. 4.2). Normal urine is almost bicarbonate-free. An amount equivalent to that filtered by the glomeruli is returned to the body by the tubular cells. The luminal surfaces of renal tubular cells are impermeable to bicarbonate. Therefore bicarbonate can only be returned to the body if first converted to CO_2 in the tubular lumina, and an equivalent amount of CO_2 converted to bicarbonate within tubular cells. The mechanism depends on the action of carbonate dehydratase, both in the brush border on the luminal surfaces and within tubular cells, and on H^+ secreted into the lumina in exchange for sodium. The sequence of events, which occurs predominantly in the proximal tubules but also in the first part of the distal tubules, is depicted in Fig. 4.2.

- Bicarbonate is filtered through the glomeruli at a plasma concentration of about 25 mmol/L.
- Filtered bicarbonate combines with H^+, secreted by tubular cells, to form H_2CO_3.
- The H_2CO_3 dissociates to form CO_2 and water. In the proximal tubules this reaction is catalysed by carbonate dehydratase in the brush border. In the distal tubules, where the pH is usually lower, H_2CO_3 probably dissociates spontaneously.
- As the luminal Pco_2 rises, CO_2 diffuses into tubular cells along a concentration gradient.
- As the intracellular concentration of CO_2 rises, carbonate dehydratase catalyses its combination with water to form H_2CO_3, which dissociates into H^+ and HCO_3^-.
- H^+ is secreted in the tubular lumina in exchange for sodium ions and so the

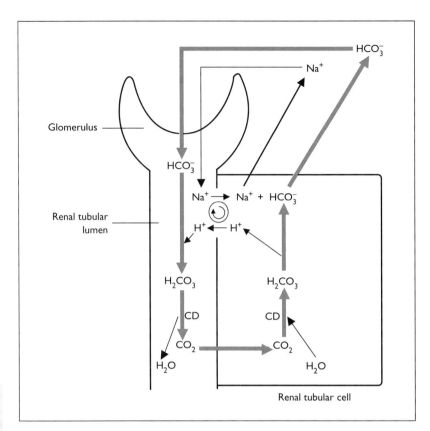

Fig. 4.2 Normal 'reabsorption' of filtered bicarbonate from the lumina of the renal tubules.

reactions start again from the second stage. As the intracellular concentration of HCO_3^- rises, HCO_3^- diffuses into the extracellular fluid accompanied by sodium, which has been reabsorbed in exchange for H^+.

This self-perpetuating cycle reclaims buffering capacity that would otherwise have been lost from the body by glomerular filtration. The secreted H^+ is derived from cellular water, and is incorporated into water in the lumina. Because there is no net change in hydrogen ion balance and no net gain of bicarbonate, *this mechanism cannot correct an acidosis but can maintain a steady state.*

Bicarbonate generation (Fig. 4.3). The mechanism in renal tubular cells for generating bicarbonate is identical with that of bicarbonate 'reabsorption', but there *is* net loss of H^+ from the body as well as a net gain of HCO_3^-. Therefore this mechanism is well suited to correct any type of acidosis.

Within tubular cells, *carbonate dehydratase may be stimulated by*:

- *a rise in* P_{CO_2}. In this case, the rise in $[CO_2]$ is the indirect result of a rise in the extracellular P_{CO_2}. Renal tubular cells, unlike erythrocytes with anaerobic pathways, constantly produce CO_2 aerobically. This diffuses out of cells into the extracellular fluid along a concentration gradient. An increase in extracellular P_{CO_2}, by reducing the gradient, slows this diffusion and the intracellular P_{CO_2} rises.
- *a fall of* $[HCO_3^-]$. Reduction of extracellular $[HCO_3^-]$, by increasing the concentration gradient across renal tubular cell membranes, increases the loss of HCO_3^- from cells.

Normally almost all the filtered bicarbonate is 'reabsorbed'. Once the luminal fluid is bicarbonate-free, continued secretion of H^+ and the intracellular generation of HCO_3^-

tion, to continue after other buffers have been depleted.

Ammonia, produced by hepatic deamination of amino acids, is rapidly incorporated into urea, with a net production of hydrogen ions. However, as the systemic hydrogen ion concentration increases, there is some shift from urea to glutamine synthesis with a slight fall in hepatic H^+ production. Glutamine ($GluCONH_2$) is taken up by renal tubular cells where it is hydrolysed by glutaminase to glutamate ($GluCOO^-$) and ammonium ion (Fig. 4.4).

$$H_2O + GluCONH_2 \longrightarrow GluCOO^- + NH_4^+$$

Ammonia and the ammonium ion form a buffer pair with a pK of about 9.8

$$pH = 9.8 + \log\frac{[NH_3]}{[NH_4^+]}$$

Because of the very high pK, at pH 7.4 and below the equilibrium is overwhelmingly in favour of NH_4^+ production. NH_3 can diffuse out of the cell into the tubular lumen much more rapidly than NH_4^+. If the luminal fluid is acidic, NH_3 will be retained within the lumen by avid combination with H^+ derived from the carbonate dehydratase mechanism. This allows H^+, produced in the kidneys, to be excreted as ammonium chloride; thus in severe acidosis, bicarbonate formation can continue even when phosphate buffering power has been exhausted. There is a *net gain of HCO_3^-*.

However, H^+ as well as NH_3 is released in renal tubular cells when NH_4^+ dissociates; this is maintained by passive diffusion of NH_3 into the luminal fluid. On the face of it there seems no advantage in buffering one H^+ secreted into the lumen if, at the same time, another is produced within the cell. Possible explanations for the role of NH_3 in the correction of acidosis include:

- *the fate of the glutamate* ($GluCOO^-$), produced at the same time as the ammonium ion. After further deamination to 2-oxoglutarate it can be converted to glucose; *gluconeogenesis uses an equivalent amount of H^+ to that of NH_4^+ produced*

from glutamine. Therefore, the H^+ liberated into the cell is probably incorporated into glucose (Fig. 4.4);
- *a shift from urea synthesis to glutamine production* in the liver with a fall in systemic H^+ production in the presence of an acidosis. This is a minor factor.

The rate of gluconeogenesis and glutamine synthesis, and glutaminase activity all increase in an acidosis.

BICARBONATE FORMATION IN THE GASTROINTESTINAL TRACT (FIG. 4.5)

Carbonate dehydratase also catalyses the formation of bicarbonate in intestinal mucosal cells. The bicarbonate may either pass into the extracellular fluid or into the intestinal lumen; in either case the mechanism can only continue if H^+ is pumped in the opposite direction. Electrochemical neutrality is maintained by one of two mechanisms:

- Na^+ exchange for H^+, by a mechanism which is the opposite of that in renal tubular cells;
- passage of Cl^- with H^+.

Acid secretion by the stomach. The parietal cells of the stomach secrete H^+ into the lumen together with Cl^-. As H^+Cl^- enters the gastric lumen, bicarbonate diffuses into the extracellular fluid, thus accounting for the postprandial 'alkaline tide'. In the normal subject this is rapidly corrected by bicarbonate secretion, mainly by the pancreas, as food passes down the intestinal tract. *This mechanism explains the metabolic alkalosis which occurs in pyloric stenosis* (p.96).

Sodium bicarbonate secretion by pancreatic and biliary cells in response to stimulation by secretin (p.**245**) accounts for the alkalinization of the duodenal fluid and occurs by the reverse process of sodium bicarbonate reabsorption in renal tubular cells (p.**84**). The pancreatic and biliary mechanisms are accelerated by the local rise in P_{CO_2} which results when H^+ is pumped into the extracellular fluid and reacts with the HCO_3^- generated by gastric parietal cells.

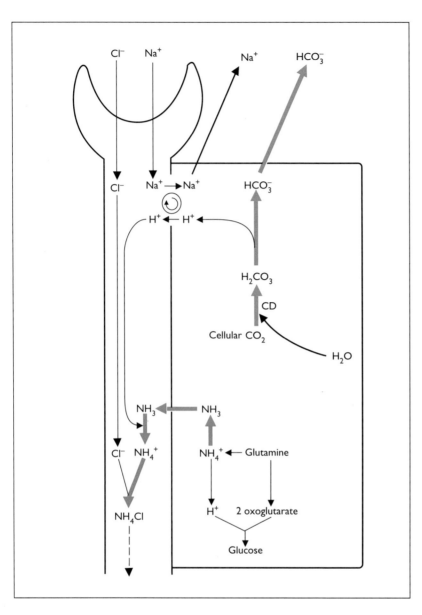

Fig. 4.4 The role of ammonia in the generation of bicarbonate by renal tubular cells. (Modified with kind permission from Williams DL, Marks V, eds. *Biochemistry in clinical practice*, London: Heinemann Medical Books, 1983.)

because the concentration of phosphate increases 20-fold to nearly 25 mmol/L as water is reabsorbed from the tubular lumen.

Even in a mild acidosis more phosphate ions are released from bone than at normal pH; the need for increased urinary H^+ secretion is linked with increased buffering capacity in the glomerular filtrate due to the increase of phosphate. At a urinary pH below 5.5, most of the filtered phosphate is converted to dihydrogen phosphate. Therefore at low pH urinary phosphate cannot maintain the essential buffering of continued hydrogen ion secretion. The predominant urinary anion is chloride, but, because hydrochloric acid is almost completely ionized in aqueous solution, it cannot act as a buffer.

The role of ammonia. As the urine becomes more acid it can be shown to contain increasing amounts of ammonium ion (NH_4^+). Urinary ammonia probably allows H^+ secretion, and therefore bicarbonate formation, to continue after other buffers have been depleted.

Ammonia, produced by hepatic deamination of amino acids, is rapidly incorporated into urea, with a net production of hydrogen ions. However, as the systemic hydrogen ion concentration increases, there is some shift from urea to glutamine synthesis with a slight fall in hepatic H+ production. Glutamine (GluCONH$_2$) is taken up by renal tubular cells where it is hydrolysed by glutaminase to glutamate (GluCOO-) and ammonium ion (Fig. 4.4).

$$H_2O + GluCONH_2 \longrightarrow GluCOO- + NH_4^+$$

Ammonia and the ammonium ion form a buffer pair with a pK of about 9.8

$$pH = 9.8 + \log \frac{[NH_3]}{[NH_4^+]}$$

Because of the very high pK, at pH 7.4 and below the equilibrium is overwhelmingly in favour of NH$_4^+$ production. NH$_3$ can diffuse out of the cell into the tubular lumen much more rapidly than NH$_4^+$. If the luminal fluid is acidic, NH$_3$ will be retained within the lumen by avid combination with H+ derived from the carbonate dehydratase mechanism. This allows H+, produced in the kidneys, to be excreted as ammonium chloride; thus in severe acidosis, bicarbonate formation can continue even when phosphate buffering power has been exhausted. There is a *net gain of HCO$_3^-$.*

However, H+ as well as NH$_3$ is released in renal tubular cells when NH$_4^+$ dissociates; this is maintained by passive diffusion of NH$_3$ into the luminal fluid. On the face of it there seems no advantage in buffering one H+ secreted into the lumen if, at the same time, another is produced within the cell. Possible explanations for the role of NH$_3$ in the correction of acidosis include:

- *the fate of the glutamate* (GluCOO-), produced at the same time as the ammonium ion. After further deamination to 2-oxoglutarate it can be converted to glucose; *gluconeogenesis uses an equivalent amount of H+ to that of NH$_4^+$ produced*

from glutamine. Therefore, the H+ liberated into the cell is probably incorporated into glucose (Fig. 4.4);
- *a shift from urea synthesis to glutamine production* in the liver with a fall in systemic H+ production in the presence of an acidosis. This is a minor factor.

The rate of gluconeogenesis and glutamine synthesis, and glutaminase activity all increase in an acidosis.

BICARBONATE FORMATION IN THE GASTROINTESTINAL TRACT (FIG. 4.5)

Carbonate dehydratase also catalyses the formation of bicarbonate in intestinal mucosal cells. The bicarbonate may either pass into the extracellular fluid or into the intestinal lumen; in either case the mechanism can only continue if H+ is pumped in the opposite direction. Electrochemical neutrality is maintained by one of two mechanisms:

- Na+ exchange for H+, by a mechanism which is the opposite of that in renal tubular cells;
- passage of Cl- with H+.

Acid secretion by the stomach. The parietal cells of the stomach secrete H+ into the lumen together with Cl-. As H+Cl- enters the gastric lumen, bicarbonate diffuses into the extracellular fluid, thus accounting for the postprandial 'alkaline tide'. In the normal subject this is rapidly corrected by bicarbonate secretion, mainly by the pancreas, as food passes down the intestinal tract. *This mechanism explains the metabolic alkalosis which occurs in pyloric stenosis (p.96).*

Sodium bicarbonate secretion by pancreatic and biliary cells in response to stimulation by secretin (p.245) accounts for the alkalinization of the duodenal fluid and occurs by the reverse process of sodium bicarbonate reabsorption in renal tubular cells (p.84). The pancreatic and biliary mechanisms are accelerated by the local rise in PCO_2 which results when H+ is pumped into the extracellular fluid and reacts with the HCO$_3^-$ generated by gastric parietal cells.

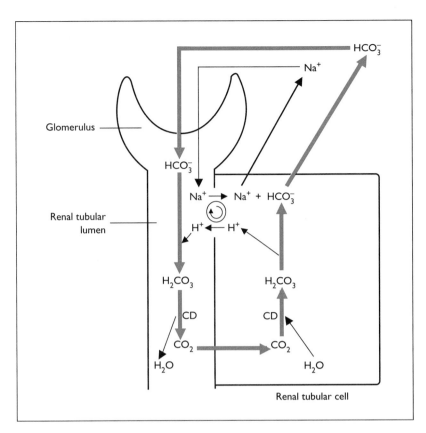

Fig. 4.2 Normal 'reabsorption' of filtered bicarbonate from the lumina of the renal tubules.

Glomerulus

Renal tubular lumen

HCO_3^-

Na^+

HCO_3^-

$Na^+ \longrightarrow Na^+ + HCO_3^-$

$H^+ \longleftarrow H^+$

H_2CO_3 H_2CO_3

CD   CD

$CO_2 \longrightarrow CO_2$

H_2O H_2O

Renal tubular cell

reactions start again from the second stage. As the intracellular concentration of HCO_3^- rises, HCO_3^- diffuses into the extracellular fluid accompanied by sodium, which has been reabsorbed in exchange for H^+.

This self-perpetuating cycle reclaims buffering capacity that would otherwise have been lost from the body by glomerular filtration. The secreted H^+ is derived from cellular water, and is incorporated into water in the lumina. Because there is no net change in hydrogen ion balance and no net gain of bicarbonate, *this mechanism cannot correct an acidosis but can maintain a steady state.*

Bicarbonate generation (Fig. 4.3). The mechanism in renal tubular cells for generating bicarbonate is identical with that of bicarbonate 'reabsorption', but there *is* net loss of H^+ from the body as well as a net gain of HCO_3^-. Therefore this mechanism is well suited to correct any type of acidosis.

Within tubular cells, *carbonate dehydratase may be stimulated by*:

- *a rise in $P\text{CO}_2$*. In this case, the rise in $[CO_2]$ is the indirect result of a rise in the extracellular $P\text{CO}_2$. Renal tubular cells, unlike erythrocytes with anaerobic pathways, constantly produce CO_2 aerobically. This diffuses out of cells into the extracellular fluid along a concentration gradient. An increase in extracellular $P\text{CO}_2$, by reducing the gradient, slows this diffusion and the intracellular $P\text{CO}_2$ rises.
- *a fall of $[HCO_3^-]$*. Reduction of extracellular $[HCO_3^-]$, by increasing the concentration gradient across renal tubular cell membranes, increases the loss of HCO_3^- from cells.

Normally almost all the filtered bicarbonate is 'reabsorbed'. Once the luminal fluid is bicarbonate-free, continued secretion of H^+ and the intracellular generation of HCO_3^-

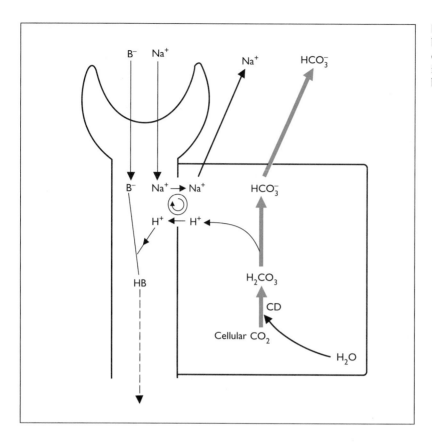

Fig. 4.3 Net generation of bicarbonate by renal tubular cells with excretion of hydrogen ions (B- = nonbicarbonate base).

depend on the presence of other filtered buffer bases (B⁻). In their absence the luminal acidity would increase so much that further H⁺ secretion would be inhibited. These buffers, unlike bicarbonate, do not form compounds capable of diffusing back into tubular cells, and nor is H⁺ incorporated into water. *There is net loss of H⁺ in urine* as HB. The bicarbonate formed in the cell is derived from cellular CO_2 and therefore represents a *net gain in bicarbonate*. Whenever a mmol of H⁺ is secreted into the tubular lumen a mmol of HCO_3^- passes into the extracellular fluid with sodium. The mechanism of bicarbonate generation is very similar to that in erythrocytes. However unlike red cells, renal tubular cells are exposed to a relatively constant PCO_2. Bicarbonate generation, coupled with H⁺ secretion, becomes very important in acidosis, when it is stimulated either by a fall in extracellular $[HCO_3^-]$ (metabolic acidosis) or a rise in extracellular PCO_2 (respiratory acidosis).

URINARY BUFFERS

The two most important urinary 'buffers', other than bicarbonate, are phosphate and ammonia; they are also involved in bicarbonate generation.

Phosphate buffer pair. At pH 7.4 most of the phosphate in plasma, and also in the glomerular filtrate, is monohydrogen phosphate (HPO_4^{2-}) which can accept H⁺ to become dihydrogen phosphate ($H_2PO_4^-$). Bicarbonate can continue to be generated within tubular cells, with H⁺ and be returned to the body after all that in the filtrate has been reabsorbed. Therefore it can help to replace that used in extracellular buffering. The pK of this buffer pair is about 6.8.

$$pH = 6.8 + \log \frac{[HPO_4^{2-}]}{[H_2PO_4^-]}$$

Phosphate is normally the most important buffer in the urine because its pK is relatively close to the pH of the glomerular filtrate and

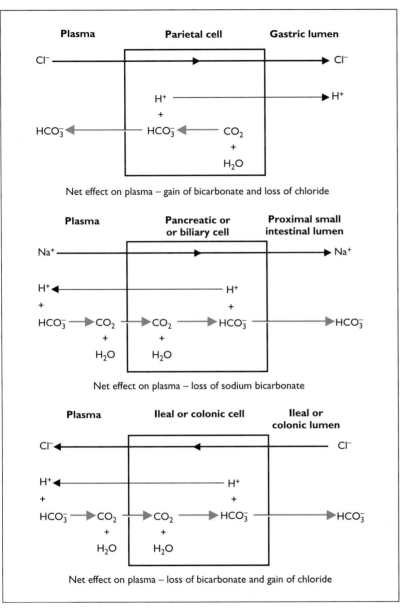

Fig. 4.5 Possible mechanism for the gastrointestinal handling of bicarbonate.

This is analogous to the stimulation of renal bicarbonate formation by the rise in luminal $P\text{CO}_2$. *Loss of large amounts of duodenal fluid may cause bicarbonate depletion* (p.**95**).

Bicarbonate secretion and chloride reabsorption by intestinal cells. As fluid passes down the intestinal tract, bicarbonate enters and chloride leaves the lumen by a reversal of the gastric mucosal mechanism.

Therefore the gastric loss of chloride and the gain of bicarbonate are finally corrected. Preferential reabsorption of urinary chloride by this mechanism after ureteric transplantation into the ileum, ileal loops or the colon explains the *hyperchloraemic acidosis associated with this operation* (p.**93**).

In summary, CO_2 is of central importance in hydrogen ion homeostasis. Despite the apparently unfavourable pK of the bicarbonate buffer system, the tendency of H_2CO_3 to form gaseous CO_2, the partial pressure of which can be controlled by the respiratory centre and lungs at about 5.3 kPa, and the ability of the renal tubular cells and erythocytes to maintain the $[HCO_3^-]$ at 25 mmol/L, enable the pH of blood to be kept above the pK of the system. *Renal or pulmonary disease may impair control of extracellular pH.*

Disturbances of Hydrogen Ion Homeostasis

Disturbances of hydrogen ion homeostasis always involve the bicarbonate buffer pair. In 'respiratory' disturbances abnormalities of CO_2 are primary, whereas in so-called 'metabolic' disturbances $[HCO_3^-]$ is affected early and changes in CO_2 are secondary.

Acidosis

Acidosis occurs if there is a fall in the ratio $[HCO_3^-] : PcO_2$ in the extracellular fluid.

$$pH = 6.1 + \log \frac{[HCO_3^-]}{PcO_2 \times 0.23}$$

Acidosis may be due to:

- *metabolic (non-respiratory) acidosis* in which the primary abnormality in the bicarbonate buffer system is a *reduction in* $[HCO_3^-]$;
- *respiratory acidosis* in which the primary abnormality in the bicarbonate buffer system is a *rise in* PcO_2.

In either metabolic or respiratory acidosis the ratio of $[HCO_3^-] : PcO_2$, and therefore the pH, can be corrected by a change in concentration of the other member of the buffer pair in the same direction as the primary abnormality. This *compensation* may be either *partial* or *complete*. The compensatory change in a metabolic acidosis is a reduction in PcO_2; in a respiratory acidosis it is a rise in $[HCO_3^-]$.

In a fully compensated acidosis the pH is normal. However, the levels of the other components of the Henderson–Hasselbalch equation are abnormal. All parameters can only return to normal if the primary abnormality is corrected.

METABOLIC ACIDOSIS

The primary disorder in the bicarbonate buffer system in a metabolic acidosis is a reduction in $[HCO_3^-]$, resulting in a fall in blood pH. The reduction in the bicarbonate may be due to:

- its use in buffering H^+ more rapidly than it can be generated by normal homeostatic mechanisms;
- loss in the urine or gastrointestinal tract more rapidly than it can be generated by normal homeostatic mechanisms;
- impaired production.

If the number of negatively charged ions (in this case HCO_3^-) is reduced, electrochemical neutrality is maintained by replacing them with an equivalent number of other anion(s). If a metabolic acidosis is classified in this way many of the associated biochemical findings can be explained. It also allows critical evaluation of the rare need to estimate the plasma chloride concentration $[Cl^-]$.

One negative charge balances one positive charge, and some substances are multivalent, having more than one charge per mole. If the molecular weight is divided by the valency the charges on each resulting *equivalent* will be the same as those on an equivalent of any other chemical. Most of the ions in the following discussion are monovalent, and hence the number of mmol is numerically the same as that of mEq. However, when calculating ion balance the latter notation should be used.

Sodium and potassium provide over 90 per cent of plasma cation concentration in the normal subject; the balance includes low concentrations of calcium and magnesium, which vary very little even in disease.

Over 80 per cent of *plasma anions* is accounted for by *chloride and bicarbonate*; the remaining 20 per cent or so (sometimes referred to as 'unmeasured anion') is made up of protein, and the normally low concentrations of urate, phosphate, sulphate, lactate and other organic anions. The protein concentration remains relatively constant, but the concentrations of other unmeasured anions can vary considerably in disease.

The 'anion gap', represented as A- in the following equations, is the difference between the total concentration of *measured cations* (sodium and potassium) and *measured* anions (chloride and bicarbonate); it is normally about 15 to 20 mEq/L. Therefore:

$$[Na^+] + [K^+] = [HCO_3^-] + [Cl^-] + [A^-]$$
$$140 \; + \; 4 \; = \; 25 \; + \; 100 \; + \; 19 \quad mEq/L$$

In the following examples, in which the abnormal figures are in **bold** type, the plasma $[HCO_3^-]$ will be assumed to have fallen by 10 mmol (mEq)/L.

Increase in [A-]. In *renal glomerular dysfunction*, even if tubular function is normal, bicarbonate generation is impaired because the amount of sodium available for exchange with H+, and the amount of filtered buffer anion B- (Fig. 4.3; p.**86**) available to accept H+, are both reduced (p.**10**). These buffer anions contribute to the unmeasured anion (A-). For each mEq of buffer anion retained, one mEq fewer H+ can be secreted, and therefore one mEq fewer

HCO_3^- is generated. The retained A- therefore replaces HCO_3^-. There is no change in chloride in uncomplicated cases.

$$[Na^+] + [K^+] = [HCO_3^-] + [Cl^-] + [A^-]$$
$$140 \; + \; 4 \; = \; \mathbf{15} \; + \; 100 \; + \; \mathbf{29} \quad mEq/L$$

The $[HCO_3^-]$ has fallen from 25 to 15 mEq/L and the anion gap, entirely due to [A-], has risen by the same amount, from 19 to 29 mEq/L. If renal bicarbonate generation is so impaired that it cannot keep pace with its peripheral utilization the pH will fall.

$$pH\downarrow \; = 6.1+ \log \frac{[HCO_3^-]\downarrow}{Pco_2 \times 0.23}$$

Compensation occurs as the respiratory centre responds to the acidosis; CO_2 is lost through the pulmonary alveoli and the pH returns towards normal. *In the partially or fully compensated case the Pco_2 is low.*

The cause of the low $[HCO_3^-]$ is usually obvious if plasma urea or creatinine concentration is estimated.

Correction can only occur if the GFR increases, for example by correction of volume depletion. Treatment of the acidosis of irreversible glomerular dysfunction, except by dialysis, is usually contraindicated because it is dangerous to give sodium salts, such as bicarbonate, if the ability to excrete sodium is impaired; it is, in any case, rarely necessary.

Increase in a single anion (X-) other than chloride such as:

- *acetoacetate and 3-hydroxybutyrate* in ketoacidosis;
- *lactate* in lactic acidosis.

In both these syndromes the rise in [X-] is due to overproduction rather than reduced excretion, with the simultaneous production of equimolar amounts of H+. The reduction of $[HCO_3^-]$ results from its use in buffering the H+ which accompanies the X-.

$$[Na^+] + [K^+] = [HCO_3^-] + [Cl^-] + [A^-] + [X^-]$$
$$140 \; + \; 4 \; = \; \mathbf{15} \; + \; 100 \; + \; 19 \; + \; \mathbf{10} \quad mEq/L$$

anion gap

In this example the $[HCO_3^-]$ has fallen from 25 to 15 mEq/L and has been replaced by

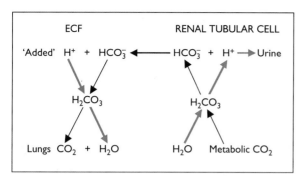

Fig. 4.6 Hydrogen ion 'shuttle' between the site of production and buffering, and the site of elimination in the kidneys.

10 mEq/L of X^-. The anion gap of 29 mEq/L is the sum of $[A^-]$ and $[X^-]$. In the uncomplicated case there is no change in chloride concentration.

Hydrogen ions are incorporated into water after being buffered by HCO_3^- and are therefore inactivated near the site of production. Water is used by renal tubular cells to replete HCO_3^-; H^+ is again liberated, but this time at a site where it can be eliminated from the body into the urine. Water can be considered as a carrier for hydrogen, transporting it in a non-toxic form from the site of production to the site of elimination (Fig. 4.6).

The CO_2 derived from buffering by bicarbonate is lost through the lungs as the respiratory centre responds to the acidosis; because of the large reserve capacity of the lungs, *the blood $P{CO_2}$ is never raised if respiratory function is normal.* The respiratory centre continues to respond to the low pH until the $P{CO_2}$ falls enough to correct the ratio of $[HCO_3^-] : P{CO_2}$; the acidosis is then *compensated.* Full renal correction is only possible if the rate of H^+ utilization is reduced enough to keep pace with production.

The diagnosis of the underlying disorder is usually obvious and includes:

- *diabetic ketoacidosis*, the commonest cause (p.**208**). Occasionally starvation ketosis can be severe enough to cause mild acidosis;

- *lactic acidosis* due to:
  impaired aerobic metabolism because of reduced tissue blood flow in the *shocked, hypotensive patient*, the commonest cause. This may aggravate acidosis due to ketoacidosis;
  drugs, such as *phenformin* or an overdosage of *salicylates* by interfering with lactate metabolism (p.**204** and p.**97**). A drug history should be taken if a low plasma $[HCO_3^-]$ is found for no immediately obvious reason.

In both keto- and lactic acidosis intravascular volume depletion may reduce the GFR, thus aggravating the acidosis. It is usually impossible to determine the relative contributions made by these different factors to the fall in plasma $[HCO_3^-]$. Treatment rarely depends on such knowledge and should always be directed at improving tissue perfusion by rehydration and by other measures designed to restore normal blood pressure. Bicarbonate infusion may sometimes be needed in very severe acidosis (pH below 7), but should be used with caution because of the danger of causing hyperosmolality and hypokalaemia (p.**53** and p.**60**). Respiratory dysfunction, which will impair compensatory CO_2 elimination, should also be treated. The management of diabetic ketoacidosis is outlined on p.**210**.

Loss of a mixture of anions and cations. In this group electrochemical neutrality is maintained by loss of cation (sodium) and anion (bicarbonate) in equivalent amounts, and the anion gap is unaffected. The losses are variable and the effects depend on fluid intake. The following is an example of a possible pattern of findings.

$$[Na^+] + [K^+] = [HCO_3^-] + [Cl^-] + [A^-]$$
$$\mathbf{130} + 4 = \mathbf{15} + 100 + 19 \quad mEq/L$$

Loss of intestinal secretions. Duodenal fluid, with a bicarbonate concentration about twice that of plasma, is alkaline. If the rate of loss, for example through small intestinal fistulae exceeds that of the renal ability to regenerate HCO_3^-, the plasma $[HCO_3^-]$ may fall enough to cause acidosis. The initial plasma electrolyte concentrations depend on the composition of the lost secretion, but are then affected by the composition of the replacement fluid. Renal generation of HCO_3^- is accelerated by the falling concentration, and only very profuse intestinal loss lowers the plasma $[HCO_3^-]$ significantly. However, if volume depletion is severe enough to reduce the GFR, impairment of renal mechanisms may precipitate acidosis.

The diagnosis is usually obvious on clinical grounds.

Treatment should aim to restore the circulating volume by administering appropriate fluid (p.**96**). If an adequate GFR is maintained the kidneys will correct the acidosis.

Generalized renal tubular dysfunction may cause a loss of a similar mixture of ions in the urine. Renal HCO_3^- reabsorption and generation are impaired due to damage to H^+ secreting mechanisms. The cause is suggested by polyuria.

Increase in [Cl⁻]. In the cases discussed so far [Cl⁻] is relatively unchanged. The combination of a low plasma $[HCO_3^-]$ and a high [Cl⁻], known as 'hyperchloraemic acidosis', is rare. The 'anion gap' in such cases is normal.

$$[Na^+] + [K^+] = [HCO_3^-] + [Cl^-] + [A^-]$$
$$140 + 4 = \mathbf{15} + \mathbf{110} + 19 \quad mEq/L$$

The causes which can usually be predicted on clinical grounds include:

- *HCO_3^- loss in a one-to-one exchange for Cl⁻.* This occurs if the *ureters are transplanted into the ileum or colon*, usually after cystectomy for carcinoma of the bladder. If chloride-containing fluid such as urine enters the ileum, ileal loops or colon, the cells exchange some of the chloride for HCO_3^- (Fig. 4.5; p.**89**). Bicarbonate depletion may occur; large doses of oral bicarbonate are needed to prevent hyperchloraemic acidosis.
- *impaired hydrogen ion secretion*, and therefore bicarbonate production, due to renal tubular disease. If the tubular ability to handle H^+ is an isolated lesion, and

other functions are relatively unimpaired, hyperchloraemic acidosis results.

In normal tubules most filtered sodium is reabsorbed with chloride; the rest is exchanged for secreted H^+ or K^+. If H^+ secretion is impaired, and yet the same amount of sodium is reabsorbed, Na^+ must be accompanied by Cl⁻ or exchanged for K^+. *This type of hyperchloraemic acidosis is therefore often accompanied by hypokalaemia* – an unusual finding in acidosis, which is usually associated with hyperkalaemia (p.**60**).

Two causes of hypokalaemic hyperchloraemic acidosis are:

- renal tubular acidosis;
- administration of carbonate dehydratase inhibitors as in the treatment of glaucoma.

Renal tubular acidosis (RTA) may be caused by either an acquired disorder or less commonly by an inherited defect, resulting in generalized tubular dysfunction (p.**17**).

Because there is no primary glomerular lesion the plasma urea and creatinine concentrations are often normal. However, chronic renal failure may develop as a consequence of nephrocalcinosis due to calcium precipitation in the kidney in untreated cases; in acidosis free-ionized calcium is released from bone more rapidly than usual (p.**174**). Increased bone breakdown also partly explains the phosphaturia often found in renal tubular acidosis.

There are two principal forms of RTA.

- The commoner, sometimes called '*classical renal tubular acidosis*' (RTA type I), is due to a *distal tubular defect*. The urinary pH cannot fall much below that of plasma even in severe acidosis. The distal luminal cells are abnormally permeable to H^+ and this impairs the ability of distal tubules to build up a $[H^+]$ gradient between the tubular lumina and cells. The re-entry of H^+ into distal tubular cells inhibits carbonate dehydratase activity at that site; proximal HCO_3^- reabsorption is normal. The inability to acidify the urine normally can be demonstrated by giving an ammonium chloride load (p.**103**).

- In the rarer form a defect in the carbonate dehydratase mechanism *impairs bicarbonate reabsorption in the proximal tubule* (RTA type II). Loss of bicarbonate may cause systemic acidosis, but *the ability to form an acid urine when acidosis becomes severe is retained*; the response to ammonium chloride loading is therefore normal.

Acetazolamide therapy is used to treat glaucoma. By inhibiting carbonate dehydratase activity in the eye, it reduces the formation of aqueous humour. Inhibition of the enzyme in renal tubular cells and erythrocytes impairs H^+ secretion and HCO_3^- formation. Hyperchloraemic acidosis sometimes complicates treatment.

The changes in anion and cation concentrations which coincide with the low plasma $[HCO_3^-]$ of metabolic acidosis are summarized in Table 4.2.

The biochemical findings in plasma in metabolic acidosis are:

- *$[HCO_3^-]$ always low;*
- Pco_2 usually low (compensatory change);
- pH low (uncompensated or partly compensated) or normal (fully compensated);
- $[Cl^-]$ unaffected in most cases; raised after ureteric transplantation, in renal tubular acidosis or during acetazolamide treatment.

Tests which may help to elucidate the cause of metabolic acidosis are:

- plasma urea or creatinine estimation;
- plasma glucose estimation;
- tests for ketones in urine or plasma.

RESPIRATORY ACIDOSIS

The findings in respiratory acidosis differ significantly from those in non-respiratory disturbances.

The primary abnormality in the bicarbonate buffer system is CO_2 retention, usually due to impaired alveolar ventilation (p.**82**) with a consequent rise in Pco_2. As in the metabolic disturbance, the acidosis is accompanied by a fall in the ratio $[HCO_3^-] : Pco_2$.

$$pH{\downarrow} = 6.1 + \log \frac{[HCO_3^-]}{Pco_2{\uparrow} \times 0.23}$$

Compensatory changes, with a rise of plasma $[HCO_3^-]$, are initiated by the high Pco_2, resulting in the acceleration of the carbonate dehydratase mechanisms in erythrocytes and renal tubular cells (Figs 4.1, p.**83** and 4.3, p.**86**). The urine becomes more acid as more H^+ is secreted.

In acute respiratory failure, for example due to bronchopneumonia or status asthmaticus, both the erythrocyte and renal tubular mechanisms increase the rate of generation

Table 4.2 Changes in the plasma concentrations of ions balancing fall in the $[HCO_3^-]$ in metabolic acidosis

	Measured ions		Unmeasured anions		
	$[Na^+]$	(Cl^-)	Mixture [A-]	Single [X-]	'Anion gap'
Glomerular dysfunction	N	N	↑	–	↑
Keto- and lactic acidosis	N	N	–	↑ (Lactate or ketoacid)	↑
Intestinal loss or renal tubular dysfunction	←———————— VARIABLE ————————→				
Ureteric transplantation renal tubular acidosis, acetazolamide	N	↑	N	N	N —

N = normal.
The last group is the rarest.
It must be stressed that these are the changes in uncomplicated cases. In many clinical situations there is more than one abnormality.

as soon as the $P\text{co}_2$ rises. In the short term renal contribution to HCO_3^- production is limited by time. A relatively large proportion of the slight rise in plasma $[HCO_3^-]$ is derived from erythrocytes because the haemoglobin buffering mechanism is not saturated. This degree of compensation is rarely adequate to prevent a fall in pH.

In chronic respiratory failure, for example due to chronic obstructive airways disease, the renal tubular mechanism is of prime importance. Haemoglobin buffering power is of limited capacity, but, as long as the glomerular filtrate provides an adequate supply of sodium for exchange with H^+ and buffers to accept H^+, tubular cells continue to generate bicarbonate until the ratio $[HCO_3^-]$: $P\text{co}_2$ is normal. In stable chronic respiratory failure the pH may be normal despite a very high $P\text{co}_2$, with a plasma bicarbonate concentration as high as twice normal.

The blood findings in respiratory acidosis are:

- $P\text{co}_2$ *always raised.*

In *acute* respiratory failure:

- pH low;
- $[HCO_3^-]$ high normal, or slightly raised.

In *chronic* respiratory failure:

- pH normal or low, depending on chronicity (time for compensation to occur);
- $[HCO_3^-]$ raised.

MIXED METABOLIC AND RESPIRATORY ACIDOSIS

If CO_2 retention occurs when there is metabolic acidosis some of the extra bicarbonate generated as a compensatory response to the high $P\text{co}_2$ is used to buffer acids other than H_2CO_3. The rise in $[HCO_3^-]$ is impaired, more CO_2 is produced during buffering, and the pH falls more than during CO_2 retention alone. This combination is common in the 'respiratory distress syndrome' of the newborn and after cardiac arrest in adults, when tissue hypoxia causes lactic acidosis. In adults or children it may

also be due to coexistence of, for example, respiratory disease with ketoacidosis or renal failure. In such cases the plasma $[HCO_3^-]$ may be high, normal or low, depending on the relative contributions from respiratory and metabolic components.

Alkalosis

Alkalosis occurs if there is a rise in the ratio $[HCO_3^-] : P\text{co}_2$ in the extracellular fluid.

In metabolic alkalosis the primary abnormality in the bicarbonate buffer system is a rise in $[HCO_3^-]$. There is little compensatory change in $P\text{co}_2$.

In respiratory alkalosis the primary abnormality is a fall in the $P\text{co}_2$. The compensatory change is a fall in $[HCO_3^-]$.

As the primary products of metabolism are hydrogen ions and CO_2, not hydroxyl ions and HCO_3^-, an alkalosis is less common than acidosis.

The presenting clinical symptom of alkalosis may be tetany despite a normal plasma total calcium concentration; this is due to a fall in the free-ionized calcium fraction in a relatively alkaline medium (p.**174**).

METABOLIC ALKALOSIS

A primary rise in plasma $[HCO_3^-]$ may occur in three situations:

- *potassium depletion* with the generation of bicarbonate by the kidney. This is the commonest cause and is discussed on p.**60**.
- *bicarbonate generation* by the gastric mucosa when hydrogen and chloride ions are lost because of *pyloric stenosis* or *gastric aspiration*. This causes *hypochloraemic alkalosis.*
- *bicarbonate administration* such as the ingestion of large amounts of bicarbonate to treat indigestion, or during intravenous bicarbonate infusion. Usually the cause and treatment are both obvious.

Pyloric stenosis. Secretion of H^+Cl^- into the gastric lumen is accompanied by the generation of equivalent amounts of HCO_3^- by the parietal cells (Fig. 4.5; p.**89**). Normally this is followed by secretion of HCO_3^- into the duodenum and, if there is free communication between the stomach and duodenum, the loss of secreted HCO_3^- in vomit counteracts the effect of its generation by the gastric mucosa. Vomiting usually causes little disturbance of hydrogen ion balance, the effects being due to volume and electrolyte losses.

The vomiting of pyloric stenosis also causes volume depletion. However, marked obstruction between the stomach and duodenum reduces loss of HCO_3^-, Na^+ and K^+. Loss of H^+ stimulates its continued production by the carbonate dehydratase mechanism in gastric mucosal cells, with generation of equivalent amounts of HCO_3^-. Hydrogen ions continue to be lost and, if duodenal secretion and renal excretion of bicarbonate are insufficient to correct for the rise in plasma $[HCO_3^-]$, alkalosis may result.

$$pH\uparrow = 6.1 + \log \frac{[HCO_3^-]\uparrow}{P_{CO_2} \times 0.23}$$

Compensation for metabolic alkalosis is relatively ineffective. Although acidosis stimulates the respiratory centre, alkalosis cannot usually depress it sufficiently to bring the pH back to normal; respiratory inhibition not only leads to CO_2 retention but also causes hypoxia, which can override the inhibitory effect of alkalosis on the respiratory centre (p.**97**). Consequently CO_2 may not be retained in adequate amounts to compensate for the rise in plasma $[HCO_3^-]$.

Correction of the alkalosis of pyloric stenosis depends on whether the rate of urinary bicarbonate loss exceeds that of gastric production. The rising extracellular $[HCO_3^-]$, derived from gastric mucosal cells, inhibits the formation of H^+ and HCO_3^- in renal tubular cells and diminished renal secretion of H^+ reduces HCO_3^- 'reabsorption' (Fig. 4.2; p.**85**). The resulting urinary HCO_3^- loss may correct for the increased generation by the gastric mucosa.

Two factors may impair this capacity to lose HCO_3^- in the urine and so may aggravate the alkalosis.

- A *reduced GFR* due to volume depletion limits the total amount of HCO_3^- which can be lost.
- The *chloride concentration in the glomerular filtrate may be reduced* if there is severe hypochloraemia due to gastric Cl- loss. Isosmotic Na^+ reabsorption in proximal tubules depends on passive reabsorption of Cl^- along the electrochemical gradient. A reduction in available chloride limits isosmotic reabsorption, and more sodium becomes available for exchange with H^+ and K^+. The urine becomes inappropriately acid, and H^+ secretion stimulates inappropriate HCO_3^- reabsorption. The increased K^+ loss aggravates the hypokalaemia due to alkalosis.

Thus, vomiting due to pyloric stenosis may cause:

- hypochloraemic alkalosis;
- hypokalaemia;
- mild uraemia and haemoconcentration due to volume depletion.

The hypokalaemia may become apparent only when the plasma volume has been repleted but it should be anticipated.

Pyloric stenosis is usually treated before severe hypochloraemic alkalosis develops. Nevertheless, the typical changes in bicarbonate and chloride may indicate the diagnosis. The plasma chloride concentration may be as much as 80, rather than the usual 40, mmol/L lower than that of sodium.

Treatment of the biochemical disorders of pyloric stenosis. If renal function is normal, water and chloride should be replaced by infusing a large volume of at least isosmolar saline. The restoration of the GFR and the correction of hypochloraemia will enable the kidney to correct the alkalosis. Potassium should be added if the plasma potassium concentration is low normal or low (p.**70**).

RESPIRATORY ALKALOSIS

The primary abnormality in the bicarbonate buffer system in respiratory alkalosis is a fall in Pco_2. This is due to abnormally rapid or deep respiration *when the CO_2 transport capacity of the pulmonary alveoli is relatively normal.* The causes are:

- *hysterical overbreathing* which overrides normal respiratory control;
- *raised intracranial pressure or brainstem lesions,* which may stimulate the respiratory centre;
- *hypoxia,* which may also stimulate the respiratory centre;
- *pulmonary oedema;*
- *lobar pneumonia;*
- *pulmonary collapse or fibrosis;*
- *excessive artificial ventilation.*

The fall in Pco_2 reduces the carbonate dehydratase activity in renal tubular cells and erythrocytes. The *compensatory fall in plasma [HCO_3^-] tends to correct the pH.*

It may be difficult to distinguish clinically between the overbreathing due to metabolic acidosis, in which the fall in plasma [HCO_3^-] is the primary biochemical abnormality, and that due to respiratory alkalosis in which it is compensatory. In doubtful cases estimation of arterial pH and Pco_2 are indicated.

The arterial blood findings in respiratory alkalosis are:

- Pco_2 *always reduced;*
- [HCO_3^-] low normal or low;
- pH raised (uncompensated or partly compensated) or normal (fully compensated).

SALICYLATE OVERDOSAGE

Salicylates stimulate the respiratory centre directly, and overdosage initially causes respiratory alkalosis. They also uncouple oxidative phosphorylation, and the consequent impairment of aerobic pathways superimposes a lactic acidosis on the respiratory alkalosis. Both these effects lower plasma [HCO_3^-], but the pH may be high if respiratory alkalosis is predominant, normal if the two 'cancel each other out', or low if metabolic acidosis is predominant. Only measurement of blood pH can reveal the true state of hydrogen ion balance.

The possible findings in disturbances of hydrogen ion homeostasis are summarized in Table 4.3.

*The student should read the section on investigation of hydrogen ion homeostasis (p.**101**) to assess how many of these tests are really needed.*

Table 4.3 Summary of findings in arterial blood in disturbances of hydrogen ion homeostasis

	pH	Pco_2	[HCO_3^-]	Plasma [K+]
Acidosis				
Metabolic				
Initial state	↓	N	↓	Usually ↑ (↓ in renal tubular
Compensated state	N	↓*	↓	acidosis and acetazolamide)
Respiratory				
Acute change	↓	↑	N or ↑	↑
Compensation	N	↑	↑↑*	
Alkalosis				
Metabolic				
Acute state	↑	N	↑	↓
Chronic state	↑	N or slightly ↑*	↑↑	
Respiratory				
Acute change	↑	↓	N or ↓	↓
Compensation	N	↓	↓↓*	

Bold arrows = primary change; * arrows = compensatory change. N = normal.

Notes: 1. Potassium depletion can cause alkalosis, or alkalosis can cause hypokalaemia. *Only the clinical history can differentiate the cause of the combination of hypokalaemia and alkalosis.*

     2. Overbreathing causes a low [HCO_3^-] in respiratory alkalosis. Metabolic acidosis, with a low [HCO_3^-], causes overbreathing. *Only measurement of blood pH and Pco_2 can differentiate these two.*

Blood Gases

Oxygen Transport by Haemoglobin

The amount of oxygen in blood is determined by the amount dissolved, the haemoglobin concentration and the affinity of haemoglobin for oxygen. Haemoglobin consists of four subunits, each made up of a haem, a porphyrin ring containing iron (p.**375**), and a polypeptide. As a haem moiety takes up an oxygen, there is a rearrangment of the subunits that facilitates the uptake of additional oxygen. This accounts for the shape of the oxyhaemoglobin dissociation curve (Fig. 4.7). Factors which affect the affinity of haem for oxygen include:

- *pH of blood.* As the pH falls the affinity for oxygen decreases. This is known as the Bohr effect. Deoxygenated haemoglobin binds H+ more avidly and accounts for the increased buffering capacity of haemoglobin in venous blood.

- *2,3-diphosphoglycerate* (DPG), which is formed during glycolysis and which is plentiful within the erythrocyte. DPG binds to haemoglobin liberating more oxygen, thus shifting the dissociation curve to the right. Increased hydrogen ion concentration (a fall in pH), decreases DPG levels, thus potentially reducing tissue oxygenation. Erythrocyte levels of DPG increase in anaemia and in some conditions associated with chronic hypoxia.

Fetal haemoglobin (HbF) has a greater affinity for oxygen than adult haemoglobin (HbA), thus facilitating the transfer of oxygen across the placenta.

Factors Affecting Blood Gas Results

In respiratory acidosis it may be important to know the partial pressure of oxygen (P_{O_2}) as well as the pH, P_{CO_2} and [HCO_3^-].

Normal gaseous exchange across the pulmonary alveoli involves loss of CO_2 and gain of O_2. However, in disease a fall in P_{O_2} and a rise in P_{CO_2} do not always coexist. The reasons are as follows.

- *Carbon dioxide is much more soluble in water than O_2* and its rate of diffusion is about 20 times as high. For example, in pulmonary oedema diffusion of O_2 across alveolar walls is hindered by oedema fluid and arterial P_{O_2} falls. The hypoxia and alveolar distension stimulate respiration and CO_2 is 'washed out'. However, the rate of oxygen transport through the

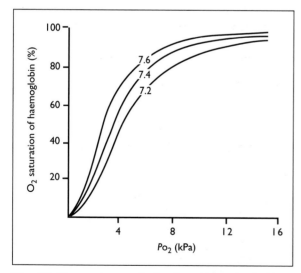

Fig. 4.7 The oxyhaemoglobin dissociation curve showing the effect of pH (Bohr effect) on oxygen saturation.

fluid cannot be increased enough to restore normal arterial Po_2. This results in a *low* or *normal* Pco_2 and a *low* Po_2. Only in very severe cases is the Pco_2 raised.

- *Haemoglobin in arterial blood is normally 95 per cent saturated with oxygen* (Fig. 4.7), and the small amount of O_2 in simple solution in the plasma is in equilibrium with oxyhaemoglobin. Increased air entry at atmospheric Po_2 cannot significantly increase oxygen carriage in blood leaving normal alveoli, but can reduce the Pco_2. Breathing pure oxygen increases arterial Po_2, but not haemoglobin saturation.

In conditions such as *lobar pneumonia, pulmonary collapse and pulmonary fibrosis or infiltration* not all alveoli are affected to the same extent, or in the same way.

- Some alveoli are unaffected. At first the gaseous composition of blood leaving them is normal. Increasing the rate or depth of respiration may later lower the Pco_2 considerably, but does not alter either the Po_2 or the haemoglobin saturation.
- Obstruction of small airways means that air cannot reach those alveoli supplied by them; the composition of blood leaving them will be near that of venous blood; there is a ventilation/perfusion mismatch with a right to left shunt. Only if gas flow, due to increased respiratory excursion, can overcome the obstruction, will it help to correct the low Po_2 and high Pco_2.
- Some alveoli may have normal air entry, but much reduced blood supply. This is 'dead space'. Increased ventilation will have no effect, because there is little blood to interact with the increased flow of gases.

Blood from unaffected alveoli and from those with obstructed airways mixes in the pulmonary vein before entering the left atrium. The high Pco_2 and low Po_2 stimulate respiration and, if there are enough unaffected alveoli, the very low Pco_2 in blood leaving them may compensate for the high Pco_2 in blood from poorly aerated alveoli; by contrast, neither the Po_2 nor the haemoglobin saturation will be significantly altered by mixing. The systemic arterial blood will then have a *low* or *normal* Pco_2 with a *low* Po_2.

If the proportion of affected to normal alveoli is very high, Pco_2 cannot adequately be corrected by hyperventilation and there will be a *high arterial* Pco_2 with a low Po_2.

If there are *mechanical or neurological lesions impairing respiratory movement or obstruction of large, or most of the small, airways* as in an acute asthmatic attack, almost all alveoli will have a normal blood supply; the poor aeration will cause a *high* Pco_2 and low Po_2 in the blood draining them, and therefore in systemic arterial blood. Occasionally stimulation of respiration by alveolar stretching can maintain a normal, or even low, Pco_2 early in an acute asthmatic attack.

In the list of examples given below the conditions marked * may fall into either group, depending on the severity of the disease.

Low arterial Po_2 with low or normal Pco_2:

- pulmonary oedema (diffusion defect);
- lobar pneumonia;
- pulmonary collapse*;
- pulmonary fibrosis or infiltration*.

Low arterial Po_2 with a high Pco_2:

- impairment of movement of the chest:
    chest injury;
    gross obesity;
    ankylosing spondylitis.
- neurological conditions affecting the respiratory drive;
- neurological conditions, for example poliomyelitis, affecting innervation of respiratory muscles;
- extensive airway obstruction: chronic obstructive airways disease; severe asthma; laryngeal spasm.
- bronchopneumonia;
- pulmonary collapse*;
- pulmonary fibrosis or infiltration*.

Summary

Hydrogen Ion Homeostasis

1. CO_2 is of central importance in hydrogen ion homeostasis. Arterial blood $P\text{CO}_2$ is controlled by the respiratory centre at about 5.3 kPa (40 mmHg).
2. At a $P\text{CO}_2$ of 5.3 kPa the carbonate dehydratase mechanism in erythrocytes and renal tubular cells maintains the plasma $[HCO_3^-]$ at about 25 mmol/L.
3. The H^+ produced in erythrocytes is buffered by haemoglobin. This mechanism is of physiological importance, but, because of its limited capacity, only plays a minor role in correcting abnormalities in H^+ balance.
4. Renal tubular cells secrete H^+ into the urine in exchange for Na^+. Hydrogen ion secretion is essential for HCO_3^- 'reabsorption' and net generation.
5. Normal urine is almost HCO_3^- free. Generation of HCO_3^- to replace its use in buffering depends on the availability of urinary buffers, especially HPO_4^{2-}.
6. Renal correction of either acidosis or alkalosis depends on a normal GFR.
7. A reduction in the ratio $[HCO_3^-]:P\text{CO}_2$ causes acidosis. Although the *ratio* is normal in compensated acidosis, both $[HCO_3^-]$ and $P\text{CO}_2$ are abnormal.
8. Acidosis may be due to excessive H^+ production, to dysfunction of the lungs or kidneys, or to excessive loss of HCO_3^-.
9. An increase in the ratio $[HCO_3^-]:P\text{CO}_2$ causes an alkalosis. In compensated alkalosis the ratio is normal but the levels of both HCO_3^- and CO_2 are abnormal.

Blood Gases

1. Oxygen is transported in blood bound to haemoglobin.
2. Factors that affect the affinity of haemoglobin for oxygen include the pH of the blood and the erythrocyte concentration of 2,3-diphosphoglycerate (DPG).

LOW $P\text{O}_2$ AND NORMAL OR LOW $P\text{CO}_2$

3. Carbon dioxide is much more soluble in water than oxygen. Arterial $P\text{CO}_2$ is therefore less affected than $P\text{O}_2$ in pulmonary oedema; it may even be low because of respiratory stimulation.
4. Arterial blood is 95 per cent saturated with oxygen. Increased respiration cannot increase oxygen carriage from normal alveoli, but can reduce the $P\text{CO}_2$. If some alveoli have a normal blood supply, but are poorly ventilated ('ventilation–perfusion mismatch') the mixture of 'shunted' blood with that from normal alveoli results in a low $P\text{O}_2$ *and a normal or low $P\text{CO}_2$ in systemic arterial blood.*

LOW $P\text{O}_2$ AND HIGH $P\text{CO}_2$

5. The $P\text{O}_2$ is low and the $P\text{CO}_2$ is high if there is widespread alveolar hypoventilation, because neither gas can be exchanged adequately.

*I*NVESTIGATION OF HYDROGEN ION DISTURBANCES

Measurements that may be used to assess Hydrogen Ion Balance

Measurement of blood pH indicates only whether there is overt acidosis or alkalosis. If the pH is abnormal the primary abnormality may be in the control of CO_2 by the lungs or respiratory centre, or in the balance between bicarbonate utilization in buffering and its reabsorption and regeneration by renal tubular cells and erythrocytes. However, a normal pH does not exclude a disturbance of these pathways: compensatory mechanisms may be maintaining it. Chemical assessment of these factors can only be made by measuring components of the bicarbonate buffer system. The concentration of dissolved CO_2 is calculated by multiplying the measured $P\text{co}_2$ by the solubility constant of the gas:

- 0.23 if $P\text{co}_2$ is in kPa;
- 0.03 if it is in mmHg.

pH and $P\text{co}_2$. There is a significant arteriovenous difference in pH and $P\text{co}_2$, and both must be measured in arterial, not venous, blood. Whole, heparinized blood must be used because the result of $P\text{co}_2$ estimation by some methods may depend on the presence of erythrocytes. The technique of sample collection is important, and details are given below.

Measurement of blood $[HCO_3^-]$. There are two methods that may be used to estimate the circulating bicarbonate concentration.

Plasma total CO_2 ($T\text{co}_2$): The 'plasma bicarbonate concentration' is probably the most commonly measured index of hydrogen ion homeostasis: the specimen tube should be full, to minimize *in vitro* loss of CO_2 into a large dead space of air during centrifugation, which will cause a falsely low result. If pH and $P\text{co}_2$ estimations are not needed the

assay has the advantage that venous blood can be used. and that it can be performed together with those for urea and electrolytes. It is an estimate of the sum of plasma bicarbonate, carbonic acid and dissolved CO_2. At pH 7.4 the ratio of $[HCO_3^-]$ to the other two components is about 20 to 1 and at pH 7.1 is still 10 to 1. Thus, if the $T\text{co}_2$ were 21 mmol/L, $[HCO_3^-]$ would contribute 20 mmol/L at pH 7.4 and just over 19 mmol/L at pH 7.1. Only 1 mmol/L and just under 2 mmol/L respectively would be due to H_2CO_3 and CO_2 respectively. Thus $T\text{co}_2$ is effectively a measure of the plasma bicarbonate concentration.

The bicarbonate concentration is calculated from the Henderson–Hasselbalch equation, using the measured values of pH and $P\text{co}_2$ (in kPa) in whole arterial blood.

$$pH = 6.1 + \log \frac{[HCO_3^-]}{P\text{co}_2 \times 0.23}$$

It is a measure of the whole blood $[HCO_3^-]$ and for the reasons discussed above, usually agrees well with plasma $T\text{co}_2$. It is the estimate of choice if the other two parameters are being measured.

COLLECTION OF SPECIMENS FOR BLOOD GAS ESTIMATIONS

1. *Arterial* specimens are preferable to capillary ones.
2. The syringe should be 'moistened' with *heparin* and the specimen well mixed.

Warning:

- Excess heparin may dilute the specimen and cause haemolysis.
- If *sodium* heparin is used do *not* estimate sodium on the same specimen. The resultant factitious hypernatraemia is often misinterpreted, and is then a danger to the patient.
3. Gas exchange with the atmosphere should be minimized by *leaving the specimen in the*

syringe and expelling any air bubbles at once. The nozzle should then be stoppered.

4. The effect on pH of anaerobic erythrocyte metabolism should be minimized by *performing the assay as soon as possible. The specimen should be kept cool.*

In newborn infants arterial puncture may be technically difficult, but should be used whenever possible. If it is really necessary to perform assays on capillary specimens the following precautions are essential:

1. In order that the composition of the blood is as near arterial as possible the area from which the specimen is taken should be warm and pink. If there is peripheral cyanosis results may be dangerously misleading.
2. The blood should flow freely. Squeezing the skin while sampling may dilute the specimen with interstitial fluid.
3. The capillary tubes must be heparinized, and mixing with the blood must be complete.
4. The tubes must be completely filled with blood. Air bubbles invalidate the results.
5. The ends of the tubes should be sealed immediately.

Suggested Diagnostic Procedure

We have discussed the mechanisms behind the abnormal findings in disorders of hydrogen ion balance. Understanding is essential for critical assessment of the value of investigation and diagnosis and management. Moreover, without such understanding the results may be dangerously misinterpreted.

INTERPRETATION OF PLASMA BICARBONATE (T_{CO_2}) CONCENTRATION

As explained above, plasma T_{CO_2} is effectively a measure of plasma [HCO_3^-]. It is safer and less unpleasant for the patient if venous rather than arterial blood is sampled. A careful assessment should always be made of whether knowledge of the other parameters will really be helpful.

The level of plasma bicarbonate *alone* tells nothing about the state of hydrogen ion balance. For example, a low concentration may be associated with compensated or uncompensated metabolic acidosis, or respiratory alkalosis. The pH is determined by the ratio of [HCO_3^-] to [CO_2], according to the Henderson–Hasselbalch equation. Nevertheless, with a little thought, the T_{CO_2} usually provides adequate information for clinical purposes.

We suggest the following procedure.

If the Plasma T_{CO_2} Concentration is Low

1. *Exclude artefactual causes* due to *in vitro* loss of CO_2 from a small specimen, or one that has been standing for some hours.
2. *Reassess the clinical picture*, particularly noting the presence of:

   • evidence suggesting renal dysfunction (Chapter 1);
   • hypotension, volume depletion or other evidence of poor tissue perfusion;
   • diarrhoea or intestinal fistulae;
   • a history of ureteric transplantation into the ileum, ileal loops or colon;
   • a drug history with special reference to biguanides such as phenformin, or acetazolamide.

3. *Estimate plasma urea and glucose concentrations* and test the urine for ketones.

In the great majority of cases the diagnosis will now be obvious. If it is not, among the few remaining possibilities are:

• respiratory alkalosis due to overbreathing;
• renal tubular acidosis.

In such rare circumstances estimation of arterial blood pH and P_{CO_2} may help to differentiate respiratory alkalosis from metabolic acidosis. If renal tubular acidosis is suspected, the finding of a high plasma chloride concentration strengthens the suspicion; an ammonium chloride loading test should be performed.

AMMONIUM CHLORIDE LOADING TEST FOR DISTAL RENAL TUBULAR ACIDOSIS

This test is not necessary if the pH of a urinary specimen, collected overnight, is already less than 5.5.

The ammonium ion (NH_4^+) is potentially acid because it can dissociate to ammonia and H^+. After ingestion of ammonium chloride the kidneys usually secrete the H^+, and the urinary pH falls.

Procedure: No food or fluid is taken after midnight.

- **08.00 hours** - ammonium chloride is given orally in a dose of 0.1 g/kg body weight.
- Urine specimens are collected hourly and the pH of each measured *immediately by the laboratory.*

Interpretation: In normal subjects the urinary pH falls to 5.5 or below between two and eight hours after the dose. In generalized tubular disease there may be a sufficient number of functioning nephrons to achieve a normal level of acidification. *In distal renal tubular acidosis* this degree of acidification does not occur. Urinary acidification is normal in proximal tubular acidosis.

If the Plasma Tco_2 Concentration is High

1. *Reassess the clinical picture*, particularly noting whether:

   - there is obstructive airways disease;
   - there is a cause for potassium depletion, such as the taking of potassium-losing diuretics;
   - bicarbonate has been ingested or infused;
   - there is severe vomiting which, especially if there is a history of dyspepsia, might indicate pyloric stenosis.

2. *Estimate plasma potassium concentration.*

Indications for Arterial pH and Pco_2 Estimations

In metabolic acidosis the fall of plasma [HCO_3^-] is the primary abnormality of the bicarbonate buffering system, and usually plasma Tco_2 concentration measurement yields adequate information for clinical purposes.

Similarly, a patient with chronic obstructive airways disease and a high plasma [HCO_3^-] undoubtedly has respiratory acidosis, which may or may not be fully compensated. Unless there is a possibility of improving air entry into the lungs by use of physiotherapy, expectorants and antibiotics, treatment on a respirator is contraindicated. Reducing the Pco_2 will lead to bicarbonate loss by a reversal of the mechanisms described on p.**85**; unless the patient continues to be artificially ventilated for life the Pco_2 will return to its initial high level once the respirator is turned off, but there will be a delay of some days before the bicarbonate reaches the previous compensatory concentration. Nothing is to be gained from the therapeutic point of view in such a case by knowing the pH and Pco_2 but occasionally it may be useful to know the Po_2. Arterial blood gas estimations may be indicated if:

- there is *doubt about the cause of the abnormal Tco_2* (for example, to differentiate metabolic acidosis from respiratory alkalosis);
- *respiratory and metabolic disturbances may coexist*, such as after cardiac arrest, in renal failure complicated by lung disease, or in salicylate overdosage. In such conditions the estimations are indicated only if the results will influence treatment;
- there is an *acute exacerbation of chronic obstructive airways disease*, or if there is *acute, potentially reversible, lung disease*. In such cases vigorous therapy or artificial respiration may tide the patient over until lung function improves; more precise information than the plasma Tco_2 concentration is needed to monitor and control treatment;
- if blood is being taken for estimation of Po_2.

Indications for Chloride Estimation

Plasma chloride concentrations are consistently affected in very few conditions. Hyperchloraemia occurs in the metabolic acidosis associated with ureteric transplantation, renal tubular acidosis and acetazolamide administration. Hypochloraemia occurs in the metabolic alkalosis of pyloric stenosis. If the procedure outlined above is followed, the level of chloride can usually be predicted, and its estimation adds nothing to diagnostic or therapeutic precision. Chloride estimation may help in two situations:

- if there is a low plasma $T\text{co}_2$ concentration of obscure origin, the finding of a high plasma [Cl⁻] (and therefore a normal 'anion gap') strengthens the suspicion of renal tubular acidosis. In most other causes of acidosis the [Cl⁻] is normal and 'anion gap' is increased;

- if a patient who is vomiting has a high plasma $T\text{co}_2$ concentration, the finding of an equivalently low [Cl⁻] favours the diagnosis of pyloric stenosis. Similar findings may be due to compensated respiratory acidosis, but the presence of severe chronic lung disease usually makes this cause obvious.

The plasma [Cl⁻] must be interpreted in relation to the plasma [Na⁺], the principal cation with which chloride is associated.

The Hypothalamus and Pituitary Gland

5

GENERAL PRINCIPLES OF ENDOCRINE DIAGNOSIS

A hormone is a substance that is secreted by an endocrine gland and is conveyed in the blood so regulating the function of another tissue or gland. Some hormones, such as insulin secreted from the pancreatic islet cells or growth hormone secreted from the anterior pituitary gland, influence tissue metabolism directly. Others, such as trophic hormones from the pituitary gland, stimulate target endocrine glands to synthesize and secrete further hormones which, in turn, partly control trophic hormone release, usually by *negative feedback inhibition*. For example, a rise in plasma thyroxine concentration inhibits secretion of thyrotrophic hormone (TSH) and hypercalcaemia inhibits that of parathyroid hormone.

Endocrine glands may secrete *excessive* or *deficient* amounts of hormone. Abnormalities of target glands may be *primary*, or *secondary* to dysfunction of the controlling mechanism, usually located in the hypothalamus or anterior pituitary gland. In the latter case the target gland is essentially normal.

Hormone secretion may vary predictably over a 24-hour (circadian) or longer period, may be episodic or may respond predictably to physiological stimuli such as stress. These physiological patterns of secretion must be understood if laboratory tests for endocrine disorders are to be correctly interpreted. It is logical to take blood samples at a time when hormone concentrations can most readily be distinguished from normal.

Accordingly, if *hypofunction* is suspected samples are taken when levels should be high, and *vice versa* when investigating *hyperfunction*.

Simultaneous measurement of both the trophic hormones and their controlling factors, whether hormones or metabolic products, may be more informative than measurement of either alone.

If results of preliminary tests are definitely abnormal the abnormality may be primary, or secondary to a disorder of one of the controlling mechanisms. If the results are near the limits of the reference range it is necessary to determine whether they are abnormal. If either of these points is not clear when the results are considered together with the clinical findings, so-called 'dynamic' tests should be carried out. In such tests the response of the gland or the feedback mechanism is assessed after stimulation or suppression by administration of exogenous hormone.

- **Suppression tests** are used mainly for the differential diagnosis of *excessive hormone secretion*. The substance (or an analogue) that normally suppresses secretion by negative feedback is administered and the response measured. *Failure to suppress* implies that secretion is not under normal feedback control (*autonomous secretion*).
- **Stimulation tests** are used mainly for the differential diagnosis of *deficient hormone secretion*. The trophic hormone that normally stimulates secretion is administered and the response measured. A normal response excludes an abnormality of the target gland whereas *failure to respond* confirms it.

In this chapter disorders of the pituitary gland and hypothalamus will be discussed. Diseases of the target endocrine organs, the adrenal cortex, gonads and thyroid gland will be considered in Chapters 6, 7 and 8. The parathyroid glands and endocrine pancreas are discussed in Chapters 9 and 12.

HYPOTHALAMUS AND PITUITARY GLAND

There is a close relation between the neural and the endocrine systems, which is most obvious in the interaction between the hypothalamus and the two lobes of the pituitary gland.

Although the anterior and posterior lobes of the pituitary gland are developmentally and functionally distinct, both depend on hormones synthesized in the hypothalamus for normal function. The hypothalamus also has extensive neural connections with the rest of the brain and stress and some psychological disorders affect secretion of pituitary hormones and those of other endocrine glands.

The Hypothalamus and the Posterior Pituitary Lobe

Two structurally similar peptide hormones, *antidiuretic hormone* and *oxytocin*, are synthesized in the hypothalamus and transported down the nerve fibres of the pituitary stalk attached to specific carrier proteins – *neurophysins*. The hormones are stored in the posterior pituitary gland and are released independently of each other into the bloodstream under hypothalamic control together with neurophysin. Neurophysin has no apparent biological function and is rapidly cleared from plasma.

- **Antidiuretic hormone (ADH: arginine vasopressin; AVP)** is synthesized primarily in the supraoptic nuclei of the hypothalamus and enhances water reabsorption from the collecting ducts in the kidneys (Chapter 2).
- **Oxytocin** is synthesized in the paraventricular nuclei of the hypothalamus. It controls the ejection of milk from the lactating breast and may have a role in initiating uterine concentrations, although normal labour can proceed in its absence. It is used therapeutically to induce labour.

The Hypothalamus and the Anterior Pituitary Lobe

There is no direct neural connection between the hypothalamus and the anterior pituitary gland. The hypothalamus synthesizes small molecules (regulating hormones or factors) that are carried to the cells of the anterior pituitary lobe by the *hypothalamic portal system*. This network of capillary loops in the median eminence forms veins which, after passing down the pituitary stalk, divide into a second capillary network in the anterior pituitary gland from where hypothalamic hormones stimulate or inhibit pituitary hormone secretion into the systemic circulation.

The cells of the anterior pituitary lobe can be classified simply by their staining reactions as acidophils, basophils or chromophobes. More sophisticated immunological techniques can identify specific hormone-secreting cells.

Acidophils are of two cell types:

- *somatotrophs* that secrete growth hormone (GH: somatotrophin);
- *lactotrophs* that secrete prolactin.

These hormones, which are *simple polypeptides* with similar amino acid sequences, mainly affect *peripheral tissues* directly. Stimulation and inhibition of secretion via the hypothalamus is influenced by neural stimuli.

Basophils secrete hormones that affect other endocrine glands. The hypothalamic control is mainly stimulatory. There are three cell types:

- *Thyrotrophs* secrete thyroid-stimulating hormone (TSH; thyrotrophin), which acts on the thyroid gland;
- *Gonadotrophs* secrete the gonadotrophins, follicle-stimulating hormone (FSH) and luteinizing hormone (LH), which act on the gonads.

These hormones are structurally similar glycoproteins consisting of two subunits α and β. The α subunit is common to all three hormones, and the β subunit is involved in receptor recognition and therefore in specific biological activity. Their secretion is influenced more by negative feedback control than by neural mechanisms.

- *Corticotrophs* synthesize a large polypeptide (pro-opiomelanocortin), which is a precursor of both adrenocorticotrophic hormone (ACTH; corticotrophin) and β-lipotrophin (β-LPH) (Fig. 5.1). Secretion of these hormones occurs in parallel:
  ACTH stimulates the synthesis and secretion of steroids, other than aldosterone, from the adrenal cortex and maintains adrenal cortical growth. Part of the molecule has melanocyte-stimulating activity and high circulating concentrations of ACTH are often associated with pigmentation;

β-LPH is inactive until rapidly converted to endorphins. These are neurotransmitters which, because they have opiate-like effects, help control of pain. They will not be considered further.

Chromophobes, once thought to be inactive, do contain secretory granules. Chromophobe adenomas often secrete hormones, particularly prolactin.

Control of Anterior Pituitary Hormone Secretion

Neural and *feedback* controls are the two most important physiological factors influencing secretion of the anterior pituitary hormones (Fig. 5.2).

- *Extrahypothalamic neural stimuli* modify and, at times override, other control mechanisms. Physical or emotional stress and mental illness may give similar findings to, and even precipitate, endocrine disease. The stress caused by insulin-induced hypoglycaemia is used to test anterior pituitary function. Stress may also stimulate secretion of ADH from the posterior pituitary.

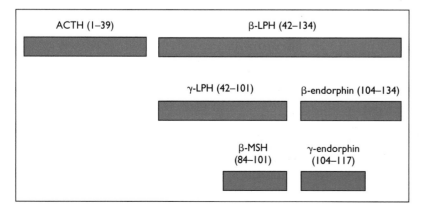

ACTH (1–39)

β-LPH (42–134)

γ-LPH (42–101)

β-endorphin (104–134)

β-MSH
(84–101)

γ-endorphin
(104–117)

Fig. 5.1 The products of pro-opiomelanocortin (POMC), ACTH, β-lipotrophin (LPH), melanocyte-stimulating hormone (MSH) and endorphin. The numbers indicate the amino acid sequence in POMC.

- *Feedback control* is mediated by the concentrations of circulating target-cell hormones; a rising concentration usually suppresses trophic hormone secretion. This negative feedback may directly suppress hypothalamic hormone secretion or may modify its effect on pituitary cells (long feedback loop). Secretion of hypothalamic hormones may also be suppressed by rising concentrations of pituitary hormone in a short feedback loop.
- *Inherent rhythms.* Hypothalamic, and consequently pituitary, hormones are released intermittently, either in pulses or in a regular circadian rhythm. Disturbances of such rhythms may be of diagnostic value. This subject will be considered further in the relevant sections.

Drugs may also stimulate or block the action of neurotransmitters, such as catecholamines, acetylcholine and serotonin, and influence the secretion of hypothalamic, and consequently pituitary, hormones. For example:

- *chlorpromazine* interferes with the action of dopamine. This results in reduced growth hormone secretion (reduced effect of releasing factor) and increased prolactin secretion (reduced inhibition).
- *bromocriptine* (2-bromo-α-ergocryptine), which has a dopamine-like action, and *L-dopa*, which is converted to dopamine, have the opposite effect in normal subjects. Bromocriptine causes a paradoxical suppression of excessive GH secretion in acromegalics; the reason for this anomalous response is unknown.

All these effects have been used both in the diagnosis and treatment of hypothalamic–pituitary disorders; they will be discussed in later sections.

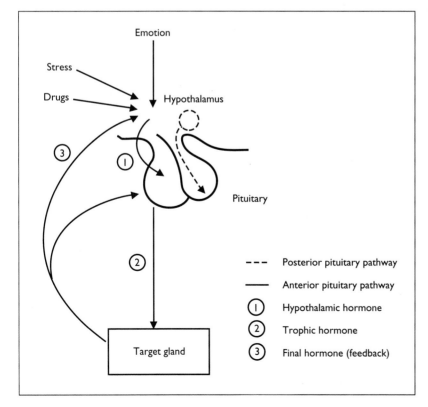

Fig. 5.2 Control of pituitary hormone secretion.

Emotion

Stress

Drugs

Hypothalamus

Pituitary

③

①

②

Target gland

- - -   Posterior pituitary pathway

———   Anterior pituitary pathway

①   Hypothalamic hormone

②   Trophic hormone

③   Final hormone (feedback)

Disorders of Anterior Pituitary Hormone Secretion

The main clinical syndromes associated with excessive or deficient anterior pituitary hormone secretion are shown in Table 5.1. Excessive secretion usually involves a single hormone, but deficiencies are often multiple. However, many pituitary tumours are non-secretory and may present clinically with eye signs or headaches (p.**114**).

Growth Hormone (GH)

Growth hormone secretion from the anterior pituitary gland is mainly controlled by hypothalamic *GH-releasing hormone* (GHRH). Secretion of GHRH, and therefore of GH, is pulsatile occurring about seven or eight times a day, usually associated with:

- exercise;
- onset of deep sleep;
- in response to the falling plasma glucose concentration about an hour after meals.

At other times plasma concentrations are usually very low or undetectable, especially in children.

Basal GH release and the GH response to such stimuli as exercise and hypoglycaemia is inhibited by another hypothalamic hormone *somatostatin* (GH-release inhibiting hormone). Somatostatin is found not only in the hypothalamus and elsewhere in the brain, but also in the gastrointestinal tract and pancreatic islet cells, where it inhibits secretion of many gastrointestinal hormones.

GH secretion may be *stimulated* by:

- stress, one cause of which is hypoglycaemia (or rapidly falling plasma glucose concentrations);

Table 5.1 Syndromes associated with primary abnormalities of anterior pituitary hormone secretion

Hormone	Excess	Deficiency
Growth hormone	Acromegaly Gigantism	Short stature
Prolactin	Amenorrhoea Infertility Galactorrhoea	Lactation failure
ACTH (corticotrophin)	Cushing's disease	Secondary adrenal hypofunction
TSH	Hyperthyroidism (very rare)	Secondary hypothyroidism
LH/FSH	Precocious puberty	Secondary hypogonadism Infertility

- glucagon;
- some amino acids, for example arginine;
- drugs such as L-dopa and clonidine.

All these stimuli have been used to assess GH secretory capacity. Oestrogens potentiate the response whereas it may be impaired in obese patients, in hypothyroidism and hypogonadism, in some cases of Cushing's syndrome and in patients receiving large doses of steroids.

GH secretion is *inhibited* by:

- hyperglycaemia in the normal subject.

ACTIONS OF GROWTH HORMONE

The main function of GH is to promote growth. Its action is mediated by *insulin-like growth factors* (IGF), polypeptides synthesized in many tissues, where they act locally. Plasma concentrations of one of these, IGF-1, correlate with GH secretion.

- *Protein synthesis* is enhanced by GH, the action of which is mediated by IGF-1 in conjunction with insulin, to stimulate amino acid uptake by cells. IGF-1 production is also influenced by other factors, the most important of which is nutritional status. In malnutrition plasma concentrations are low whereas GH concentrations are elevated, suggesting that plasma IGF-1 may influence GH secretion by negative feedback. Other factors, such as adequate nutrition and thyroxine, are also needed for normal growth. The growth spurt during puberty is probably enhanced by androgens.

- *Carbohydrate metabolism* is affected by GH. GH antagonizes the insulin-mediated cell uptake of glucose and excess secretion may produce glucose intolerance.
- *Fat metabolism* is stimulated by GH. Lipolysis is stimulated with a consequent increase in circulating free-fatty acids (FFA). FFA antagonizes insulin release and action.

Abnormalities of Growth Hormone Secretion

During childhood, GH excess causes gigantism and deficiency short stature. In adults GH excess causes acromegaly but deficiency very rarely causes symptoms.

GROWTH HORMONE EXCESS: GIGANTISM AND ACROMEGALY

Most patients with GH excess have acidophil adenomas of the anterior pituitary gland. These may be secondary to excessive hypothalamic stimulation. The condition may therefore recur after removal of the pituitary adenoma. The clinical manifestations depend on whether the condition develops before or after fusion of the bony epiphyses.

Gigantism is caused by excess GH secretion in childhood before fusion of the epiphyseal plates which may be delayed by accompanying hypogonadism. Heights of up to 7 feet

(2.1 m) may be reached. Acromegalic features may develop after bony fusion, but these giants often die in early adult life from infection, cardiac failure or as a consequence of progressive pituitary tumour growth.

Acromegaly results from GH excess in adults, after epiphyseal fusion; this may cause:

- an increase in bulk of *bone* and *soft tissues* with *enlargement* of, for example, the hands, jaw and heart. Changes in facial appearance are often marked, due to the increasing size of the jaw and sinuses; the gradual coarsening of the features may pass unnoticed for many years. Thyroid gland enlargement may be clinically detectable, but the patient is usually euthyroid;
- excessive hair growth and *sebaceous gland secretion.*
- *menstrual disturbances* which are common;
- *impaired glucose tolerance*, present in about 25 per cent of cases, about half of whom develop symptomatic diabetes mellitus. In most cases the pancreas can secrete enough insulin to overcome the antagonistic effect of GH. Probably only those with a diabetic tendency develop the disease under these conditions.

A different group of symptoms may occur due to the encroachment of a pituitary tumour on surrounding structures.

- Compression of the optic chiasma may cause visual field defects.
- If destruction of the gland progresses other anterior pituitary hormones may become deficient. Plasma prolactin concentrations may, however, be raised (p.**114**).

Acromegaly is sometimes one of the manifestations of multiple endocrine neoplasia (p.**397**).

Diagnosis. The diagnosis of GH excess is suggested by the clinical presentation and radiological findings. Plasma GH concentrations are usually higher than normal and may reach several hundred mU/L, but, because of the wide reference range, results from ambulant patients may fail to distinguish those with only moderately raised plasma concentrations from normal subjects.

The diagnosis is confirmed by demonstrating a *raised plasma GH concentration that is not suppressed by a rise in plasma glucose concentration.* In normal subjects plasma GH concentrations fall to very low levels after a glucose load. In acromegalics secretion of GH is effectively autonomous and this fall may not occur, be only slight, or there may even be a rise.

Plasma IGF-1 concentrations are raised and may be used in diagnosis. Plasma concentrations correlate with the activity of the disease. Measurement of plasma concentrations of GH, or IGF-1, may be used to monitor the efficacy of treatment.

GROWTH HORMONE DEFICIENCY

In adults, GH deficiency rarely causes clinical symptoms.

A small percentage of normally proportioned dwarfed children have growth hormone deficiency. The birth weight may be normal but the rate of growth is subnormal. Other causes of growth retardation and short stature must be excluded before a diagnosis of GH deficiency is made (Table 5.2).

Emotional deprivation may be associated with growth hormone deficiency indistinguishable by laboratory tests from that due to organic causes.

It is important to investigate children with reduced growth rate to identify those who may benefit from GH replacement treatment.

Isolated GH deficiency is most commonly secondary to idiopathic deficiency of hypothalamic GH-releasing hormone. In some cases the secretion of other hormones is also impaired. Sometimes there may be an organic disorder of the anterior pituitary gland or hypothalamus; rare inherited forms have been described.

Diagnosis. Plasma GH concentrations in normal children are usually low and assays under basal conditions rarely exclude the diagnosis. If blood *is taken at a time when physiologically high concentrations are expected* the need for the more unpleasant stimulation tests may be avoided. Such times are 60 to 90 minutes after the onset of sleep and about 20 minutes after vigorous exercise.

If GH deficiency is not excluded by the above measurements, it is necessary either to measure the overnight urinary GH excretion or to perform one or more *stimulation tests* (p.**148**). An unequivocally normal response to a stimulation test excludes the diagnosis and a clearly impaired one confirms it.

Once GH deficiency is established a cause should be sought by appropriate clinical and radiological means.

Table 5.2 Some causes of growth retardation and short stature

Familial short stature
Emotional deprivation
Malnutrition and chronic disease
   coeliac disease
   rickets
Endocrine disorders
   GH deficiency, congenital or acquired
   hypothyroidism
   Cushing's syndrome
   congenital adrenal hyperplasia
Chromosomal abnormalities
   Turner's syndrome (45,X)
Skeletal disorders
   achrondroplasia

Hypopituitarism

The anterior pituitary gland has considerable functional reserve. Clinical features of deficiency are usually absent until about 70 per cent of the gland has been destroyed, unless there is associated hyperprolactinaemia, when amenorrhoea and infertility may be early symptoms (p.**139**).

Causes of hypopituitarism include:

- destruction of, or damage to, the anterior pituitary gland or the hypothalamus by a primary or a secondary tumour. Secondary deposits originate most commonly from the breast or bronchus;

- infarction, most commonly postpartum (Sheehan's syndrome) or, rarely, after other major vascular catastrophes;
- pituitary surgery or irradiation;
- less common causes include:
  head injury;
  infections or granulomas.

Failure of all anterior pituitary functions (panhypopituitarism) with the full clinical picture described below, is uncommon. Suspicion of anterior pituitary hypofunction usually arises in patients presenting with:

- hypogonadism or adrenocortical insuffi-ciency which is shown by preliminary testing to be secondary in origin;
* clinical and radiological evidence of a pituitary or localized brain tumour;
- short stature caused by GH deficiency.

Although isolated hormone deficiency, particularly of GH, may occur, several hormones are usually involved. If a deficiency of one hormone is demonstrated it is important to establish whether the secre-tion of others is also abnormal. This evidence is needed, not only to manage replacement therapy, but also to assess the ability of the pituitary gland to respond to stress, such as that due to infection or surgery.

Consequences of Hormone Deficiencies

Progressive pituitary damage usually presents with evidence of deficiencies of gonadotrophins and GH. Plasma ACTH and/or TSH concentrations may remain normal, or become deficient months or even years later. The clinical and biochemical consequences of the target gland failure include:

- *secondary hypogonadism* due to gonadotrophin deficiency, presenting as amenorrhoea, infertility, atrophy of secondary sexual characteristics with loss of axillary and pubic hair and impotence or loss of libido. Puberty is delayed in children;
- *growth retardation in children* may be due to deficiency of GH. TSH and therefore thyroid hormone deficiency may contribute;
- *secondary hypothyroidism* (TSH de-ficiency) which may sometimes be clinic-ally indistinguishable from primary hypothyroidism;
- *secondary adrenocortical hypofunction* (ACTH deficiency). In contrast to the primary form (Addison's disease) patients are *not hyperpigmented* because ACTH secretion is deficient, not excessive. Sodium and water deficiency and hyper-kalaemia, characteristic of Addison's disease, do not occur because aldosterone secretion, which is controlled by angiotensin and not by ACTH, is normal. However, cortisol is needed for normal free water excretion, and consequently there may be a *dilutional hyponatraemia* due to cortisol deficiency. Cortisol is also necessary for maintenance of normal blood pressure. Hypotension may be associated with ACTH deficiency. Cortisol and/or growth hormone deficiency may cause increased insulin sensitivity with fasting hypoglycaemia;
- *prolactin deficiency* with failure to lactate may occur after postpartum pituitary infarc-tion (Sheehan's syndrome). However, in hypopituitarism due to a tumour plasma prolactin concentrations are often raised and may cause galactorrhoea (secretion of breast fluid).

Patients with hypopituitarism, like those with Addison's disease, may die because of an inability to secrete an adequate amount of cortisol in response to stress caused by, for example, infection or surgery. Other life-threatening complications are hypogly-caemia, water intoxication severe enough to cause gross hyponatraemia and hypother-mia.

EVALUATION OF ANTERIOR PITUITARY FUNCTION

Interpretation of results of basal pituitary hormone assays is often difficult. Low plasma concentrations are not necessarily abnormal and plasma concentrations within the reference range do not exclude pituitary disease. The diagnosis of suspected hypopituitarism is best excluded by *direct measurement of pituitary hormones after stimulation* (p.**148**) or by demonstrating target-gland hyposecretion after administration of the relevant trophic hormone (Chapters 6, 7 and 8). However, prolonged hypopituitarism may result in secondary failure of the target gland with diminished response to stimulation.

Laboratory tests only establish the presence or absence of hypopituitarism. The *cause* must be sought by clinical and radiological means.

HYPOTHALAMUS OR PITUITARY DYSFUNCTION?

It is frequently difficult to distinguish between hypothalamic and pituitary causes of pituitary hormone deficiency or, more correctly, between deficient releasing factor and a primary deficiency of pituitary hormone secretion. Isolated hormone deficiencies are more likely to be of hypothalamic than of pituitary origin. The coexistence of diabetes insipidus suggests a hypothalamic disorder, but symptoms of water loss may not occur at first because of ACTH, and therefore of cortisol, deficiency causing water retention.

Some biochemical investigations evaluate both hypothalamic and pituitary function and some only the latter although it may be possible to distinguish the anatomical site of the lesion. For example, the TSH response to TRH may differ in hypothalamic and pituitary causes of secondary hypothyroidism (p.**168**). In cases of hypogonadism due to gonadotrophin deficiency the differentiation on the basis of the response to gonadotrophin-releasing hormone (GnRH) is less clear cut.

Pituitary Tumours

The clinical presentation of pituitary tumours depends on the types of cell involved and on the size of the tumour.

Tumours of secretory cells may produce the clinical effects of excess hormone secretion. Excess:

- prolactin causes infertility, amenorrhoea and varying degrees of galactorrhoea;
- GH causes acromegaly or gigantism;
- ACTH causes Cushing's syndrome.

Large tumours may present with:

- visual disturbances caused by pressure on the optic chiasma or headache due to raised intracranial pressure;
- deficiency of some or all of the pituitary hormones due to destruction of secretory cells in the gland.

Nonsecreting tumours are difficult to diagnose using biochemical tests although the combined pituitary stimulation test (insulin stimulation, TRH and GnRH tests; p.**148**) may indicate subclinical impairment of function. *Hyperprolactinaemia* (p.**139**), which may be asymptomatic, is a valuable biochemical marker of the presence of a pituitary tumour. Prolactin may be secreted by the tumour cells or it may be secreted by unaffected lactotrophs if tumour growth interferes with the normal inhibition of prolactin secretion.

Summary

1. The anterior pituitary gland secretes growth hormone (GH), prolactin, adrenocorticotrophic hormone (ACTH; corticotrophin), β-lipotrophin (β-LPH), thyroid-stimulating hormone (TSH) and the two gonadotrophins, follicle-stimulating hormone (FSH) and luteinizing-hormone (LH). The posterior lobe secretes antidiuretic hormone (ADH; arginine vasopressin, AVP) and oxytocin.

2. The secretion of anterior pituitary hormones is controlled by regulating hormones secreted by the hypothalamus. These, in turn, are controlled by circulating levels of hormones or metabolic products (feedback), or respond to stimuli from higher cerebral centres.

3. GH controls growth and has a number of effects on intermediary metabolism. *Excessive GH* secretion causes gigantism or acromegaly. Laboratory evidence of autonomous GH secretion is obtained by failure of suppression of plasma levels of GH during a glucose tolerance test. *GH deficiency* in childhood leads to short stature. Diagnosis of such deficiency is made by demonstrating a subnormal GH response to appropriate stimuli.

4. Anterior pituitary hormone deficiency usually involves several hormones. Less commonly an isolated deficiency occurs. The clinical features of hypopituitarism are those of gonadotrophin and sex hormone deficiencies and of secondary hypofunction of the adrenal cortex and thyroid gland. Diagnosis is made by demonstrating reduced anterior pituitary reserve after stimulation.

5. Pituitary tumours may produce excess of GH, ACTH or prolactin, or may cause hypopituitarism. In patients without obvious endocrine disturbance hyperprolactinaemia may be found.

Adrenal Cortex

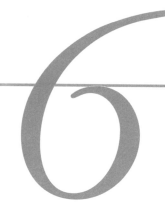

The adrenal glands are divided into two embryologically and functionally distinct units.

- *The adrenal cortex* is part of the hypothalamic–pituitary–adrenal endocrine system. Morphologically, the adult adrenal cortex consists of three layers. The outer thin layer (*zona glomerulosa*) secretes only aldosterone. The inner two layers, the *zona fasciculata* and the *zona reticularis*, form a functional unit and secrete most of the adrenocortical hormones. In the fetus there is a wider fourth layer which disappears soon after birth. During fetal life, one of its most important functions is, together with the adrenal cortex, to synthesize oestriol, in association with the placenta (p.**138**).
- *The adrenal medulla* is part of the sympathetic nervous system. Glucocorticoids are probably needed for the synthesis of adrenalin (epinephrine) (p.**394**).

CHEMISTRY AND BIOSYNTHESIS OF STEROIDS

Steroid hormones are derived from cholesterol. Figure 6.1 shows the internationally agreed numbering of the 27 carbon atoms of steroid molecules and the lettering of the four rings. The products of cholesterol are also indicated. If the molecule contains 21 carbon atoms it is referred to as a C_{21} steroid. The carbon atom at position 21 of the molecule is written as C-21. The side chain on C-17 is the main determinant of the type of hormonal activity (Fig. 6.1) but substitutions in other positions modify activity within a particular group.

The first hormonal product of cholesterol is pregnenolone. Several important synthetic pathways diverge from it (Fig. 6.1). The final product depends on the tissue and the enzymes that it contains.

Adrenal Cortex

The zonae fasciculata and reticularis synthesize and secrete two groups of steroid:;

- *cortisol*, a glucocorticoid (the most important C_{21} steroid) is formed by progressive addition of hydroxyl groups at C-17, C-21 and C-11;
- *androgens* (for example androstenedione) are formed after the removal of the side chain to produce C_{19} steroids.

Synthesis of these two steroids is stimulated by ACTH, secreted by the anterior pituitary gland (p.**108**). ACTH secretion is influenced by negative feedback from changes in plasma cortisol concentrations. Impaired cortisol synthesis, due, for example, to an inherited 21α- or 11β-hydroxylase deficiency (congenital adrenal hyperplasia) results in increased ACTH stimulation with increased activity of both pathways. The resultant excessive androgen production causes virilization (p.**128**).

The zona glomerulosa secretes:

- *aldosterone* produced by 18-hydroxylation. Synthesis of this steroid is controlled by the renin–angiotensin system and not normally by ACTH (p.**27**). Although ACTH is important for maintaining growth of the zona glomerulosa, deficiency does not significantly reduce output.

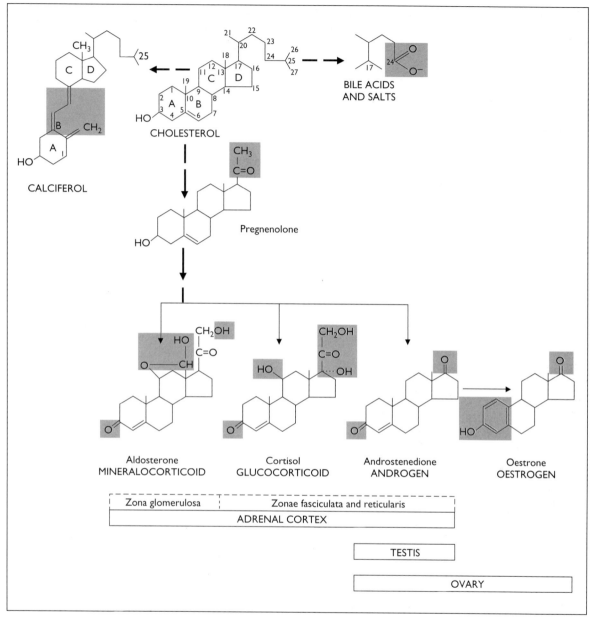

Fig. 6.1 Numbering of the steroid carbon atoms of cholesterol and the synthetic pathway of steroid hormones; those chemical groups highlighted determine the biological activity of the steroid (For oestrogens see p.134).

*P*HYSIOLOGY

The adrenocortical hormones can be classified into groups depending on their predominant physiological effects.

Glucocorticoids

Cortisol and *corticosterone* are naturally occurring glucocorticoids. They stimulate gluconeogenesis and the breakdown of protein and fat. Therefore, they oppose some of the actions of insulin. In excess they impair glucose tolerance and alter the distribution of adipose tissue. Cortisol helps maintain the extracellular fluid volume and normal blood pressure.

Circulating cortisol is bound to cortisol-binding globulin (CBG; transcortin) and to albumin. At normal concentrations, only about 5 per cent of the total is unbound and is physiologically active (compare with thyroxine, p.**159**). Plasma CBG is almost fully saturated so that increased cortisol secretion causes a disproportionate rise in the free active fraction.

Glucocorticoids are conjugated with glucuronate and sulphate in the liver to form inactive metabolites which, because they are more water soluble than the mainly protein-bound parent hormones, can be excreted in the urine.

Cortisone, sometimes used therapeutically, is not secreted in significant amounts by the adrenal cortex. It is biologically inactive until it has been converted *in vivo* to cortisol (hydrocortisone).

Mineralocorticoids

Aldosterone, in contrast to other steroids, is not transported in plasma bound to specific proteins. It stimulates the *exchange of sodium for potassium and hydrogen ions* across cell membranes and its renal action is especially important for sodium and water homeostasis. It is discussed more fully on p.**27**. Like the glucocorticoids it is inactivated by hepatic conjugation and excreted in the urine.

There is overlap in the actions of C_{21} steroids. Cortisol, in particular, may have a significant mineralocorticoid effect at high plasma concentrations when the free fraction is significantly increased.

Adrenal Androgens

The main adrenal androgens are dehydroepiandrosterone (DHA), its sulphate (DHAS) and androstenedione. They promote protein synthesis and are only mildly androgenic at physiological concentrations. *Testosterone, the most powerful androgen*, is synthesized in the testes or ovaries but not in the adrenal cortex. Most circulating androgens, like cortisol, are protein bound, mainly to *sex-hormone-binding globulin* (SHBG) and albumin.

There is extensive peripheral interconversion of adrenal and gonadal androgens. The end products, androsterone and aetiocholanolone, together with DHA, are conjugated in the liver and excreted as glucuronides and sulphates in the urine.

CONTROL OF ADRENAL STEROID SECRETION

The hypothalamus, anterior pituitary gland and adrenal cortex form a functional unit – the hypothalamic–pituitary–adrenal axis, (Fig. 6.2).

Cortisol is synthesized and secreted in response to ACTH from the anterior pituitary gland. ACTH secretion is dependent on corticotrophin (CRH), released from the hypothalamus. At least three mechanisms influence CRH secretion.

Negative feedback. High plasma free-cortisol concentrations suppress CRH secretion and alter the ACTH response to CRH, thus acting on both the hypothalamus and on the anterior pituitary gland (Fig. 6.2). The melanocyte-stimulating effect of high plasma concentrations of ACTH, or related peptides, cause pigmentation in two conditions associated with low plasma cortisol concentrations:

- *Addison's disease*;
- *after bilateral adrenalectomy* for Cushing's disease. Removal of the previously marked cortisol feedback causes a further rise in plasma ACTH concentrations from already high levels (Nelson's syndrome).

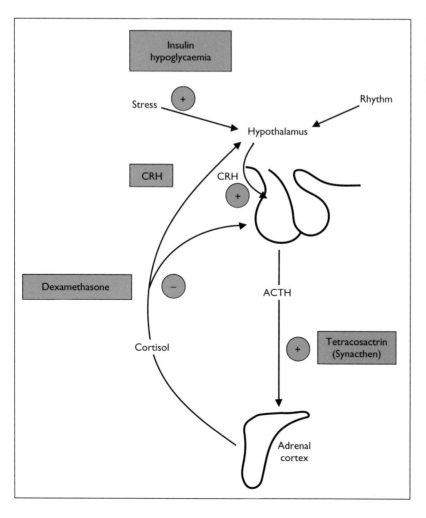

Fig. 6.2 Factors controlling the secretion of cortisol from the adrenal gland, including the site of action of dynamic function tests (shaded) (+ = stimulates; – = inhibits).

Inherent rhythms. ACTH is secreted episodically, each pulse being followed five to 10 minutes later by cortisol secretion. These episodes are more frequent in the early morning (between the fifth and eighth hour of sleep) and least frequent in the few hours before sleep. Plasma cortisol concentrations are usually high between about 07.00 and 09.00 hours and low between 23.00 and 04.00 hours.

ACTH and cortisol secretion usually vary inversely and the almost parallel circadian rhythm of the two hormones may be due to cyclical changes in the sensitivity of the hypothalamic feedback centre to cortisol levels. Inappropriately high plasma cortisol concentrations at any time of day suppress ACTH secretion. This effect can be tested by the dexamethasone suppression test (p.**124**). Loss of circadian rhythm is one of the earliest features of Cushing's syndrome.

Stress, either physical or mental, may override the first two mechanisms and cause sustained ACTH secretion. The consequent diagnostic difficulties are discussed on p.**125**. An inadequate stress response may cause acute adrenal insufficiency. Stress caused by insulin-induced hypoglycaemia can be used to test the axis.

ACTH (corticotrophin)

ACTH is a single-chain polypeptide made up of 39 amino acids with biological activity at the N-terminal end of the peptide (p.**108**). A peptide consisting of this sequence has been synthesized (tetracosactrin, 'Synacthen') and can be used for diagnosis and treatment in place of ACTH. ACTH stimulates cortisol synthesis and secretion by the adrenal cortex. It has much less effect on adrenal androgen production and, at physiological concentrations, virtually no effect on aldosterone production.

Disorders of the Adrenal Cortex

The main disorders of adrenocortical function are shown in Table 6.1.

Adrenocortical Hyperfunction

Cushing's syndrome

Cushing's syndrome is caused by an excess of circulating cortisol. Many of the clinical and metabolic disturbances can, at least partly, be explained by the known actions of cortisol. The clinical and metabolic features include:

- *obesity*, mild to moderate, typically involving the trunk and face. It is the commonest presenting symptom of patients with classical Cushing's disease. Like the round red 'moon' face, this type of obesity is characteristic, but not diagnostic, of cortisol excess; the reason for these features is not understood;

- *impaired glucose tolerance*, which occurs in about two-thirds of the patients, many of whom have *hyperglycaemia* and therefore *glycosuria*. As cortisol has an opposite action to insulin, the resultant picture in some ways resembles diabetes mellitus. Protein breakdown is accelerated and the carbon chains of the liberated amino acids

Table 6.1 Disorders of adrenocortical function

Altered hormone secretion	Associated clinical disorder
Hypersecretion of:	
cortisol	Cushing's syndrome
aldosterone	Primary aldosteronism (Conn's syndrome)
androgens	Adrenocortical carcinoma
	Congenital adrenal hyperplasia
Hyposecretion of:	
cortisol and aldosterone	Primary adrenal disorders
	Addison's disease
	congenital adrenal hyperplasia
ACTH and cortisol	Adrenal insufficiency

may be converted to glucose (gluconeogenesis) (p.**200**);

- *increased protein catabolism*, which also increases urinary protein loss. Thus there is a negative nitrogen balance associated with muscle wasting with weakness, thinning of the skin and osteoporosis. The tendency to *bruising*, and the *purple striae*, most obvious on the abdominal wall, are probably due to this thinning;

- *hypertension*, caused by urinary retention of sodium and therefore of water, which are due to the mineralocorticoid effect of cortisol. Increased urinary potassium loss may cause *hypokalaemia* and so aggravate muscle weakness;

- *androgen excess* which may account for the common findings of greasy skin with *acne vulgaris* and *hirsutism* and menstrual disturbances in women;

- *psychiatric disturbances*, particularly agitated depression.

The typical presenting clinical features depend on the cause of the cortisol excess.

Causes of Cushing's Syndrome

Excessive cortisol production may be due to hyperstimulation of the adrenal gland by ACTH, either from the pituitary gland or from an 'ectopic' source or due to largely autonomous secretion by an adrenal tumour (Fig. 6.3). ACTH secretion is increased in:

- *Cushing's disease*, which is, although very rare, the commonest form of Cushing's syndrome. It usually occurs in women of

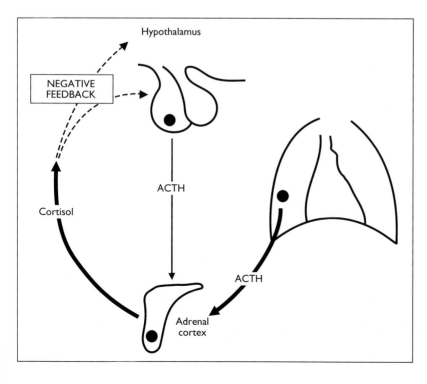

Fig. 6.3 Cushing's syndrome, indicating excess cortisol production caused either because of hyperstimulation of the adrenal gland by ACTH, from either the pituitary or an ectopic source or by autonomous hormone secretion from an adrenal tumour.

Hypothalamus

NEGATIVE FEEDBACK

ACTH

Cortisol

ACTH

Adrenal cortex

reproductive age. It is associated with bilateral adrenal hyperplasia, often secondary to a basophil adenoma of the anterior pituitary gland. It is not known whether the pituitary tumour is the primary lesion, or whether there is excessive CRH secretion from the hypothalamus;

- *ACTH producing tumours*, other than those of the anterior pituitary gland, causing bilateral adrenal hyperplasia.

  In overt ectopic ACTH secretion, usually from a small-cell carcinoma of the bronchus, ACTH concentrations may be high enough to cause pigmentation. The patient may have weight loss with cachexia and not have the clinical features of Cushing's disease. The most striking metabolic complication is often hypokalaemic alkalosis.

  In occult ectopic ACTH secretion, often from slow growing pulmonary or mediastinal carcinoid tumours, the clinical features may be indistinguishable from those of Cushing's disease.

ACTH secretion is appropriately *suppressed* in:

- *primary cortisol secreting tumours of the adrenal cortex.* The tumour may be benign or malignant. Benign adenomas occur in the same sex and age group as Cushing's disease and produce a similar clinical picture. Carcinomas secrete a variety of steroids, some of which may cause virilization.

Cushing's syndrome may also be caused by excessive steroid treatment.

Basis of Investigation of Suspected Cushing's Syndrome

Untreated patients with Cushing's syndrome have a high morbidity and mortality rate. Any suspected case must be adequately investigated. Obese, red-faced, hairy, hypertensive women usually *do not* have Cushing's syndrome. The diagnosis is more often one of exclusion than of confirmation. However, as the tests available are not specific, it is essential to apply them in a logical sequence.

The following questions should be asked:

- is there abnormal cortisol secretion?
- if so, does the patient have any other condition that may cause it?
- if Cushing's syndrome is confirmed, what is the cause?

Is there abnormal secretion? Blood is easy to collect but plasma cortisol concentrations reflect adrenocorticotrophic activity at that moment and, because of the episodic nature of cortisol secretion, such isolated values may be misleading. The measurement of steroids in a 24 hour urine sample reflects the overall daily secretion.

One of the earliest features of Cushing's syndrome is the *loss of the diurnal variation in cortisol secretion* with high concentrations in the late evening, when secretion is normally at a minimum. However, it is not a diagnostic finding because it can also be caused by, for example, stress and endogenous depression. Assessment of diurnal rhythm is not a practical outpatient procedure. Outpatient screening tests therefore include:

- *24-hour urinary free-cortisol estimation.* Only the unbound fraction of cortisol in plasma is filtered at the glomeruli and excreted in the urine (*urinary 'free'-cortisol*). In Cushing's syndrome, because of the loss of circadian rhythm, raised plasma values are present for longer than normal and daily urinary cortisol excretion is further increased. The urinary free-cortisol excretion will be more markedly raised than plasma concentrations. Plasma and urinary cortisol concentrations are much higher when Cushing's syndrome is due to adrenocortical carcinoma or overt ectopic ACTH secretion.
- *low-dose overnight dexamethasone suppression test.* A small dose of this synthetic steroid inhibits ACTH, and therefore cortisol, secretion by negative feedback (p.**121**). Suppression does not occur in patients with:

  Cushing's disease in whom the feedback centre is less sensitive than normal;
  ectopic ACTH secretion;

Table 6.2   Usual test results in patients with Cushing's syndrome

Diagnosis	Adrenocortical hyperplasia			Adrenocortical tumour	
	Pituitary-dependent (Cushing's disease)	Ectopic ACTH		Carcinoma	Adenoma
		Occult	Overt		
Plasma cortisol morning	Raised, may be N			Raised	Raised, may be N
evening	← ————————————— Raised ————————————— →				
after 2 mg dexamethasone	← ———————————— No suppression ———————————— →				
Urinary cortisol	Raised		Usually very high		Raised

Aetiology

	Pituitary-dependent (Cushing's disease)	Ectopic ACTH		Carcinoma	Adenoma
Plasma ACTH	High normal or moderately raised		Raised	Very low	
Plasma cortisol after 8 mg dexamethasone	Suppression	← ——————————— No suppression ——————————— →			

N = normal.

adrenal tumours in whom ACTH secretion is already suppressed.

The overnight dexamethasone suppression test is a sensitive, but not completely specific test in evaluating such patients. A normal fall in cortisol concentrations makes the diagnosis of Cushing's syndrome very unlikely, but failure to fall does not confirm it with certainty.

Is there another cause for the abnormal cortisol secretion? The following non-Cushing's causes of abnormal cortisol secretion are of particular importance:

- *Stress* overrides the other mechanisms controlling ACTH secretion, with loss of the normal circadian variation of plasma cortisol and a reduced feedback response. Urinary free cortisol excretion may be increased even in relatively minor physical illness or mental stress.
- *Endogenous depression* is often associated with sustained high plasma cortisol and

ACTH concentrations that may not be suppressed even by a high dose of dexamethasone. However, these patients usually have a normal cortisol response to insulin-induced hypoglycaemia, whereas those with Cushing's syndrome do not.

- *Severe alcohol abuse* can cause hypersecretion of cortisol that mimics Cushing's syndrome clinically and biochemically. The abnormal findings revert to normal when alcohol is stopped.

What is the cause of Cushing's syndrome? Unless Cushing's syndrome is proven, tests to establish its cause cannot be interpreted. Because of the timing of these tests, they should be carried out on an in-patient basis.

The stress caused by hospital admission may be enough to reduce the circadian rhythm of hormone secretion. For this reason tests should not be started until 48 hours later. The following biochemical investigations should help to elucidate the cause (Table 6.2):

- *assessment of circadian rhythm.*
- *plasma ACTH* is detectable only in ACTH dependent Cushing's syndrome and plasma concentrations are very low in patients with secreting adrenocortical tumours. In patients with Cushing's disease or with occult ectopic ACTH production plasma concentrations may be either high normal or moderately raised but inappropriate for the high plasma cortisol concentration. Plasma ACTH concentrations are markedly raised in patients with 'ectopic' ACTH production.
- *high-dose dexamethasone suppression test.* The principal of this test is the same as that described earlier, but a higher dose may suppress the relatively insensitive feedback centre of pituitary-dependent Cushing's disease. In the other two categories, ectopic ACTH production or adrenal tumours, when pituitary ACTH is already suppressed, even this high dose will usually have no effect although there may be some suppression in cases of 'ectopic' ACTH secretion.
- *insulin tolerance test.* Elevated plasma cortisol concentrations suppress the stress response to hypoglycaemia and this test may be of value in differentiating Cushing's syndrome from hypercortisolaemia due to depression or obesity.

Adrenocortical Hypofunction

PRIMARY ADRENOCORTICAL HYPOFUNCTION (ADDISON'S DISEASE)

Addison's disease is caused by bilateral destruction of all zones of the adrenal cortex, usually as the result of an autoimmune process. Tuberculosis is an important cause in some countries where this disease is common. Rare causes of bilateral destruction of the adrenal glands include amyloidosis, mycotic infections and secondary deposits often originating from a bronchial carcinoma.

The clinical presentation of Addison's disease depends on the degree of adrenal destruction. The patient may be shocked, with volume depletion; this adrenal crisis should be treated as a matter of urgency. It may be difficult to make a diagnosis if destruction is less extensive; a prolonged period of vague ill health, tiredness, weight loss, mild hypotension and pigmentation of the skin and buccal mucosa are common in many severe chronic diseases. The cause of these vague symptoms may only become evident if an Addisonian crisis is precipitated by the stress of some other, perhaps mild, illness or of surgery.

Mineralocorticoid (aldosterone) deficiency causes sodium and water depletion with serious consequences, as described on p.**43**.

Glucocorticoid deficiency contributes to the hypotension and causes marked sensitivity to insulin; hypoglycaemia may be a presenting feature. Addisonian crisis is described fully on p.**44**.

Androgen deficiency is not clinically evident because testosterone production by the testes is unimpaired, and because androgen deficiency does not produce obvious effects in women.

Pigmentation that develops in some cases of Addison's disease is probably due to the high circulating levels of ACTH or related peptides resulting from the lack of cortisol suppression of the feedback mechanism.

SECONDARY ADRENAL HYPOFUNCTION (ACTH DEFICIENCY)

ACTH release may be impaired by disorders of the hypothalamus or the anterior pituitary gland, most commonly due to a tumour or infarction. Corticosteroids suppress ACTH release and, if such drugs have been taken for a long time, the ACTH releasing mechanism may be slow to recover. There may be temporary adrenal atrophy after prolonged lack of stimulation.

Extensive destruction of the anterior pituitary gland may cause *panhypopituitarism* (p.**112**) but, if it is only partial, ACTH secretion may be adequate for basal requirements. Adrenocortical deficiency may then only become clinically evident under conditions of stress, which may precipitate acute adrenal insufficiency. The most usual causes of stress are infection and surgery.

Patients may present with non-specific symptoms such as weight loss and tiredness. Hypoglycaemia may occur because of marked insulin sensitivity. Pigmentation is absent because plasma ACTH concentrations are low.

Patients with acute cortisol deficiency may present with nausea, vomiting and hypotension. Dilutional hyponatraemia may be present because cortisol is needed for sodium-free water excretion by the kidneys. The biochemical changes therefore resemble those of inappropriate ADH secretion. Because aldosterone secretion is normal, hyperkalaemia does not occur.

BASIS OF INVESTIGATION OF SUSPECTED ADRENOCORTICAL HYPOFUNCTION

If a diagnosis of acute adrenal insufficiency is suspected clinically, blood should be taken so that the plasma cortisol concentration can be measured later; treatment must be started at once. If possible a short tetracosactrin ('Synacthen') test should be performed; this will only delay the onset of treatment by up to one hour.

Results of the plasma cortisol assay on the initial sample should distinguish between adrenocortical insufficiency with inappropriately low values and clinically similar crises when concentrations are markedly raised due to stress. However, adrenocorticol hypofunction may not be excluded on the results of estimation of a random plasma cortisol concentration alone as it may be at the upper end of the reference range but, nevertheless, be inappropriate for the degree of stress. The results of a plasma cortisol estimation will not distinguish between primary and secondary adrenal failure.

The essential abnormality in adrenocortical hypofunction is that the adrenal gland cannot adequately increase cortisol secretion in response to stress. Because this may be due to adrenal (primary) or hypothalamic–pituitary (secondary) pathology, it may be necessary to test the whole axis.

- *Insulin-induced hypoglycaemia* should cause ACTH secretion from the anterior pituitary gland. This can be assessed by demonstrating a rise in plasma cortisol concentrations, indicating adrenocortical stimulation. An impaired response only indicates pituitary dysfunction if the adrenal cortices have already been shown to be capable of responding to exogenous ACTH. Tetracosactrin (for example, 'Synacthen') has the same biological action as ACTH but, because it lacks the antigenic part of the molecule, there is much less danger of an allergic reaction. If the patient cannot stop using steroids, then a steroid such as dexamethasone, which does not interfere with the assay, should be prescribed.
- *Plasma ACTH assay* is of value in some cases. When inappropriately low plasma cortisol concentrations have been found, a raised plasma ACTH concentration indicates primary, and a low level secondary, insufficiency. This will distinguish between true adrenocortical disease (when mineralocorticoid replacement is needed) and reversible atrophy due to prolonged ACTH deficiency.

CORTICOSTEROID THERAPY

There is a risk of adrenocortical hypofunction when long term corticosteroid treatment is stopped suddenly. This may be due to either secondary adrenal atrophy or impaired ACTH release.

A simple means of testing the feedback centre and the responsiveness of the pituitary–adrenal axis is to estimate the morning plasma cortisol concentration two or three days after stopping steroid treatment. A plasma concentration within the reference range indicates a functioning adrenal, pituitary and feedback centre. It must be emphasized, however, that this does not test the all-important stress pathway (p.**122**).

*A suggested sequence of testing is described on p.**147***.

Congenital Adrenal Hyperplasia

All forms of congenital adrenal hyperplasia are rare. An inherited deficiency of one of the enzymes involved in the biosynthesis of cortisol, with a low plasma concentration, causes a high rate of secretion of ACTH from the anterior pituitary gland (Fig. 6.4). This results in hyperplasia of the adrenal cortex, with increased synthesis of cortisol precursors before the enzyme block. The precursors may then be metabolized by alternative pathways, especially those of androgen synthesis.

Increased androgen production may cause:

- *female pseudohermaphroditism* by affecting the development of the female genitalia *in utero*;
- *virilization in childhood* with phallic enlargement in either sex, development of pubic hair and a rapid growth rate;
- *milder virilization in females at or after puberty*, with amenorrhoea.

Aldosterone synthesis may be markedly reduced in more than half of the infants with 21α-hydroxylase deficiency and may cause an Addisonian-like picture with marked renal

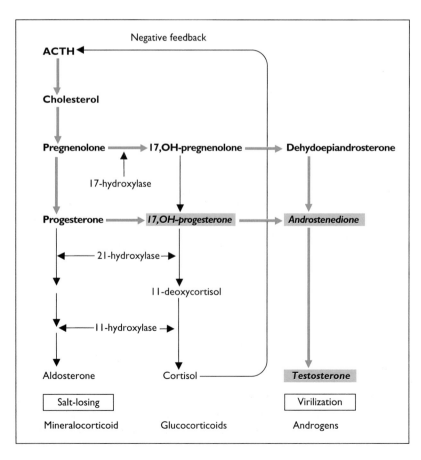

Fig. 6.4 The abnormalities occurring in congenital adrenal hyperplasia. Substances highlighted are of diagnostic importance; those shown in bold are increased in 21α-hydroxylase deficiency.

sodium loss during the first few weeks of life. Vomiting is severe. Volume depletion may be accompanied by hyponatraemia and hyper-kalaemia. Even if plasma sodium concentrations are within the reference range, demonstrably increased plasma renin activity may suggest lesser degrees of sodium and water depletion.

All female infants with ambiguous genitalia should have plasma electrolytes estimated. In male infants with no obvious physical abnormalities the diagnosis may not be suspected.

Diagnosis. The investigation of suspected congenital adrenal hyperplasia is best undertaken in special centres. Only the principles of the diagnosis of 21α-hydroxylase deficiency will be outlined here (Fig. 6.4).

- *17-hydroxyprogesterone* can only be metabolized by the cortisol pathway in the presence of 21α-hydroxylase. Plasma concentrations are raised in patients with congenital adrenal hyperplasia.

- *Plasma androstenedione* concentrations are raised in those patients with excessive androgen synthesis.

Some indication of which enzyme is deficient may be suggested by evaluating the pattern of steroid excretion in a random urine sample.

Treatment. Congenital adrenal hyperplasia is treated by giving cortisol or one of the glucocorticoid analogues with, if necessary, a mineralocorticoid. This treatment not only replaces the deficient hormones but, by negative feedback, suppresses ACTH secretion and therefore androgen production.

The efficacy of treatment is monitored by measuring 17-hydroxyprogesterone and androstenedione concentrations in plasma or saliva. Salivary steroid concentrations correlate well with those in plasma and collection of saliva may be more acceptable to some patients than repeated venepunctures. The adequacy of mineralocorticoid replacement may be assessed by measuring the plasma renin activity.

Summary

1. The steroids of the adrenal cortex may be classified into three groups:

   - *glucocorticoids*, for example cortisol, which influence intermediary metabolism, fluid balance and blood pressure. Secretion is controlled by ACTH from the anterior pituitary gland;
   - *mineralocorticoids*, for example aldosterone, which influence sodium balance and secondarily that of water and potassium. Secretion is controlled by the renin–angiotensin system;
   - *androgens*, for example androstenedione, which have an anabolic action on protein synthesis.

2. ACTH (and therefore cortisol) secretion is stimulated by CRH from the hypothalamus. The important controlling factors are:

   - an inherent rhythm which produces an overall circadian variation in plasma cortisol levels. These are lowest at around midnight and highest in the morning;
   - negative feedback by circulating free cortisol concentrations;
   - stress which may override both the above controls.

3. Estimations of plasma and urinary cortisol concentrations are the most useful tests. Plasma ACTH measurements are of value

in the differential diagnosis of Cushing's syndrome and, more rarely, to distinguish between primary and secondary adrenal failure.

4. Cushing's syndrome is due to inappropriately high circulating cortisol concentrations. The causes are hyperplasia or a tumour of the adrenal cortex. Hyperplasia is due to excess ACTH, either from the pituitary (pituitary-dependent) or from a non-endocrine tumour. There are three stages in investigation.

   • Is there abnormal cortisol secretion?
   • If so, can it be accounted for by a condition other than Cushing's syndrome?
   • If not, what is the cause of the Cushing's syndrome?

5. Primary adrenocortical hypofunction (Addison's disease) is due to destruction of the adrenal cortex with deficiency of all its hormones. Aldosterone deficiency causes sodium and consequent water depletion. Diagnosis is made by demonstrating that the adrenal cortex cannot respond to stimulation by exogenous ACTH (or an analogue).

6. Secondary adrenal insufficiency is caused by diminished ACTH secretion by the anterior pituitary gland. This may be due to a disorder of the hypothalamus or of the pituitary, or may be the result of corticosteroid treatment.

   It is usually diagnosed by demonstrating a definite but impaired response to tetracosactrin (synthetic ACTH) stimulation. In cases without adrenal atrophy the hypothalamic–pituitary–adrenal axis may be assessed by the insulin stress test.

7. Congenital adrenal hyperplasia is due to an inherited enzyme deficiency in cortisol synthesis. Symptoms are due to a deficiency of cortisol and to excessive androgen secretion. Diagnosis of the commonest form, 21α-hydroxylase deficiency, is made by estimating plasma 17-hydroxyprogesterone concentration. Plasma androgen concentrations are raised.

The Reproductive System

7

The study of the endocrinology of the male and female reproductive systems is a specialized field. However, many disorders can be assessed using the general principles of endocrine diagnosis based on a knowledge of normal function. This chapter deals only with such principles.

HYPOTHALAMIC–PITUITARY–GONADAL AXIS

The reproductive system is responsible, not only for the production of hormones, but also for maturation of the germ cells in the gonads. It is essential to understand the relations between hormones with respect to these two functions if the results of tests are to be correctly interpreted.

HYPOTHALAMIC HORMONES

The hypothalamus secretes two hormones concerned with the reproductive system:

- *gonadotrophin-releasing hormone (GnRH)*, which regulates the secretion of the pituitary gonadotrophins, luteinizing hormone (LH) and follicle stimulating hormone (FSH);
- *dopamine*, a neurotransmitter, which also controls prolactin secretion.

ANTERIOR PITUITARY HORMONES

The pituitary gonadotrophins (LH and FSH), secreted by basophil cells, control the function and secretion of hormones by the testes and ovaries. The secretion of GnRH, and consequently of LH and FSH, is pulsatile. Although there is only one releasing hormone, secretion of LH and FSH does not always occur in parallel and may be modified by feedback from the circulating concentrations of gonadal androgens or oestrogens. The actions of the gonadotrophins overlap:

- LH primarily stimulates the production of hormones by the gonads;
- FSH stimulates the development of the germ cells.

Prolactin, secreted by acidophil cells, is important during pregnancy and the postpartum period (p.**138**). It differs from all other pituitary hormones in the method of its control.

- secretion is *inhibited*, not stimulated, by dopamine; therefore impairment of hypothalamic control causes hyperprolactinaemia.
- secretion is regulated by a *short feedback loop* between pituitary prolactin and hypothalmic dopamine;
- Oestrogens enhance secretion; circulating prolactin concentrations are normally higher in women.

Although thyrotrophin-releasing hormone (TRH) stimulates secretion of prolactin, as well as of thyroid-stimulating hormone (TSH), this action does not seem to be of physiological importance; it may, however, be important in pathological conditions (p.**139**).

Similar factors affect prolactin and growth hormone (GH) secretion. Secretion of both increases during sleep and in response to physical and psychological stress.

Abnormally high plasma concentrations may affect gonadal function.

TESTICULAR HORMONES

Testosterone is secreted by the *Leydig cells*, which lie in the interstitial tissue of the testes between the seminiferous tubules. Its production is stimulated by LH and it, in turn, inhibits LH secretion by negative feedback.

Inhibin is a hormone produced by the *Sertoli cells*, part of the basement membrane of the seminiferous tubules, during germ cell differentiation and spermatogenesis. These processes require testosterone and are stimulated by FSH. Inhibin controls FSH secretion by negative feedback (Fig. 7.1).

Testosterone is involved in sexual differentiation, development of secondary sexual characteristics, spermatogenesis and anabolism. In the male, the effects of testosterone depend on intracellular conversion to the even more potent androgen, *dihydrotestosterone* by the enzyme 5α-reductase in target cells (Fig. 7.2).

Testosterone and, to a lesser extent, oestradiol circulate bound to a carrier protein, *sex-hormone binding globulin* (SHBG) as well as albumin. As with other hormones, only the free fraction is metabolically active.

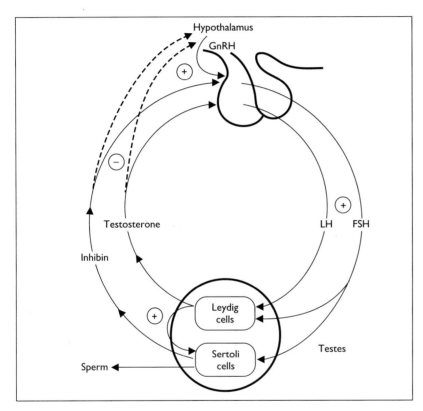

Fig. 7.1 The effect of gonadotrophins, LH and FSH, on testicular function. LH stimulates testosterone production from the Leydig cells. The Sertoli cells are involved in germ cell differentiation and spermatogenesis. These functions depend on testosterone and are stimulated by FSH.

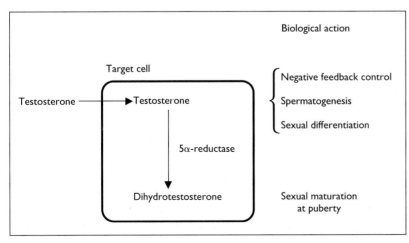

Fig. 7.2 The relation between the biological actions of testosterone and dihydrotestosterone.

OVARIAN HORMONES

Oestrogens, progesterone and *androgens* are secreted by the ovarian follicles of the ovaries, which consist of germ cells (ova) surrounded by granulosa and theca cells. Androgens (C_{19} steroids), synthesized by theca cells, are converted into oestrogens (C_{18} steroids) in the granulosa cells, a process which involves aromatization of the A ring and the loss of the C-19 methyl group (Fig. 6.1; p.**119**). Oestradiol is the most important ovarian oestrogen. The liver and subcutaneous fat convert ovarian and adrenal androgens to oestrone. Both oestradiol and oestrone are metabolized to the relatively inactive oestriol

Oestrogens are essential for the development of female secondary sex characteristics and for normal menstruation. Their concentration in plasma in children is very low.

Androstenedione is the main androgen secreted by the ovaries. It is converted to oestrone and to the more active testosterone in extraovarian tissue. A small amount of testosterone is secreted directly by the ovaries. Plasma concentrations in women are about a tenth of those in men.

Progesterone is secreted by the corpus luteum during the luteal phase of the menstrual cycle. It prepares the endometrium of the uterus to receive a fertilized ovum and is necessary for the maintenance of early pregnancy.

SEXUAL DEVELOPMENT FROM CONCEPTION

The complex series of events leading to the development of sexual competence depends on many steps occurring at the correct time. The following simplified account aims to provide a background for the discussion of abnormalities of the system.

Chromosomal sex is determined at fertilization by the chromosomes present in the ovum and sperm, each of which contributes 22 autosomes and one sex chromosome, X or Y (p.**350**). Normal males have a 46,XY

karyotype, and normal females 46,XX. Abnormalities occurring at this stage may result in defective gonadal development, as occurs in Klinefelter's syndrome in males (47,XXY) or Turner's syndrome in females (45,X).

The sex chromosomes determine whether the primitive gonads become testes or ovaries. The development and disorders of gonadal function in the male and female will be considered separately.

THE MALE

Development of Male Characteristics

In the presence of the Y chromosome the fetal gonads develop into testes at about seven weeks gestation. The testes secrete:

- a factor that causes degeneration of the potential female genitalia;
- testosterone that stimulates development of the potential male internal genitalia.

The intracellular conversion of testosterone to dihydrotestosterone by the enzyme 5α-reductase is essential for the development of male external genitalia. If this enzyme is deficient, varying degrees of feminization may occur, causing male pseudo-hermaphroditism. Genetic males with almost complete tissue insensitivity to the action of testosterone develop female sex characteristics despite normal testosterone secretion (*testicular feminization syndrome*). The very rare true hermaphrodite has both testicular and ovarian tissue.

PUBERTY

During childhood the rate of secretion of gonadotrophins from the anterior pituitary gland is low. As puberty approaches the pulse amplitude and frequency of LH secretion in particular increase. Initially, this occurs during sleep but later continues throughout the day. Leydig cell function and testosterone secretion increase and so stimulate the development of secondary male characteristics.

Gonadotrophin secretion also stimulates meiosis of previously dormant germ cells in the seminiferous tubules and so the production of sperm.

- *Deficient* secretion of either pituitary or gonadal hormones may cause *delayed puberty*.
- *Premature* secretion of gonadotrophins may cause early (*true precocious*) puberty.
- *Abnormally high* androgen secretion, such as from gonadal tumours, leads to the development of secondary sex characteristics before maturation of the testes (*pseudoprecocious puberty*).

The Adult Male

The male germ cells produce spermatozoa continuously after puberty. Spermatogenesis is dependent on both normal Sertoli cell function and on testosterone secretion by Leydig cells. Therefore, both LH and FSH are needed for normal spermatogenesis, but

testosterone secretion can occur in the absence of normal seminiferous tubules.

Disorders of Gonadal Function in Males

Gonadal dysfunction in men may present with the symptoms of androgen deficiency, infertility or with both. Hormone measurement has a limited but important role in the assessment of these patients. Only the principles will be discussed here.

Androgen deficiency is the result of impaired testosterone secretion by Leydig cells. The patient may present with delayed puberty or with regression of previously established male characteristics that are dependent on testosterone (hair distribution, potency and libido). There may be:

- *primary testicular dysfunction*, in which case the low plasma testosterone concentration is accompanied by raised plasma LH concentrations (hypergonadotrophic hypogonadism);
- *dysfunction secondary pituitary or hypothalamic disease*, with low plasma LH concentrations (hypogonadotrophic hypogonadism).

Infertility may be caused by androgen deficiency, but most infertile men have normal plasma androgen concentrations. Sertoli cell function is dependent on both FSH and on testosterone produced locally. Semen analysis is the most important investigation for male infertility. However, biochemical tests may sometimes help:

- if the cause is primary testicular failure the plasma testosterone concentration is low, and reduced inhibin production by Sertoli cells causes a rise in FSH concentrations;
- if there is evidence of a failure of spermatogenesis the plasma FSH concentration should be measured. If the cause is secondary to anterior pituitary failure, both plasma testosterone and FSH concentrations are low;

• if Leydig cell function is normal neither testosterone nor LH secretion is affected.

Hyperprolactinaemia is much less common in males than in females, but its presence may indicate a pituitary tumour.

Clinical features may suggest a chromosomal abnormality, such as Klinefelter's syndrome.

The investigation of male gonadal dysfunction is considered on p.**154**.

THE FEMALE

Development of Female Characteristics

In the absence of a Y chromosome the fetus starts to develop female characteristics at about 12 weeks of gestation. If androgens are produced at this stage as, for example, in congenital adrenal hyperplasia (p.**128**), masculinization of the external genitalia may occur (*female pseudohermaphroditism*).

Proliferation of fetal germ cells produces several million oocytes. By late fetal life all the germ cells have degenerated and no more oocytes can be produced. Those present enter the first stage of meiosis and their numbers decline throughout the rest of the intrauterine period and childhood; the inability to replenish them explains the limit to the span of reproductive life in women in contrast to the continuous ability of men to produce sperm. If the rate of decline is abnormally high there is premature menopause.

PUBERTY

At the onset of puberty gonadotrophin secretion increases, as it does in the male. Ovarian oestrogen secretion rises and stimulates the development of female secondary sex characteristics and the onset of menstruation (menarche).

As in the male, abnormal hormone secretion may cause delayed puberty, true precocious puberty, or pseudoprecocious puberty (p.**135**).

The Adult Female

NORMAL GONADAL FUNCTION

At puberty the ovaries contain between 100 000 and 200 000 primordial follicles. During each menstrual cycle a small number develop but only one reaches maturation, with extrusion of the ovum from the ovary (ovulation), and is ready for fertilization. The menstrual cycle is regulated by changing hormone concentrations (Fig. 7.3) and by changing sensitivity of ovarian tissue.

FOLLICULAR (PREOVULATORY) PHASE

At the beginning of the menstrual cycle ovarian follicles are undeveloped and plasma oestradiol concentrations are low. LH and FSH secretion increases because of diminished negative feedback by oestrogens.

LH and FSH together cause growth of a group of follicles. By about the seventh day of the cycle one follicle becomes especially sensitive to FSH and matures while the rest atrophy. LH also stimulates oestradiol secretion, the plasma concentrations of which rise steadily. This stimulates the regeneration of the endometrium.

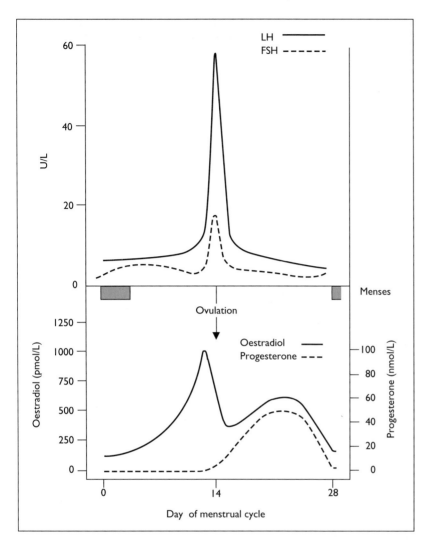

Fig. 7.3 Example of plasma hormone concentrations during the menstrual cycle.

OVULATION

The dominant follicle develops rapidly and plasma oestradiol concentrations rise; this triggers a surge of LH release from the anterior pituitary gland by 'positive feedback'. Ovulation occurs about 16 hours later.

LUTEAL (POSTOVULATORY OR SECRETORY) PHASE

The high concentration of LH after ovulation stimulates the granulosa cells of the ruptured follicle to luteinize and to form the *corpus luteum* which synthesizes and secretes progesterone and oestradiol. Progesterone is the principal hormone of the luteal phase and prepares the endometrium for the implantation of the fertilized ovum.

The subsequent events depend on whether the released ovum is fertilized. If it is not, the corpus luteum regresses and plasma ovarian hormone concentrations fall; the menstrual cycle takes its course with sloughing of the endometrium and menstrual bleeding. As the plasma ovarian hormone concentrations fall, the concentrations of LH and FSH in plasma begin to rise and the cycle recommences. If fertilization does occur pregnancy may super-vene.

Interpretation of plasma sex hormone concentrations must be made in relation to the stage of the cycle. It may be important to establish whether a patient, complaining of infertility, has ovulated, either spontaneously or as a result of treatment to induce ovulation. The plasma progesterone concentration should be measured on a blood sample taken during the second half of the menstrual cycle. A value within the reference range for the time of the cycle is good presumptive evidence of ovulation (Fig. 7.3), whereas a value in the range expected in the follicular phase indicates the absence of a corpus luteum, and therefore of ovulation. Ovulation may also be detected by ultrasound examination of the ovaries.

Progesterone secretion is associated with a rise in body temperature, which may be monitored serially to determine the time of ovulation.

Plasma prolactin concentrations do not change cyclically during the menstrual cycle.

PREGNANCY AND LACTATION

If the ovum is fertilized it may implant in the endometrium which has been prepared by progesterone during the luteal phase. The function of LH is taken over by *human chorionic gonadotrophin (HCG)*, produced by the chorion and developing placenta. HCG is similar in structure and action to LH and prevents the involution of the corpus luteum as circulating pituitary gonadotrophin concentrations fall. Consequently, plasma oestrogen and progesterone concentrations continue to rise and endometrial sloughing is prevented. After the first trimester these hormones are produced by the placenta. *During pregnancy the predominant oestrogen is oestriol.*

Prolactin secretion increases progressively after the eighth week of pregnancy, probably because of the high plasma oestrogen concentrations. At term it may be 10 to 20 times that of non-pregnant women.

Prolactin, oestrogens, progesterone and (human) placental lactogen (HPL, p.**142**) stimulate breast development in preparation for lactation. High plasma oestrogen concentrations inhibit milk secretion. Lactation can only start when plasma concentrations fall after delivery of the placenta.

Initially lactation depends on prolactin and in its absence, for example, due to pituitary damage by infarction or to inhibition of prolactin secretion by administration of bromocriptine, milk production ceases. Suckling stimulates secretion of the hormone but, even during lactation, plasma prolactin concentrations fall progressively postpartum and reach non-pregnant levels after two or three months. Apart from the effects on the breast, the high plasma concentration of prolactin interferes with gonadotrophin-ovarian function and produces a period of relative infertility.

THE MENOPAUSE

The menopause occurs when all the follicles have atrophied. Plasma concentrations of oestrogens fall and those of FSH and, to a lesser extent, LH increase after removal of the negative feedback to the pituitary. These findings are identical with those of primary gonadal failure (p.**153**).

Disorders of Gonadal Function in Females

Gonadal dysfunction in women may present with any or all of the following:

- delayed puberty and primary amenorrhoea;
- infertility with or without amenorrhoea;
- hirsutism;
- virilism.

The investigation of these disturbances cannot be covered in detail here and the student should consult a textbook on endocrinology.

AMENORRHOEA

Amenorrhoea is defined as the absence of menstruation; it may be due to hormonal abnormalities. If there is ovarian failure pituitary gonadotrophin concentrations in plasma are high (*hypergonadotrophic hypogonadism*); if the cause is in the hypothalamus or anterior pituitary gland gonadotrophin secretion is reduced (*hypogonadotrophic hypogonadism*). Amenorrhoea may be classified as either primary or secondary; note that 'primary' and 'secondary' used here have different meanings from those used in other endocrine disorders.

- *Primary amenorrhoea occurs when the patient has never menstruated* and is most commonly associated with delayed puberty. The age of the menarche is very variable. Extensive investigation should probably be postponed until the age of 18 unless there are other clinical features either of endocrine disturbances, such as hirsutism and virilization, or of chromosomal abnormalities. Turner's syndrome and testicular feminization (p.**135**) usually present with primary amenorrhoea.
- *Secondary amenorrhoea occurs when previously established menstrual cycles have stopped* and is most commonly due to physiological factors such as pregnancy and the menopause. Other causes include severe illness, excess or rapid weight loss for any reason, or stopping oral contraceptives. These causes should be considered before extensive and potentially dangerous investigations are started. Endocrine disorders, such as hyperprolactinaemia, hyperthyroidism, Cushing's syndrome and acromegaly may present with amenorrhoea.

Hyperprolactinaemia is an important cause of amenorrhoea and infertility. High plasma prolactin concentrations inhibit the normal pulsatile release of GnRH and inhibit gonadal steroid hormone synthesis directly. Plasma gonadotrophin and oestrogen concentrations are therefore low and the symptoms of oestrogen deficiency may occur. About a third of patients with hyperprolactinaemia have galactorrhoea.

The finding of hyperprolactinaemia should be interpreted with caution. Samples for prolactin estimations should be taken at least two to three hours after waking in order to eliminate the misleading elevated plasma concentrations found during sleep; the stress of venepuncture may also cause prolactin secretion.

Pathological causes of hyperprolactinaemia include:

- *a prolactin-secreting microadenoma of the pituitary gland*, the most important cause. Patients with no apparent cause of hyperprolactinaemia should be examined at regular intervals and lateral skull X-rays, and possibly CT scanning, of the pituitary fossa should be performed, in case an obvious pituitary adenoma develops. The higher the plasma prolactin concentration the greater the likelihood that a tumour is present;
- *failure of hypothalamic inhibitory factors to reach the anterior pituitary gland:*
    damage to the pituitary stalk by non-prolactin-secreting tumours of the pituitary gland or hypothalamus;
    surgical section of the pituitary stalk.
- *other pituitary tumours;*
- *drugs* such as:
    oestrogens;
    dopaminergic antagonists:
        phenothiazines;
        haloperidol;
        metoclopramide.
    drugs that deplete dopamine stores; these are less frequently prescribed than they used to be:
        methyldopa;
        reserpine.
- *chronic renal failure*, (possibly due to reduced plasma clearance);
- *severe primary hypothyroidism* (possibly due to anterior pituitary stimulation by high TRH concentrations).

The investigation of amenorrhoea is considered on p.**153**.

HIRSUTISM AND VIRILISM

Increased plasma free androgen concentrations, or increased tissue sensitivity to androgens, produce effects ranging from *increased hair growth (hirsutism)* to marked *masculinization (virilism)*. Testosterone is the most important androgen, although a marked increase in others may produce similar clinical symptoms. In normal women about half the plasma testosterone comes from the ovaries, both by direct secretion and by peripheral conversion of androstenedione. The rest is derived from peripheral conversion of adrenal androgens, androstenedione and dehydroepiandrosterone (DHA). Because of the extensive interconversion of androgens, the source of a slightly raised plasma testosterone concentration may be difficult to establish. In general, markedly raised plasma concentrations of DHA or DHAS indicate an adrenocortical origin, and of testosterone an ovarian origin.

The biological activity of testosterone depends on the plasma free hormone concentration. The plasma total concentration is also influenced by the concentration of the binding protein *sex-hormone binding globulin* (SHBG). Conditions associated with altered plasma concentrations of SHBG are shown in Table 7.1.

Hirsutism is defined as an *excessive growth of hair in a male distribution* and is common. Extensive investigations should not be started until the possibility of a familial or racial origin has been excluded. Plasma *testosterone* concentrations may be *slightly* raised but are often within the female reference range. However, the plasma concentration of free hormone may be significantly increased if that of SHBG is low. Causes include:

- *polycystic ovary syndrome.* This is a common cause of hirsutism. Presenting clinical symptoms may also include obesity, menstrual disturbances and infertility. Plasma testosterone concentrations are usually at the upper end of the female reference range. Because plasma SHBG

Table 7.1 Conditions associated with altered plasma levels of sex-hormone binding globulin (SHBG)

Increased SHBG	Decreased SHBG
Oestrogens	Androgens
Hyperthyroidism	Hypothyroidism
	Obesity

concentrations are reduced in obese individuals the plasma concentration of free testosterone is frequently increased. The plasma prolactin concentrations may also be high. Multiple small subcapsular ovarian cysts may be demonstrated on ultrasound scanning of the ovaries.

- *congenital adrenal hyperplasia* of late onset. This disorder may present with hirsutism, with or without amenorrhoea. It is most frequently caused by 21α-hydroxylase deficiency. The diagnosis may be confirmed by demonstrating raised plasma concentrations of 17α-hydroxyprogesterone, either under basal conditions or after stimulation by ACTH, and of testosterone.

Virilism is characterized by additional evidence of *excessive androgen secretion* such as an *enlarged clitoris* (clitoromegaly), increased hair growth of the male distribution, *receding temporal hair, deepening of the voice* and breast atrophy. It is uncommon but much more serious that hirsutism. It is always associated with increased plasma androgen concentrations. The main causes are:

- *ovarian tumours* (such as arrhenoblastomas and hilus-cell tumours) which secrete androgens, mainly testosterone;
- *adrenocortical disorders:*
    tumours, usually carcinomas;
    hyperplasia:
        pituitary-dependent Cushing's disease (rarely);
        congenital adrenal hyperplasia.

Plasma DHA and DHAS concentrations are increased.

SOME DRUG EFFECTS ON THE FEMALE HYPOTHALAMIC–PITUITARY GONADAL AXIS

Oral contraceptives contain synthetic oestrogens and/or progestogens. They suppress pituitary gonadotrophin secretion and therefore inhibit ovulation. Withdrawal mimics involution of the corpus luteum and results in menstrual bleeding.

Clomiphene blocks oestrogen receptors in the hypothalamus and so prevents negative feedback. It may stimulate gonadotrophin release even when circulating oestrogen concentrations are high. Clomiphene may be used to induce ovulation in patients with amenorrhoea or infertility.

Gonadotrophin treatment may be used if clomiphene fails to induce ovulation. Human menopausal gonadotrophin (FSH and LH, 'Pergonal') or pure FSH ('Metrodin') is given to mimic the follicular phase. This treatment may cause dangerous follicular enlargement due to hyperstimulation, or may stimulate many follicles and so cause multiple pregnancy. Treatment must therefore be monitored either by frequent plasma or urinary oestrogen estimations or by ovarian ultrasound examination. Human chorionic gonadotrophin (HCG) is then given to induce ovulation by mimicking the midcycle LH surge. Ovulation may be assessed by demonstrating rising plasma progesterone concentrations or by ultrasound. Gonadotrophins may also be used to stimulate the production of enough oocytes to enable them to be 'harvested' for use in *in vitro* fertilization (IVF) or gamete intrafallopian transfer (GIFT).

GnRH treatment is the treatment of choice for patients with infertility secondary to hypogonadotrophic hypogonadism. It is given subcutaneously in pulses, usually every 90 minutes, using a portable syringe pump. Continuous GnRH infusion suppresses pituitary gonadotrophin release and may be used to treat hormone dependent tumours, such as carcinoma of the prostate.

Bromocriptine may rapidly reduce high plasma prolactin concentrations, whatever the cause, to normal after which menstruation restarts and fertility is restored.

Monitoring Pregnancy

The change from the hormonal pattern of the luteal phase of the menstrual cycle into that of pregnancy has been outlined (p.**138**). The changes that occur during pregnancy fall into two types:

- substances produced by the fetus or placenta may be measured to detect fetal abnormalities or to monitor the progress of the pregnancy;
- changes in the maternal plasma that result from pregnancy which need to be recognized so as to avoid misdiagnosis. There may be similar changes in the newborn infant, who has been exposed *in utero* to the mother's hormonal background.

Fetoplacental Products

Substances secreted by the fetoplacental unit may be detected throughout pregnancy and are usually measured in those patients known to be at risk of miscarriage. Changes in the composition of maternal plasma or urine often reflect changes in fetal and placental metabolism. Such sampling is safe and simple. Occasionally there are indications for testing amniotic fluid obtained by amniocentesis. However, the ability to visualize the fetus using ultrasound has reduced the need for this invasive procedure.

MONITORING PREGNANCY (PLACENTAL FUNCTION)

Human choriogonadotrophin (HCG) secretion by the placenta reaches a peak at about 13 weeks of pregnancy and then falls. The fetoplacental unit then takes over hormone production and secretion of both oestrogen and progesterone rises rapidly.

Relatively crude tests for plasma or urinary HCG, which give positive results at one or two weeks after the first missed menstrual period, are most commonly used to diagnose pregnancy. However, by using more sensitive immunoassay techniques plasma HCG may be detected soon after implantation of the ovum and before the first missed period. Such early diagnosis may be of value if an ectopic pregnancy is suspected, or if the patient is being treated for infertility.

Serial HCG measurements may be used to assess the progress of early pregnancy; single values are difficult to interpret because of the wide reference range. As a rough guide levels should double in two days.

Human placental lactogen (HPL) is a peptide hormone of unknown biological function synthesized by the placenta. It is detectable in maternal plasma after about the eighth week of gestation and has been used to assess the likelihood of threatened abortion and to monitor late pregnancy.

Assessment of fetal well-being and of placental function may indicate the need for early obstetric intervention. *Biochemical tests* during late pregnancy, such as estimation of placental total oestrogen (oestriol) and HPL output, *have largely been replaced by ultrasound examination.*

Detection of Fetal Abnormalities

Some fetal abnormalities may be diagnosed by tests carried out on maternal plasma or amniotic fluid. Amniocentesis is a procedure by which amniotic fluid is obtained through a needle inserted into the uterus through the maternal abdominal wall and is usually carried out after about 14 weeks gestation. The procedure carries a small risk to the fetus. Both the safety and the reliability of the procedure can be improved if combined with ultrasound examination in order to locate the position of the fetus, placenta and maternal bladder. It should *only be performed for very strong clinical indications and if the diagnosis cannot be made by noninvasive procedures.* Analytical results may be dangerously misleading if, for example, the specimen is contaminated with maternal or fetal blood or maternal urine, is not fresh or is not properly preserved. Close liaison between the clinician and the laboratory staff helps to ensure the suitability of the specimen and the speed of the assay.

Amniotic fluid is probably derived from both maternal and fetal sources, but its value in reflecting abnormalities arises from its intimate contact with the fetus and from the increasing contribution of fetal urine in later pregnancy.

DETECTION OF NEURAL TUBE DEFECTS

Alpha-fetoprotein (AFP) is a low molecular weight glycoprotein synthesized mainly in the fetal yolk sac and liver. Its production is almost completely repressed in the normal adult. AFP can diffuse slowly through capillary membranes and appears in the fetal urine, and hence in the amniotic fluid, and in maternal plasma. Severe fetal neural tube defects, such as open spina bifida and anencephaly, are associated with abnormally high concentrations in these fluids. The reason for this is not clear but the protein may leak from the exposed neural tube vessels. Causes of raised AFP concentration in amniotic fluid and maternal plasma include:

- multiple pregnancy;
- serious fetal abnormalities:
  neural tube defects;
  exomphalos.

In some countries all pregnant women attending for antenatal care have plasma AFP concentrations measured between 16 and 18 weeks of gestation to screen for the presence of a fetus with a neural tube defect. The gestational age should be confirmed by ultrasound, which should also exclude multiple pregnancy as a cause of high concentrations. Positive results must be confirmed on a fresh sample and, if still high and if the diagnosis has not been confirmed by ultrasound, should be followed by AFP estimation on amniotic fluid. This is a more precise diagnostic test and yields fewer false positive results than plasma assays if sampling is properly performed. It should be reserved for subjects known to be at risk either because of a family history of neural tube defects, or because of the finding of a high concentration in maternal plasma with a normal or equivocal ultrasound scan. Amniocentesis should not usually be performed for this purpose unless the parents are willing to consider termination of pregnancy if the result is positive.

Amniotic fluid acetylcholinesterase assay may be used to detect many serious fetal malformations, including neural tube defects and exomphalos. It gives reliable results up to about 23 weeks of gestation. The interpretation of the result is less dependent on fetal age than that of AFP, but is equally invalidated by contamination with fetal or maternal blood. The assay is less widely available than that for AFP.

DETECTION OF DOWN'S SYNDROME

A low maternal plasma AFP, and a raised HCG, concentration, measured between the 16 and 18 weeks of gestation, is associated with an increased risk of the fetus having Down's syndrome (p.**355**). The use of this combination of tests to screen for the congenital disorder is available in specialized laboratories because, at the time of writing, the investigation is still under evaluation.

DETECTION OF OTHER FETAL ABNORMALITIES

Chromosomal abnormalities and some inborn errors of metabolism may be detected by cytogenetic, biochemical or enzymatic assays on cells cultured from amniotic fluid or after biopsy of chorionic villi. These tests are performed only in special centres and only on subjects with a family history of a genetic condition.

ASSESSMENT OF FETOMATERNAL BLOOD GROUP INCOMPATIBILITY

Rhesus or other blood group incompatibility has effects on the fetus which may be assessed by measuring amniotic fluid concentrations of bilirubin in conjunction with maternal antibody titres. Normally bilirubin concentrations in amniotic fluid decrease during the last half of pregnancy. The concentrations at any stage correlate with the severity of haemolysis. Used with tests of fetal maturity, the optimum time for induction of labour or the need for intrauterine transfusion may be assessed.

ASSESSMENT OF FETAL LUNG MATURITY

Examination of amniotic fluid may be useful to assess pulmonary maturity. Immature lungs do not expand normally at birth and may cause neonatal *respiratory distress syndrome* (*hyaline membrane disease*) with the need for respiratory support (p.**341**). It is therefore important to have evidence of pulmonary maturity before labour is induced.

At about 32 weeks of gestation the cells lining the fetal alveolar walls start to synthesize a surface tension lowering complex ('surfactant'), 90 per cent of which is the phospholipid, lecithin, which contains palmitic acid. Surfactant is probably washed from, or secreted by, the alveolar walls into the surrounding amniotic fluid, in which both lecithin and palmitic acid concentrations steadily increase. The concentration of lecithin, relative to another lipid, sphingomyelin, which remains constant in amniotic fluid, can be measured. A rise in the *lecithin/sphingomyelin (L/S)* ratio may help determine pulmonary maturity. Other estimates used have included total lecithin and total palmitic acid concentrations. The predictive value of all these parameters is similar. This test is rarely indicated now as steroids, which induce surfactant synthesis, are usually given to those patients who have premature rupture of the membranes.

MATERNAL BIOCHEMICAL CHANGES IN PREGNANCY

The concentrations of many plasma constituents are affected by steroid hormones. For example, the reference ranges of plasma urate and iron differ in males and females after puberty. Therefore, it is not surprising to find that during pregnancy, the very high circulating concentrations of oestrogens and progesterone alter the concentrations of many substances in plasma (Table 7.2).

The plasma concentrations of many specific carrier proteins increase during pregnancy. If this fact is not recognized an erroneous diagnosis may be made. In most cases the rise in the concentration of the carrier protein is accompanied by a proportional increase of the substance bound to it, without any change in the unbound free fraction. Because the protein-bound fraction is a transport form and because, in all cases, it is the free substance that is physiologically active, this rise in concentration is of importance in the interpretation of the results of such assays as those of plasma *thyroxine.*

Many of these changes may also be found in newborn infants and in subjects taking oral contraceptives, particularly those with a high oestrogen content.

Other changes in maternal plasma are due to progressive haemodilution by fluid retained during pregnancy. This is maximal at about the 30th week and the effects are most evident in reduced concentrations of *albumin*, and of *calcium*, which is bound to albumin. These changes are more marked in pre-eclamptic toxaemia, in which fluid retention may be greater than normal.

Renal *glycosuria* is common both in pregnancy and in subjects taking oral contraceptives. The glomerular filtration rate increases by about 50 per cent during

Table 7.2 Some biochemical changes that occur during pregnancy and that may confuse the diagnosis

Test	Effect	Comment
Plasma		
Total T_4*	Increased	Increased TBG. Free T_4 usually normal
Cortisol*	Increased	Increased CBG. Free cortisol probably normal
Transferrin or TIBC*	Increased ⎫	
Iron*	Increased ⎬	See Chapter 20
Alkaline phosphatase	Increased	Placental isoenzyme
Total protein and albumin	Decreased	Dilution by fluid retention
Urea and urate	Decreased	Anabolism due to fetal growth and increased GFR
Urine		
Glucose	Glycosuria	Increased GFR

*These changes may also occur in women taking oestrogen oral contraceptives.

pregnancy and glycosuria may partly be due to an increased glucose load in normal tubules.

The positive protein and purine balance during growth of the fetus, and the increase in glomerular filtration rate that occurs during pregnancy, result in lowered maternal plasma urea and urate concentrations. These findings are of little clinical significance, but must be recognized to avoid diagnostic confusion. A raised plasma *urate* concentration may be found in patients with pre-eclamptic toxaemia.

Plasma *alkaline phosphatase* activity rises during the last three months of pregnancy due to the presence of the placental iso-enzyme (p.**306**) and should not be misinterpreted. Placental alkaline phosphatase does not cross the placenta and therefore it is not present in the plasma of the newborn infant.

DETECTION AND FOLLOW-UP OF TROPHOBLASTIC TUMOURS

Trophoblastic tumours (*hydatidiform mole, choriocarcinoma*), which may follow abnormal pregnancy or a miscarriage and some *teratomas*, secrete HCG. For diagnostic purposes the simple pregnancy tests are usually adequate but they are not sensitive enough for follow up studies. HCG estimation in plasma or urine by sensitive tests allows early detection and treatment of recurrence. It will not differentiate pregnancy from recurrence of a tumour because in both cases plasma HCG concentrations rise.

Summary

Reproductive System

1. The secretion of gonadal hormones and the development of the germ cells are controlled by pituitary gonadotrophins, LH and FSH. These, in turn, are influenced by hypothalamic-releasing factors and by circulating gonadal hormone levels by negative feedback.
2. The main gonadal hormones are testosterone, secreted by the Leydig cells of the testes, and oestradiol, secreted by the cells of the ovarian follicles. There is extensive interconversion of these hormones with androgens secreted from the adrenal cortex.
3. In the male LH stimulates testosterone secretion from the testicular Leydig cells, and FSH stimulates spermatogenesis. Testicular failure may be confined to failure of spermatogenesis (raised FSH only) or may also involve the Leydig cells when plasma concentrations of testosterone are low and those of both LH and FSH are raised.
4. In the female, cyclical hormonal changes prepare the endometrium for implantation of a fertilized ovum. In the first half of the menstrual cycle LH and FSH stimulate ovarian follicle development and oestrogen secretion. A mid-cycle LH surge induces ovulation from one follicle, which is converted into a corpus luteum secreting

oestrogens and progesterone. In the absence of successful implantation the corpus luteum involutes and, as hormone concentrations fall, there is endometrial breakdown and shedding (menstruation). If implantation occurs the developing placenta produces HCG, which maintains the corpus luteum and prevents menstruation.

5. Plasma gonadal hormone concentrations must be interpreted in relation to the stage of the menstrual cycle.

6. In primary ovarian failure, and at the menopause, plasma oestrogen concentrations are low and gonadotrophin concentrations are high (loss of negative feedback). In secondary ovarian failure both oestrogen and gonadotrophin concentrations are low.

7. Hyperprolactinaemia is commonly due to a pituitary adenoma. In females it may cause amenorrhoea and infertility and is sometimes accompanied by galactorrhoea. Reducing prolactin secretion by bromocriptine restores fertility.

8. Gonadal hormones and gonadotrophin estimations are of value in:

- detection of ovulation;
- monitoring of treatment designed to induce ovulation;
- assessment of amenorrhoea;
- evaluation of hypogonadism and infertility;
- evaluation of delayed puberty.

Pregnancy

1. The measurement of HCG is of value in diagnosing pregnancy and in monitoring the progress during the early stages in selected cases.

2. Tests on amniotic fluid may be used to assess fetal development. These include:

- α-fetoprotein (AFP), which is raised in cases of severe neural tube defect. Maternal plasma AFP concentrations may also be abnormally high;
- bilirubin, to assess the severity of maternofetal blood group incompatibility;
- the lecithin/sphingomyelin (L/S) ratio, or similar assay, to assess fetal lung maturity.

3. Several biochemical parameters alter in maternal plasma and urine during pregnancy, and in the newborn infant. Amongst the most obvious is the increase in carrier protein, thyroxine-binding globulin (TBG), which causes increases in plasma total thyroxine concentrations. It is important to recognize these, and other changes, as physiological rather than pathological.

*I*NVESTIGATION OF PITUITARY, ADRENAL AND GONADAL DISORDERS

This section includes the investigations covered in the last three chapters because pituitary disorders, particularly hypofunction, may present with features of adrenal or gonadal deficiency.

SPECIMEN COLLECTION

The laboratory should always be consulted before any complex investigation or uncommon test is performed, in order to check details of specimen collection and handling and whether there are local variations in test protocols. This should also ensure a more efficient and speedy analytical service.

Most hormones are stable in blood for several hours or even days. However, others, including those listed below must be kept cool and sent to the laboratory without delay; these include:

Insulin	Renin	ACTH
PTH	Calcitonin	

Gut peptides (p.**245**) must be collected into special tubes containing trasylol which prevents protein digestion.

The time of sampling must always be recorded on the request form and on the specimen.

FACTORS AFFECTING PLASMA CORTISOL CONCENTRATIONS

Plasma cortisol is usually measured by immunoassay, in which the antibody may cross-react with other steroids or drugs. Examples of factors that may affect results are:

- hydrocortisone (cortisol) and cortisone (converted to cortisol by metabolism);
- prednisolone, which will contribute to the 'cortisol' concentration using most immunoassay methods. It is recommended either that the patient is prescribed dexam-ethasone or that the prednisolone is gradually reduced and stopped for about three days before sampling. However this may not always be possible;
- dexamethasone, which does not affect the plasma assay, but metabolites of which may interfere with some immunoassay methods in urine;
- oestrogens and some oral contraceptives that increase the plasma CBG concentration, and therefore protein-bound cortisol concentration.

PROCEDURE FOR REPEATED SAMPLING

For many 'dynamic' tests of endocrine function several blood samples should be taken over a short period of time. Repeated venepuncture is unpleasant for the patient and may cause enough stress to affect the results. Insertion of an indwelling needle or cannula helps to minimize these problems and enables intravenous therapy to be given without delay if there should be an untoward reaction, such as hypoglycaemia. We recommend the following procedure:

- a needle or cannula, at least as large as a 19G, is inserted into a vein at a site that preferably will not be subjected to movement, especially flexion, and secured in position with adhesive strapping;
- isotonic saline is infused slowly, or the cannula flushed with sodium citrate, to keep the needle open. Heparin should not be used because it interferes with some assays;
- the first specimen should not be taken for at least 30 minutes after insertion of the needle, so that stress-induced elevation of hormones may fall to basal concentrations.

All samples may be taken through this needle as follows:

- disconnect the saline infusion, or use a three way tap between the infusion set and the needle;
- aspirate and discard about 2 ml of the saline– or citrate–blood mixture, which will dilute the specimen;
- using a different syringe aspirate the specimen for the hormone assay;
- reconnect and restart the saline flow.

Investigation of Suspected Hypopituitarism

Deficiency of pituitary hormones causes hypofunction of the target endocrine glands. Investigation aims to confirm such deficiency, to exclude disease of the target gland and then to test pituitary hormone secretion after maximal stimulation of the gland.

1. Measure plasma concentrations of:

- LH, FSH and oestradiol (female) or testosterone (male);
- total or free T_4 and TSH;
- prolactin, to test for hypothalamic or pituitary stalk involvement;
- cortisol at 09.00 hours, to assess the risk of adrenocortical insufficiency during later testing.

2. If the plasma concentration of the target gland hormone is low and the trophic hormone is raised, investigate the affected target gland.
3. If the plasma concentrations of both the target gland and trophic hormones are low or low normal, proceed to a combined hypothalamic–pituitary stimulation test.
4. Investigate the pituitary region using radiological techniques, such as CT scanning.

COMBINED PITUITARY STIMULATION TEST

This test is potentially dangerous and must be done under direct medical supervision. It is contraindicated in patients with:

- ischaemic heart disease;
- epilepsy.

Glucose for intravenous administration must be immediately available in case severe symptomatic hypoglycaemia develops. Care should be taken not to induce hyperglycaemia during infusion, as it may cause hyperosmolality (p.**35**) *this is especially dangerous in children. After the test the patient must be given something to eat.*

The plasma concentrations of anterior pituitary hormones are measured after stimulation by stress, TRH and GnRH. Plasma cortisol is usually measured as an index of ACTH secretion; the entire hypothalamic–pituitary–target gland axis is therefore tested. It will be referred to again when discussing investigations of individual target glands. If glucose needs to be given, continue with the sampling. The hypoglycaemic stress has certainly been adequate to stimulate hormone secretion.

Procedure. After an overnight fast:

- insert an indwelling intravenous cannula;
- after at least 30 minutes, take basal samples;

Table 7.3 Protocol for a combined pituitary stimulation test

	Time (minutes) related to injection					
	-10	0	30	60	90	120
Insulin						
Glucose	√		√	√	√	√
Cortisol	√		√	√	√	√
Growth hormone	√		√	√	√	√
TRH						
T₄	√					
TSH	√		√	√		
Prolactin	√		√	√		
GnRH						
LH	√		√	√		
FSH	√		√	√		

√ indicates when blood should be analysed for specific hormones.

- inject soluble insulin in a high enough dose to lower plasma glucose concentrations to less than 2.5 mmol/L (45 mg/dl) and to cause symptomatic hypoglycaemia. The recommended dose of insulin must be adjusted for the patients bodyweight (BW) and for the suspected clinical condition under investigation.

    The usual dose is 0.15 U/kg BW.

    If either pituitary or adrenocortical hypofunction is suspected, or if a low fasting glucose concentration has been found, reduce the dose to 0.1 or 0.05 U/kg BW.

    If there is likely to be resistance to the action of insulin because of Cushing's syndrome, acromegaly or obesity, 0.2 or 0.4 U/kg BW may be needed.

- immediately inject 200 µg of TRH and 100 µg of GnRH.
- take blood samples at least 30, 60, 90 and 120 minutes after the injections and request hormone assays as indicated in Table 7.3.

Interpretation. Methods of hormone assay vary and results should not be compared with reference values issued by other laboratories. The following is intended as a guide only.

If hypoglycaemia has been adequate:

- plasma cortisol concentrations should rise by more than 200 nmol/L (7 µg/dl) and exceed 550 nmol/L (20 µg/dl).
- plasma GH concentrations should exceed 20 mU/L.
- plasma TSH concentrations should increase by at least 2 mU/L and exceed the upper limit of the reference range;
- plasma prolactin and gonadotrophin concentrations should rise significantly (p.**153**) for the reference range for the method.

If the plasma cortisol concentration does not rise a tetracosactrin test (p.**152**) should be performed to exclude primary adrenocortical hypofunction. In Cushing's syndrome, neither plasma cortisol nor GH concentrations rise.

Investigation of Suspected Growth Hormone Deficiency

The finding of a single high plasma GH concentration excludes deficiency. The initial sample should be taken when the highest physiological concentrations occur – immediately after exercise or during sleep.

An insulin stimulation test, similar to the combined stimulation test (see above), can be used if plasma GH concentrations do not exclude deficiency.

Interpretation. Plasma GH concentrations should rise and should exceed 20 mU/L.

At least two different types of tests should be performed on different occasions before GH deficiency is diagnosed.

Investigation of Suspected Acromegaly or Gigantism

A raised plasma GH concentration that fails to suppress normally in response to a rising plasma glucose concentration suggests autonomous hormone secretion. Basal plasma GH concentrations may be, but are not always, high enough to confirm the diagnosis. It saves time to start with a glucose suppression test.

GLUCOSE SUPPRESSION TEST

Procedure. After an overnight fast:

- Insert an indwelling intravenous cannula.
- After at least 30 minutes take basal samples for plasma glucose and GH estimation.
- The patient should drink 75 g of glucose dissolved in 300 ml of water, or an equivalent glucose load (p.**218**).

- Take samples for glucose and GH assay at 30, 60, 90 and 120 minutes after the glucose load has been taken.

Interpretation. In normal subjects, plasma GH concentrations fall to less than 4 mU/L. Although failure to suppress suggests acromegaly or gigantism, it may be found in some patients with severe liver or renal disease, in heroin addicts or in those taking L-dopa.

The plasma glucose concentrations may demonstrate impaired glucose tolerance (p.**219**).

Investigation of Suspected Cushing's Syndrome

Because of the serious nature of Cushing's syndrome, and because it may be treatable, the diagnosis must be excluded even when clinical features are only suggestive. Initial tests may exclude the diagnosis, but may yield some 'false positive' results.

Has the patient got Cushing's syndrome?

The following tests can be carried out initially without admitting the patient into hospital:

- *overnight dexamethasone suppression test.* Dexamethasone (2 mg) is given as a single oral dose at 23.00 hours. Plasma cortisol concentrations are measured on a specimen taken at 09.00 hours the next morning. Suppression is defined as a plasma cortisol of less than 190 nmol/L (7 mg/dl).
- *24 hour urinary free-cortisol estimation.* Cortisol is assayed on a 24-hour urine collection. An increased excretion is suggestive of Cushing's syndrome.

If these tests are normal, it is unlikely that the patient has Cushing's syndrome. If either is abnormal, or if there is a strong clinical suspicion, further tests should be carried out in hospital.

- *Loss of the circadian rhythm of plasma cortisol* may be demonstrated by measuring cortisol on blood samples collected at 09.00 hours and 23.00 hours. This test must be performed in hospital and may be followed by repeating the overnight dexamethasone test.

If all these tests are normal, follow up the patient in the outpatient clinic. The manifestations of Cushing's syndrome may be intermittent and tests may have to be repeated later.

If the results show abnormal cortisol secretion consider alternative causes such as:

- stress, even that associated with admission to hospital;
- alcoholism;
- endogenous depression.

If the latter is likely, perform an insulin stimulation test (p.**148**). A normal cortisol response to this suggests endogenous depression rather than Cushing's syndrome.

Once the diagnosis of Cushing's syndrome has been made, proceed to the next step.

What is the cause of Cushing's syndrome?

1. *Extremely high plasma cortisol or urinary free-cortisol concentrations* are suggestive of either adrenocortical carcinoma, especially if the patient is virilized, or of ectopic ACTH production. Investigate clinically and using other investigations, bearing in mind the possibility of carcinoma of the adrenal gland or bronchus. Severe hypokalaemic alkalosis suggests ectopic ACTH secretion.
2. *Estimate plasma ACTH concentrations.* Moderately raised plasma concentrations, even when within the upper limit of the reference range, are suggestive of either Cushing's disease or occult ectopic ACTH secretion. Very high plasma concentrations are found with overt ectopic ACTH secreting tumours, while in patients with adrenocortical tumours the plasma ACTH concentration is low. Remember that stress increases the plasma ACTH and cortisol concentrations.

3. *The high-dose dexamethasone suppression test* may distinguish between Cushing's disease and adrenocortical tumour or overt ectopic ACTH production.

Procedure. Dexamethasone (2 mg) is given orally every six hours for two days, starting at 09.00 hours. Plasma cortisol concentration is measured in specimens taken at 09.00 hours on the first and third days.

Interpretation. Anticonvulsant drugs, particularly phenytoin, may interfere with dexamethasone suppression tests. They induce liver enzymes that increase the rate of metabolism of dexamethasone. Plasma concentrations may therefore be too low to suppress the feedback centre.

Suppression is defined as a plasma cortisol concentration of less than 50 per cent of previously measured values. Suppression suggests either pituitary-dependent Cushing's disease or an occult ACTH secreting tumour. Failure to suppress suggests either an adrenocortical tumour (low ACTH concentrations) or overt ectopic ACTH production (very high ACTH concentrations).

4. *Estimate plasma androgens,* especially DHAS, if there is virilization. High plasma concentrations suggest adrenocortical carcinoma.

The distinction between occult ectopic ACTH secreting tumours and Cushing's disease may be difficult. CT scans of the chest and abdomen may detect a tumour.

Investigation of Suspected Adrenal Hypofunction

SUSPECTED ADDISONIAN CRISIS

1. Take blood *before starting treatment* for immediate plasma urea and electrolyte estimations, and for cortisol which can be stored and analysed later.

2. Start steroid treatment at once. Do not wait for the laboratory results.

Interpretion. Hyponatraemia, hyperkalaemia and uraemia, although compatible with an Addisonian crisis, are common in many clinically similar acute conditions. Treat appropriately (see Chapters 2 and 3). The plasma cortisol concentration may be estimated later:

- if the cortisol is very high an Addisonian crisis is excluded;
- if it is very low or undetectable, and if there is no reason to suspect severe CBG deficiency, for example due to the nephrotic syndrome (p.**17**), an Addisonian crisis is confirmed.

Plasma cortisol concentrations, which would be 'normal' under basal conditions, may be inappropriately low for the degree of stress. Perform a short tetracosactrin test (see below).

SUSPECTED CHRONIC ADRENAL HYPOFUNCTION

1. Measure plasma cortisol concentrations. A high concentration at any time of day excludes Addison's disease.
2. If the plasma cortisol concentrations are equivocal, perform a short tetracosactrin test. A normal result excludes Addison's disease and makes long-standing secondary adrenal insufficiency unlikely. Prolonged ACTH deficiency causes reversible adrenal insensitivity to trophic stimulation.
3. If the results of the short tetracosactrin test are equivocal, send a blood specimen to the laboratory before proceeding further, in case plasma ACTH assay seems indicated later (see 7).
4. Admit the patient to hospital and perform a five-hour tetracosactrin test. A normal result excludes primary adrenal hypofunction; if there was a subnormal response to the short tetracosactrin test it suggests secondary adrenal hypofunction.

5. If doubt remains perform a three-day tetra-cosactrin test. The same impaired response to the short, five-hour and three-day tetra-cosactrin tests would confirm *primary adrenal hypofunction*.
6. An increasing response to the short, five-hour and three-day tetracosactrin tests indicates gradual recovery of the adrenal cortex following prolonged lack of ACTH, and suggests *hypothalamic or pituitary hypofunction*. Perform a combined pituitary stimulation test (p.**148**).
7. If doubt remains, assay ACTH on the plasma specimen taken earlier. If the cortisol concentration is low or low normal:

   * *a high ACTH concentration confirms primary adrenal hypofunction*;
   * *a low ACTH concentration suggests secondary adrenal hypofunction*, and a combined pituitary stimulation test should be performed.

TETRACOSACTRIN TEST OF ADRENAL FUNCTION

Tetracosactrin is marketed as 'Synacthen' (Ciba).

Short Tetracosactrin Stimulation Test
Procedure. The patient should be resting quietly.

* Blood is taken for basal cortisol assay.
* 250 µg of tetracosactrin, dissolved in about 1 ml of sterile water or isotonic saline, is given by intramuscular injection.
* 30 and 45 minutes later blood is taken for cortisol assay.

Interpretation. Normally the plasma cortisol concentration increases by at least 200 nmol/L (7 µg/dl), to a concentration of at least 550 nmol/L (20 µg/dl).

Five-hour Tetracosactrin Stimulation Test
Procedure.

* Blood is taken for basal cortisol assay.
* 1 mg of depot tetracosactrin is injected intramuscularly.

* Blood is taken 1 and 5 hours later for cortisol assay.

Interpretation. Normally plasma cortisol concentrations rise to between 600 and 1300 nmol/L (22 and 46 µg/dl) at one hour and to between 1000 and 1800 nmol/L (37 and 66 µg/dl) at five hours.

Three-day Tetracosactrin Stimulation Test
Repeated injections of depot tetracosactrin are painful and may cause sodium and water retention. Therefore this test is contraindicated in those patients in whom sodium retention may be dangerous, such as those with congestive cardiac failure. The test is rarely indicated if a basal plasma ACTH concentration is known.

Procedure.

* 1 mg of depot tetracosactrin is given daily, at 09.00 hours, by intramuscular injection for three days.
* Plasma cortisol concentration is estimated in blood withdrawn five hours after each injection.

Interpretation. The plasma cortisol concentrations should rise to between 1000 and 1800 nmol/L (37 and 66 µg/dl) at five hours and remain in excess of this concentration for the duration of the test.

PATIENTS ON STEROID TREATMENT WITH SUSPECTED ADRENAL HYPOFUNCTION

It is not uncommon for patients to be treated before adrenal hypofunction has been proved. Steroids, such as hydrocortisone, may interfere with the assays and should be stopped. If there is a danger that this may precipitate an adrenal crisis stimulation tests may be performed while the biologically active dexamethasone, which does not interfere with the assays, is given. *Consult your laboratory staff to find out which steroids interfere with their assays.*

Investigation of Amenorrhoea

A full clinical assessment should be made and the patient should be questioned carefully to determine whether the amenorrhoea is primary or secondary. It may accompany any severe disease.

The aim of laboratory investigations is to detect hypogonadism and to distinguish between pituitary and ovarian causes. Before embarking on such investigations it is essential to test for pregnancy. If the pregnancy test is negative proceed as follows.

1. Measure plasma LH, FSH and oestradiol concentrations:

   - raised plasma gonadotrophin (especially FSH) with low oestradiol concentrations indicate ovarian failure. If the amenorrhoea is primary, chromosome studies are indicated;
   - normal plasma gonadotrophin with low oestradiol concentrations suggest the possibility of testicular ferminization syndrome. Plasma testosterone should be measured. A plasma concentration within the male reference range supports the diagnosis, which may be confirmed by chromosomal analysis;
   - low plasma oestradiol with low normal or low gonadotrophin concentrations suggest a hypothalamic or pituitary cause.

2. Measure the plasma prolactin concentration at least three hours after waking (p.**132**).

   - a high plasma concentration supports a hypothalamic or pituitary cause. Because prolactin concentrations respond variably to stress, a raised value should be confirmed on a specimen taken on a different occasion. Exclude drugs as a cause (p.**139**).

3. Perform a gonadotrophin-releasing hormone (GnRH) test:

   - a normal gonadotrophin response suggests a probable hypothalamic cause, perhaps involving only GnRH;

   - a subnormal response suggests a pituitary lesion.

4. Proceed to a combined pituitary stimulation test (p.**148**).

GONADOTROPHIN RELEASING HORMONE (GnRH) TEST

Synthetic GnRH stimulates the release of the gonadotrophins LH and FSH from the normal anterior pituitary gland.

Procedure.

- 100 µg of GnRH is given by rapid intravenous injection.
- Plasma LH and FSH concentrations are measured in blood drawn before and at 30 and 60 minutes after the injection.

Interpretation. In normal subjects plasma LH rises by at least 5 U/L, but this rise fails to occur in patients with pituitary hypofunction.

Other endocrine disorders such as hyperthyroidism and Cushing's syndrome must be considered as causes of amenorrhoea and, if necessary, excluded by appropriate tests. If there is hirsutism or virilism, proceed as below.

Investigation of Hirsutism and Virilism

The aim of investigation, after full clinical assessment, is to detect cases with significant elevation of plasma androgen concentrations and to identify the source as the ovary or the adrenal cortex.

Depending on the clinical presentation, some of the following plasma assays may help:

- total- and assessment of the free-testosterone concentration;
- DHA or DHAS;
- 17α-hydroxyprogesterone if *late onset* congenital adrenal hyperplasia (CAH) is suspected. In some cases, there may be an

Table 7.4 Interpretation of biochemical tests in the diagnosis of hirsutism

Plasma findings					
Testosterone	**DHAS**	**LH**	**FSH**	**17-OH-progesterone**	
N or slightly ↑	N or slightly ↑	N	N	N	Simple hirsutism
↑	N	↑	N or ↓	N	Polycystic ovaries
↑↑	N	N or ↓	N or ↓	N	Ovarian tumour
N or slightly ↑	↑↑	N or ↓	N or ↓	N	Adrenocortical tumour
↑	↑	N or ↓	N or ↓	↑	Congenital adrenal hyperplasia

N = normal.

exaggerated response of 17α-hydroxyprogesterone to tetracosactrin;
- LH and FSH.

The interpretation of these tests is outlined in Table 7.4. They may be supplemented with other investigations, such as ovarian ultrasound.

Investigation of Infertility

It is important to make a full clinical assessment of, and to investigate, both partners if a woman complains of infertility.

FEMALE INFERTILITY

A woman may be infertile despite having a clinically normal menstrual cycle, or may have amenorrhoea or oligomenorrhoea. Even if the cycle seems to be regular it is important to determine whether ovulation is occurring and if luteal development is normal.

1. If the patient is menstruating regularly measure plasma progesterone concentration during the luteal phase on day 21 or 22 of cycle.

   - A normal plasma concentration is strong evidence that the patient has ovulated.

   - A low plasma concentration suggests either ovulatory failure or impaired luteal function. This investigation should be repeated on more than one occasion.

2. Follicular development and ovulation may be monitored by ovarian ultrasound examination.
3. Histological examination of an endometrial biopsy specimen should indicate whether luteal function is normal.

   Discussion of the complete investigation of female infertility is beyond the scope of this book.

MALE INFERTILITY

Laboratory investigations may detect early hormonal deficiency or distinguish between testicular and pituitary causes.

1. Measure plasma testosterone, LH and FSH concentrations and perform a semen analysis.

   Interpretation.

   - A raised plasma LH with a low testosterone concentration indicates Leydig cell failure.
   - A raised plasma LH with a normal testosterone concentration suggests a lesser degree of damage with a compensatory increase in LH secretion (compare TSH in primary hypothyroidism).

- Low plasma LH and testosterone concentrations suggest pituitary or hypothalamic disease.
- A raised plasma FSH concentration indicates seminiferous tubular failure, irrespective of the plasma testosterone concentration. There is usually oligospermia.
- Oligospermia with a low plasma FSH concentration suggests pituitary or hypothalamic disease and the paitent should be investigated for the condition.

2. Measure plasma prolactin.

Interpretation. If the plasma prolactin is markedly raised this is suggestive of a pituitary tumour. Perform a combined pituitary stimulation test if clinically indicated.

Thyroid Function

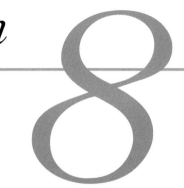

Thyroxine (T$_4$), triiodothyronine (T$_3$) and calcitonin are secreted by the thyroid gland. T$_4$ and T$_3$ are products of the follicular cells and influence the rate of all metabolic processes. Calcitonin is produced by the specialized C-cells and influences calcium metabolism. This is an anatomical rather than a functional relationship and in some lower animals the calcitonin-secreting cells are completely separated from the thyroid gland. Calcitonin is discussed briefly on p.**174**.

PHYSIOLOGY

Thyroid hormones are synthesized in the thyroid gland by iodination and coupling of two molecules of the amino acid tyrosine, a process that is dependent on an adequate supply of iodide.

Iodide in the diet is absorbed rapidly from the small intestine. Most foods contain adequate amounts. In areas where the iodide content of the soil is very low there used to be a high incidence of enlargement of the thyroid gland (*goitre*), but the general use of artificially iodized salt has made this a less common occurrence. Sea foods have a high iodide content. Fish and iodized salt are the main dietary sources of the element.

Normally about a third of dietary iodide is taken up by the thyroid gland, a little by the mammary and salivary glands and the gastric mucosa. The rest is excreted by the kidneys.

SYNTHESIS OF THYROID HORMONES

A knowledge of the biosynthesis and secretion of the thyroid hormones is essential for the understanding of the mode of action of drugs, whether used to diagnose or treat thyroid disorders, and of the effects of congenital enzyme deficiencies (p.**164**).

- *Iodide is actively taken up by the thyroid gland* under the control of thyroid stimulating hormone (TSH). Uptake is blocked by thiocyanate and perchlorate. The concentration of iodide in the gland is at least 20 times that in plasma and may exceed it by a hundred times or more.

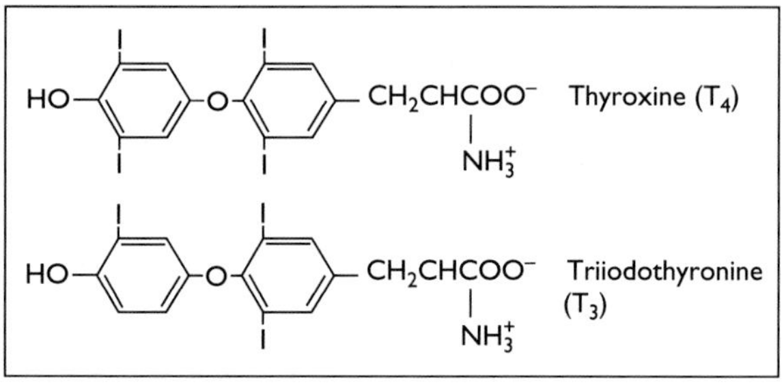

Fig. 8.1 Chemical structure of the thyroid hormones.

- *Iodide is rapidly converted to iodine*, within the thyroid gland.
- *Iodination of tyrosine residues* in a large glycoprotein, thyroglobulin, takes place to form mono- and diiodotyrosine (MIT and DIT). This step is inhibited by carbimazole and propylthiouracil.
- *Iodotyrosines are coupled to form thyroxine (T$_4$)* (DIT and DIT) and triiodothyronine (T$_3$) (DIT and MIT) (Fig. 8.1). Normally much more T$_4$ than T$_3$ is synthesized but if there is an inadequate supply of iodide the ratio of T$_3$ to T$_4$ in the gland increases. The thyroid hormones, still incorporated in thyroglobulin, are stored in the colloid of the thyroid follicle.

Before secretion of thyroid hormones, thyroglobulin is taken up by the follicular cells and T$_4$ and T$_3$ are released by proteolytic enzymes into the bloodstream. This process is stimulated by TSH and inhibited by iodide. The thyroid hormones are immediately bound to plasma proteins. Mono- and diiodotyrosine, released at the same time, are deiodinated and the iodine is reused.

Each step is controlled by specific enzymes and congenital deficiency of any of these enzymes can lead to enlargement of the thyroid gland (goitre) and, if severe, hypothyroidism. The uptake of iodide, as well as the synthesis and secretion of thyroid hormones, is regulated by TSH, secreted from the anterior pituitary gland.

PROTEIN BINDING OF THYROID HORMONES IN PLASMA

More than 99 per cent of plasma T_4 and T_3 is protein bound, mainly to an α-globulin, thyroxine-binding globulin (TBG) and, to a lesser extent, to albumin and thyroxine-binding prealbumin. *The free unbound fraction is the physiologically active form* which also regulates TSH secretion from the anterior pituitary (compare cortisol, p.**120**).

Changes in the plasma concentrations of the binding proteins, particularly TBG, alter plasma total T_4 and T_3 concentrations but not those of the free hormones.

PERIPHERAL CONVERSION OF THYROID HORMONE

Some of the circulating T_4 is deiodinated by enzymes in peripheral tissues, especially in the liver and kidneys. About 80 per cent of the plasma T_3 is produced by the removal of an iodine atom from the outer (β) ring; the remaining 20 per cent is secreted by the thyroid gland. Deiodination of the inner (α) ring produces reverse T_3 which is probably inactive. T_3 binds more avidly to thyroid receptors than T_4 and is the main active form. The conversion of T_4 to T_3 may be:

- *reduced* by many factors, of which the most important are:
    systemic illness;
    prolonged fasting;
    drugs such as:
        β-blockers, for example propranolol;
        amiodarone.
- *increased* by drugs, such as phenytoin, which induce hepatic enzyme activity.

The plasma T_3 concentration is a poor indicator of thyroid hormone secretion because it is influenced by many non-thyroidal factors and consequently its measurement is rarely indicated.

ACTION OF THYROID HORMONES

Thyroid hormones affect many metabolic processes, increasing oxygen consumption. By binding to specific receptors in cell nuclei, they change the expression of some genes. Thyroid hormones are essential for normal growth, mental development and sexual maturation. They also increase the sensitivity of the cardiovascular and central nervous systems to catecholamines and so influence cardiac output and heart rate.

CONTROL OF TSH SECRETION

TSH stimulates the synthesis and release of thyroid hormones from the thyroid gland.

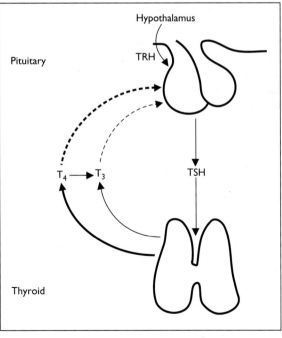

Fig. 8.2 Secretion, and control of thyroid hormones. Solid lines indicate secretion and interconversion of hormones. Dotted lines indicate negative feedback.

The secretion of TSH from the anterior pituitary gland is controlled by:

- circulating concentrations of thyroid hormones;
- thyrotrophin-releasing hormone (TRH).

Effects of thyroid hormones in control of TSH secretion. Thyroid hormones reduce TSH secretion by negative feedback. T_3 binds to anterior pituitary nuclear receptors. In the anterior pituitary gland most of the intracellular T_3 is derived from circulating free T_4. Therefore this gland is more sensitive to changes in plasma T_4 than to T_3 concentra-

tions. For example, in early hypothyroidism plasma T_3 concentrations are often normal; their effect on peripheral tissue minimizes the clinical effects of low plasma T_4 concentrations but TSH secretion may be increased in response to falling plasma T_4 concentrations.

Effect of TRH. TSH secretion is stimulated by TRH, produced in the hypothalamus. Its stimulatory effect can be overridden by high circulating free-T_4 concentrations. This is why exogenous TRH has little effect on TSH secretion in hyperthyroidism (TRH test; p.**168**).

The metabolism and control of thyroid hormones are summarized in Fig. 8.2.

THYROID FUNCTION TESTS

Treatment of thyroid disease may need to be prolonged and, in the case of primary hypothyroidism, life long. Therefore, before treatment is started it is essential to confirm the diagnosis by laboratory tests. During treatment the original clinical picture disappears and therefore laboratory tests are necessary to confirm the biochemical response and also to assess treatment compliance.

Assessment of thyroid hormone secretion can be made either by measuring the plasma total- or free-hormone concentration or by assessing the degree of negative feedback by thyroid hormone on TSH secretion by the pituitary. Each test has its advantages and disadvantages. Students must know which investigations have been chosen by their local laboratory and the reasons why such thyroid hormone tests have been adopted.

PLASMA TOTAL THYROXINE (T₄)

Plasma T_4 is more than 99 per cent protein bound; therefore measurement of plasma total T_4 assays reflect the protein bound rather than the free-hormone fraction. Changes in thyroid secretion produce parallel changes in plasma

total and free T_4 levels. Total T_4 reflects free T_4 concentrations unless there are abnormalities of binding proteins (Table 8.1).

- *In the euthyroid state,* about a third of the binding sites on TBG are occupied by T_4 and the remainder are unoccupied, irrespective of the concentration of the binding protein.
- *In hyperthyroidism,* both plasma total and free T_4 concentrations are increased and the number of unoccupied binding sites on TBG are decreased.
- *In hypothyroidism* the opposite occurs.

An increase in plasma TBG concentration causes an increase in both bound T_4 and unoccupied binding sites but no change in plasma free T_4 concentrations. Such an increase may occur because of:

- *a high oestrogen concentration* during pregnancy or in the newborn infant;
- *oestrogen therapy,* or taking oral contraceptives;
- *inherited TBG excess* (rare).

A decrease in plasma TBG concentration decreases both bound T_4 concentrations and unoccupied binding sites but does not alter

Table 8.1   Interpretation of thyroid function tests

	Total T_4	Free T_4	TBG	Bound T_4 Unoccupied binding sites	
Euthyroid	N	N	N		Total T_4 / Free T_4
Hyperthyroid	↑	↑	N		
Hypothyroid	↓	↓	N		
TBG excess	↑	N	↑		
TBG deficiency	↓	N	↓		
T_4 displacement by drug	↓	N	N		Drug

N = normal.

the plasma free T_4 concentration. Such changes may occur because of:

- *severe illness*, but this is frequently temporary;
- *loss of low molecular weight proteins*, usually in the urine (nephrotic syndrome);
- *androgens or danazol* treatment;
- *inherited TBG deficiency* (rare).

These changes might be misinterpreted as being diagnostic of hyperthyroidism or hypothyroidism respectively if only plasma total T_4 concentrations were measured. If there is doubt about the true thyroid status, additional investigations must be requested, such as plasma TSH or free T_4 concentrations, and these are discussed later in the chapter.

Displacement of T_4 by drugs (Table 8.1). Some drugs, such as salicylates and danazol, bind to TBG and displace T_4. The change in unoccupied binding sites is variable and TBG concentrations are unaffected. Low plasma T_4, with normal TSH, concentrations can only be interpreted with a knowledge of which drugs are being taken by the patient.

Measurement of plasma TBG concentrations may occasionally be indicated to confirm either congenital TBG excess or deficiency.

PLASMA FREE THYROXINE (FREE T_4)

True free thyroxine assays are technically difficult to develop and are expensive compared with total hormone assays. In uncomplicated situations, they perform well but they are not always reliable when abnormal binding proteins or abnormal albumin levels are present. The user must be aware of which 'free T_4' assay is being used and of its limitations.

PLASMA TSH

TSH assays are useful in diagnosing, not only primary hypothyroidism, but also hyperthyroidism in which the high plasma T_4 concentration suppresses TSH release from the pituitary, resulting in very low or undetectable plasma TSH concentrations.

PLASMA TOTAL OR FREE TRIIODOTHYRONINE (T_3)

T_3 concentrations may help in the diagnosis of hyperthyroidism, but should not be used to diagnose hypothyroidism because normal plasma concentrations are very low. In hyperthyroidism, the increase in plasma T_3 concentrations are greater, and usually occur earlier than that of T_4.

Occasionally, only the plasma T_3 concentrations are elevated (T_3 toxicosis). T_3, like T_4, is bound to protein. It is preferable to measure the plasma concentration of free rather than total T_3 as the latter may be altered by changes in the plasma concentrations of thyroxine-binding globulin.

TRH TEST

The normal anterior pituitary gland responds to administration of TRH by increasing the secretion and therefore the plasma concentrations of TSH. The rise in plasma TSH concentration, in response to TRH, is exaggerated in:

- *hypothyroidism*, when negative feedback is reduced because plasma T_4 concentrations

are low. This test may occasionally be useful to diagnose early or 'preclinical' primary hypothyroidism.

The response is reduced in:

- *hypopituitarism* with secondary hypothyroidism when the anterior pituitary gland is unable to respond normally to TRH. In these cases the plasma T_4 concentrations will tend to be low;
- *hyperthyroidism*. Negative feedback due to increased plasma T_4 concentrations overrides the stimulatory effect of TRH. Sensitive TSH assays have replaced the TRH test in the diagnosis of early hyperthyroidism when plasma T_4 concentrations may still be within the upper reference range.

Disorders of the Thyroid Gland

The most common presenting clinical features of thyroid disease are the result of:

- hyperthyroidism, due to excessive thyroid hormone secretion;
- hypothyroidism, due to deficient thyroid hormone secretion;
- goitre, either diffuse or due to one or more nodules within the gland. There may or may not be abnormal thyroid hormone secretion.

Increased or reduced plasma thyroid hormone concentrations produce characteristic clinical changes. However, disease of the thyroid gland may be present without hyper- or hypofunction.

Table 8.2 Common causes of hyperthyroidism

Autonomous secretion
Graves' disease
toxic multinodular goitre or a single functioning nodule
(occasionally an adenoma)
Ingestion of thyroid hormones
Rare causes
TSH secretion by tumours of trophoblastic origin
struma ovarii (thyroid tissue in an ovarian teratoma)
administration of iodine to a subject with iodine
deficiency goitre
TSH secreting tumour of the pituitary (extremely rare)

Hyperthyroidism (Thyrotoxicosis)

Hyperthyroidism, produced by sustained high plasma concentrations of thyroid hormone,

may be easy to diagnose clinically or may remain unsuspected for a long time. There is a generalized increase in the metabolic rate, evidenced clinically by, for example, a fine tremor, tachycardia and sometimes cardiac arrhythmias, weight loss, tiredness, sweating and diarrhoea. There may be severe anxiety and emotional symptoms. In some cases, particularly in the elderly, a single feature predominates, such as weight loss, diarrhoea, tachycardia or atrial fibrillation. Some common causes of hyperthyroidism are shown in Table 8.2.

Graves' disease may occur at any age. It is commoner in females than in males. It may be caused by relatively autonomous secretion from a diffuse goitre and is characterized by:

- exophthalmos, due to lymphocytic infiltration and swelling of retro-orbital tissues of the eyes;
- sometimes localized thickening of the subcutaneous tissue over the shin ('pretibial myxoedema').

Graves' disease is an autoimmune thyroid disease. Thyroid antibodies are detectable in some cases, as well as *thyroid stimulating immunoglobulins* that probably cause hyperfunction.

Toxic nodules, either single or multiple, in a nodular goitre may secrete thyroid hormones *autonomously. TSH secretion is suppressed* by negative feedback, as in Graves' disease. These nodules may be detected by their uptake of radioactive iodine or technetium with suppression of uptake in the rest of the thyroid tissue ('*hot nodules*'). Toxic nodules are found most commonly in older patients who may present with only one of the features of hyperactivity, usually cardiovascular symptoms such as atrial fibrillation.

PATHOPHYSIOLOGY

Plasma T_4 and T_3 concentrations are usually both increased in hyperthyroidism. Much of the T_3 is secreted directly by the thyroid gland and the increase in plasma T_3 levels is greater, and usually evident earlier, than that of T_4. Rarely only plasma T_3 concentrations are elevated (T_3 toxicosis). In both situations TSH secretion is suppressed by negative feedback and plasma TSH concentrations are either very low or undetectable.

The diagnostic approach to hyperthyroidism is considered on p.167.

TREATMENT

The aetiology of hyperthyroidism must be fully investigated before treatment is started. Various forms of treatment are available, the selection of which depends on the cause, the clinical presentation and the age of the patient. β-blocker drugs such as propranolol, which inhibit the peripheral conversion of T_4 to T_3, may be used initially. Additional treatment includes the use of such drugs as carbimazole, propylthiouracil or radioactive iodine; surgery is rarely indicated. Thyroid function must be monitored regularly as some patients may become hypothyroid or may relapse.

Hypothyroidism

Hypothyroidism is caused by suboptimal circulating concentrations of thyroid hormones. The presenting signs and symptoms depend to some extent on the aetiology of the disorder.

The condition may develop insidiously and in its early stages may cause only vague symptoms. Many of the features of severe hypothyroidism which, because of better methods of diagnosis, are less commonly found than previously, are the opposite to those of hyperthyroidism. There is a generalized slowing down of metabolism, with mental dullness, lethargy and physical slowness.

If the hormone deficiency is caused by a primary disorder of the thyroid gland the patient may present with weight gain, menstrual disturbances, such as oligomenorrhoea, and menorrhagia. The skin is dry, the hair may fall out and the voice becomes hoarse. The face is puffy and subcutaneous tissues are thickened; this pseudo-oedema, with a histological myxoid appearance, accounts for the term myxoedema which is used to describe advanced primary hypothyroidism. In the most severe cases myxoedema coma, with profound *hypothermia*, may develop.

Congenital thyroid hormone deficiency, either due to thyroid dysgenesis or 'dyshormonogenesis', leads to cretinism and impaired growth.

Primary hypothyroidism. *The common causes are:*

- atrophic autoimmune thyroiditis;
- Hashimoto's disease;
  (in both these conditions there is progressive destruction of thyroid tissue. Circulating thyroid antibodies are usually present, often in high concentration).
- other inflammatory diseases of the gland;
- following treatment of hyperthyroidism:
    post-thyroidectomy;
    post radioiodine treatment.
- drugs:
    carbimazole;
    propylthiouracil;
    lithium carbonate.

Rare causes of primary hypothyroidism are:

- exogenous goitrogens;
- 'dyshormonogenesis'. This term includes inherited deficiencies of any of the enzymes involved in thyroid hormone synthesis. Although the biochemical and clinical features differ, the end result is hypothyroidism. In most cases prolonged TSH stimulation, due to reduced negative feedback, causes goitre. The commonest form is due to failure to incorporate iodine into tyrosine.

Secondary hypothyroidism is due to anterior pituitary or hypothalamic deficiency and is much less common than primary hypothyroidism. In long-standing secondary hypothyroidism the thyroid gland may atrophy irreversibly.

The essential biochemical difference between primary and secondary hypothyroidism is in the plasma TSH concentration which is high in primary and inappropriately low in secondary hypothyroidism.

PATHOPHYSIOLOGY

As *primary hypothyroidism* develops TSH secretion from the anterior pituitary gland increases as the negative feedback, associated with the falling plasma T_4 concentration, decreases. Initially, the plasma T_4 concentration may be within the population reference range, although abnormally low for the individual. For this reason the plasma TSH concentration is the most sensitive index of early disease. T_3 assays are of no help in making the diagnosis as plasma T_3 concentrations are often normal.

Secondary hypothyroidism may be caused by impaired TSH secretion, due either to a disorder of the pituitary gland itself, or to reduced hypothalamic secretion. In the former case there is a subnormal rise in plasma TSH concentrations after administration of exogenous TRH (TRH test).

*The diagnosis of hypothyroidism is considered on p.**167**.*

SPECIAL PROBLEMS IN THE DIAGNOSIS OF HYPOTHYROIDISM

Two situations merit special consideration:

- *neonatal hypothyroidism*. The incidence of neonatal hypothyroidism in most populations is about 1 : 3500. The routine screening for inborn errors of metabolism and, in particular, for congenital hypothyroidism are outlined in Chapter 18 (p.**353**). Thyroid function fluctuates considerably during the immediate postpartum period. These changes are discussed in more detail in Chapter 17 (p.**347**);
- *'sick euthyroid'*. Any severe illness may be associated with low plasma total T_4 concentrations and may make the interpretation of thyroid function tests very difficult. Unless primary hypothyroidism is also present, plasma TSH concentrations are usually normal or slightly high. There may be impaired conversion of T_4 to T_3 with low plasma T_3 levels. The TSH response to TRH may also be impaired. Consequently, the assessment of thyroid function is best deferred until the patient has recovered from the illness. If hypo- or hyperthyroidism is suspected as a part of

the illness, the results must be interpreted in the context of the changes outlined above.

Euthyroid Goitre

If plasma T_4 concentrations fall enlargement of the thyroid gland (goitre) may be caused by TSH stimulation resulting in cellular hyperplasia. Thyroxine synthesis may be impaired by iodide deficiency, by drugs such as para-aminosalicylic acid, or possibly by partial deficiency of enzymes involved in thyroxine synthesis. Under the influence of prolonged stimulation by TSH the number of thyroid cells increases and plasma thyroid hormone concentrations are maintained at the expense of the development of a goitre. In areas with a low soil iodide content iodine deficiency goitres were endemic before the prophylactic iodinization of salt was introduced.

Inflammation of the thyroid gland (thyroiditis), whether acute or subacute, may produce marked but temporary aberrations of thyroid function tests. These conditions are relatively uncommon.

Other Biochemical Findings in Thyroid Disease

The following biochemical changes, of no diagnostic significance, may be associated with *hypothyroidism*, particularly if severe:

- *plasma cholesterol concentration.* In hypothyroidism the clearance of plasma LDL-cholesterol is impaired and plasma cholesterol concentrations may be moderately high;
- *plasma creatine kinase (CK)* activity is often raised in hypothyroidism. It may also be increased in patients with thyrotoxic myopathy;
- *hyponatraemia* may occasionally be present in patients with profound hypothyroidism or myxoedema coma. It is caused by increased ADH release with excessive water retention, occasionally precipitated by a constrictive pericardial effusion that some patients develop.

The following may be caused by *hyperthyroidism*.

- *Hypercalcaemia* is very rarely found in patients with severe thyrotoxicosis. There is an increased turnover of bone cells, probably due to a direct action of thyroid hormone (p.**177**).

Summary

1. There are two naturally occurring thyroid hormones (apart from calcitonin), thyroxine and triiodothyronine. Their synthesis depends on an adequate supply of iodine, and is controlled by negative feedback of circulating thyroid hormone concentrations on TSH secretion from the anterior pituitary gland.

2. Circulating thyroid hormone concentrations may be assessed by estimating plasma total T_4 and TSH concentrations.

3. An excess of circulating thyroid hormones produces the syndrome of hyperthyroidism. This may be due to generalized thyroid hyperplasia as in Graves' disease, or to hyperfunctioning thyroid nodule(s).

In primary hyperthyroidism, basal plasma TSH concentrations are usually undetectable and plasma thyroid hormone concentrations raised.

4. A decreased circulating thyroid hormone concentration produces the syndrome of hypothyroidism. This may be primary, due to disease of the thyroid gland, or be secondary to pituitary or hypothalamic disease. Plasma TSH concentrations are raised in the former group and low in the latter.

The diagnosis of primary hypothyroidism is made by finding a high plasma TSH associated with a low-normal or usually low T_4 concentration. If both plasma T_4 and TSH concentrations are low TRH may be administered to stimulate TSH secretion. This will confirm secondary hypothyroidism and may help to distinguish between pituitary and hypothalamic causes.

5. Euthyroid goitre represents compensated thyroid disease. Biochemical thyroid function tests may be normal.

*I*NVESTIGATION OF THYROID FUNCTION

Investigation of Suspected Hyperthyroidism

Measure plasma total T_4 and TSH concentrations (Table 8.3).

1. If the plasma T_4 concentration is clearly high and the TSH concentration suppressed in a clinically thyrotoxic patient, no further tests are necessary.
2. If the plasma T_4 concentration is normal and the TSH suppressed, measure plasma free T_3. A clearly elevated plasma free T_3 concentration confirms the diagnosis of hyperthyroidism.
3. If the plasma T_4 concentration is raised and the TSH concentration normal, this is suggestive of biochemical euthyroidism and an increase in plasma TBG concentration. This can be confirmed by measuring plasma TBG concentrations. However, this is rarely necessary as the cause is usually apparent from the clinical history.

MONITORING TREATMENT OF HYPERTHYROIDISM

The progress of a patient being treated for hyperthyroidism is monitored by estimating plasma total T_4 concentrations, or free T_3 if the latter is the predominant abnormality, and plasma TSH concentrations. Overtreatment may induce hypothyroidism, with a rise in plasma TSH concentrations. In some patients with severe prolonged hyperthyroidism, such a rise in plasma TSH may be delayed because of the prolonged feedback suppression of T_4 on the pituitary.

Investigation of Suspected Hypothyroidism

Measure plasma TSH and total T_4 concentrations (Table 8.3). The lower limit of 'normal' for plasma T_4 is poorly defined. Levels within the reference range may be suboptimal for

Table 8.3 Results of thyroid function tests

	True T_4 abnormalities			TBG abnormalities	
	Hyperthyroidism	**Hypothyroidism**		**Increased**	**Decreased**
		Primary	**Secondary**		
Plasma					
Total T_4	↑	↓	↓	↑	↓
Free T_3	↑	↓	↓	N	N
TSH	↓	↑	↓	N	N
TRH response	Absent	Increased	See text	N	N

N = normal.

Table 8.4 Drug effects on thyroid function tests.

Drug	Total T_4	Free T_4	T_3	Remarks
Oestrogens	↑	N	↑	↑ TBG
Oral contraceptives	↑	N	↑	↑ TBG
Some radiocontrast media (e.g. ioponoate)	↑	N	↓	Blocking $T_4 \rightarrow T_3$ (transient effect)
Amiodarone	↑	N or ↑	N	Blocking $T_4 \rightarrow T_3$
Propranolol	N	N	↓	Blocking $T_4 \rightarrow T_3$
Carbimazole	↓	↓	↓	Therapeutic effect
Propylthiouracil	↓	↓	↓	Therapeutic effect
Androgens	↓	N	↓	↓ TBG
Danazol	↓	N		Reduced TBG binding
Salicylates	↓	N		Reduced TBG binding
Phenytoin	↓	↓	N	Increased $T_4 \rightarrow T_3$
Carbamazepine	↓	↓	N	Increased $T_4 \rightarrow T_3$

N = normal

the patient under investigation. A very low plasma T_4 concentration indicates either hypothyroidism or gross TBG deficiency. In most cases of primary hypothyroidism the plasma TSH concentration will be high. If it is low, proceed to a TRH test to exclude pituitary or hypothalamic hypothyroidism. If the patient is very ill investigations should be deferred ('sick euthyroid'). A borderline low plasma T_4 concentration with a:

- *slightly elevated plasma TSH concentration* may indicate early hypothyroidism. Measure circulating thyroid antibodies to assess the presence of autoimmune thyroiditis. Note, however, that their presence does not confirm hypothyroidism. Replacement treatment is probably not indicated at this stage, but the tests should be repeated after three to six months. Rarely, a TRH test may be indicated;
- *normal plasma TSH concentration* is suggestive of either competition by a drug for binding sites on TBG, or TBG deficiency. In most cases this is apparent from the clinical history but occasionally plasma TBG concentrations may be measured, for example to confirm inherited TBG deficiency and so prevent unnecessary investigations in the future;
- *low plasma TSH concentration* suggests that the hypothyroidism is caused by a hypothalamic or pituitary disorder. Proceed to a TRH test (see below).

MONITORING TREATMENT OF HYPOTHYROIDISM

The progress and drug compliance of a patient with primary hypothyroidism taking thyroid hormone replacement should be monitored by estimating plasma TSH and T_4 concentrations.

TSH assays are of no value in monitoring secondary hypothyroidism.

TRH TEST

The TRH test is used to confirm the diagnosis of secondary hypothyroidism, or occasionally to diagnose early primary hypothyroidism. Since the development of sensitive TSH assays, it is no longer used to diagnose hyperthyroidism. You must contact your laboratory before starting the test.

Procedure.

- A basal blood sample is taken.
- 200 μg of TRH is 2 ml saline is injected intravenously over about a minute.

- Further blood samples are taken 20 and 60 minutes after the TRH injection. TSH is measured on all samples.

Interpretation. In normal subjects plasma TSH concentrations increase by at least 2 mU/L and exceed the upper limit of the reference range. The maximum response occurs at 20 minutes

- A high normal basal plasma TSH concentration, with an exaggerated response at 20 minutes and a slight fall at 60 minutes is suggestive of early primary hypothyroidism;
- A subnormal rise of TSH confirms the diagnosis of secondary hypothyroidism of pituitary origin;
- A normal or exaggerated increment but delayed response, with plasma TSH concentrations higher at 60 minutes than at 20 minutes suggests secondary hypothyroidism due to hypothalamic dysfunction. If clinically indicated, pituitary and hypothalamic function should be investigated (p.**147**).
- A flat response is compatible with hyperthyroidism.

Investigation of a Patient Already on Treatment

No patient should be given thyroid hormone replacement therapy until the clinical diagnosis has been confirmed and documented by laboratory tests. If it is necessary to confirm the diagnosis in a patient already on treatment, but without adequate laboratory confirmation of the disease, plasma T_4 and TSH concentrations should be measured and, unless hypothyroidism is confirmed by a low T_4 and raised TSH, treatment should be stopped. The tests should then be repeated at intervals, but the diagnosis cannot be excluded until at least six weeks after stopping treatment.

Drug Effects of Thyroid Function Tests

Drugs may alter plasma total T_4 and total T_3 concentrations. The more common effects are summarized in Table 8.4. If the primary change is in binding protein concentrations, plasma free hormone concentrations are usually normal.

Calcium, Phosphate and Magnesium Metabolism

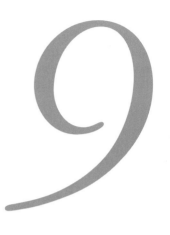

Most calcium is in bone and prolonged calcium deficiency may cause disorders of bone. The extraosseous fraction, although amounting to only one per cent of the total, is of great importance because of its effect on neuromuscular excitability and on cardiac muscle.

Phosphate is the most important anion associated with calcium; a knowledge of its plasma concentration is needed to interpret disturbances of calcium metabolism. Net renal tubular secretion of hydrogen ion and generation of bicarbonate depend on the presence of phosphate and sodium in the glomerular filtrate (p.**86**). Cellular 'high energy' phosphate compounds are of great biological importance.

More than half the magnesium is in bone. Most of the remainder is intracellular, but about one per cent is extracellular and, like calcium, is important because of its effect on neuromuscular activity.

CALCIUM METABOLISM

Total Body Calcium

The total body calcium depends on that absorbed from the dietary intake and that lost from the body (Fig. 9.1).

FACTORS AFFECTING INTAKE

About 25 mmol (1 g) of calcium is ingested per day, of which there is a net absorption of between 6 and 12 mmol (0.25–0.50 g). The active metabolite of vitamin D, 1,25-dihydroxy-vitamin D (1,25-dihydroxycholecalciferol), is needed for adequate calcium absorption.

FACTORS AFFECTING LOSS

Calcium is lost in faeces and urine.

- *Faecal calcium* is derived from the diet and that portion of the large amount of intestinal secretions that has not been reabsorbed and is therefore lost from the body. Calcium in the intestine, whether endogenous or exogenous in origin, may form insoluble, poorly absorbed complexes with phosphate or fatty acids. Orally administered phosphate may be used therapeutically to reduce calcium absorption and reabsorption (p.**186**). An excess of fatty acids in the intestinal lumen in steatorrhoea may contribute to calcium malabsorption.
- *Urinary calcium* excretion depends on the amount of calcium reaching the glomeruli, the glomerular filtration rate and on renal tubular function (p.**185**). Parathyroid hormone and 1,25-dihydroxyvitamin D increase calcium and, to a lesser extent, urinary phosphate reabsorption.

Plasma Calcium

The mean plasma calcium concentration in healthy subjects is about 2.50 mmol/L (10 mg/dl). Calcium is present in plasma in two main forms:

- *that bound to proteins, mainly albumin.* This accounts for a little less than half the total calcium concentration as measured by routine analytical methods. It is a physiologically inactive transport form, comparable with iron bound to transferrin (p.**378**);
- *free-ionized calcium* (Ca^{2+}), which comprises most of the rest. It is the physiologically active fraction, comparable with free thyroxine (p.**159**).

Changes in plasma protein concentration, particularly of albumin, alter the most

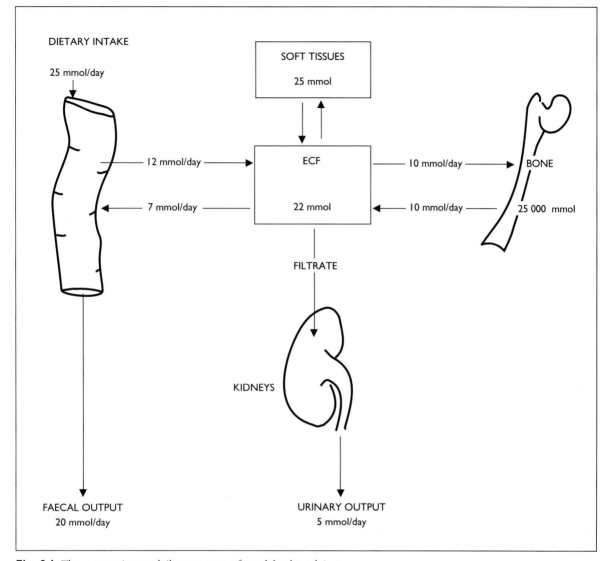

DIETARY INTAKE

25 mmol/day

SOFT TISSUES

25 mmol

12 mmol/day

ECF

22 mmol

7 mmol/day

10 mmol/day — BONE

10 mmol/day — 25 000 mmol

FILTRATE

KIDNEYS

FAECAL OUTPUT
20 mmol/day

URINARY OUTPUT
5 mmol/day

Fig. 9.1 The approximate daily turnover of total body calcium.

commonly measured concentration, that of plasma total calcium but not that of the free-ionized fraction. The plasma total, but not free-ionized, calcium concentration is lower in the supine than in the erect position because of the effect of posture on fluid distribution and therefore on plasma protein concentration (p.**423**). Although direct measurement of the physiologically active free-ionized fraction is, for technical reasons, confined to special cases, it is possible to interpret it if the plasma albumin concentration on the same specimen

is known. Formulae, incorporating the albumin concentration, have been devised in an attempt to calculate the active fraction of the plasma total calcium concentration but, because binding is not simple, these are not always reliable and give a spurious sense of accuracy.

Changes in plasma hydrogen ion (H^+) concentration affect binding of calcium to plasma proteins because H^+ competes with Ca^{2+} for binding sites. The plasma total calcium concentration is unaltered by changes in that of H^+. If the H^+ concentration falls as in alkalosis, tetany may occur despite a normal plasma total calcium concentration. By contrast, acidosis decreases binding and so increases the proportion of plasma calcium in the free-ionized form; by increasing calcium solubility, it also increases the rate of release of calcium from bones into the extracellular fluid. The increased load reaching the kidneys increases the renal calcium loss. Prolonged acidosis may cause osteomalacia despite a normal dietary calcium intake.

CONTROL OF PLASMA CALCIUM

Bone provides a reservoir from which both parathyroid hormone and calcitonin control plasma free-ionized calcium concentrations.

- *Parathyroid hormone (PTH)*, secreted by the parathyroid glands, increases the circulating level of free-ionized calcium and is the most important controlling factor.
- *Calcitonin*, produced in the C-cells of the thyroid gland, by decreasing osteoclastic activity, slows calcium release from bone and has the opposite effect on plasma concentrations to PTH. It is less important than PTH in physiological homeostasis. Plasma concentrations may be very high in patients with medullary carcinoma of the thyroid, although hypocalcaemia has not been reported in this condition. Calcitonin has been used to treat hypercalcaemia (p.**186**) and Paget's disease of bone.
- *1,25-dihydroxyvitamin D* increases calcium absorption from the intestine and, at physiological concentrations, is necessary for PTH activity.

Action and Control of Parathyroid Hormone Secretion

Parathyroid hormone is a single-chain polypeptide containing 84 residues, of which the 34 N-terminal amino acids determine biological activity. The hormone is metabolized by renal, hepatic and bone cells. Renal clearance from plasma of the physiologically inert C-terminal fragment is slower than that of the N-terminal fragment. The C-terminal fragment may accumulate in plasma in renal

glomerular dysfunction and this may complicate the intepretation of results of some PTH assays. The biological actions of PTH include:

- *stimulation of osteoclastic bone resorption*, so releasing both free-ionized calcium and phosphate into the extracellular fluid. This action *increases the plasma concentrations of both calcium and phosphate.*
- *decreased renal tubular reabsorption of phosphate*, causing phosphaturia and *increased reabsorption of calcium*. This action tends to *increase the plasma calcium concentration but to decrease the phosphate.*

The control of PTH secretion depends on the concentration of free-ionized calcium circulating through the parathyroid glands. A fall increases the rate of PTH secretion which, under physiological conditions, continues until the calcium concentration returns to normal. PTH secretion is also affected by the extracellular magnesium concentration and is decreased by severe, chronic hypomagnesaemia. It is not known to be controlled by any other endocrine gland.

Parathyroid hormone-related protein (PTHRP) is a peptide hormone that has a similar amino acid sequence at the biologically active end of the peptide, therefore activating the same receptors as PTH. The function of PTHRP is uncertain but it may be important in mineral metabolism in the fetus. The gene that codes for PTHRP is widely distributed in body tissues but is normally repressed. However it may become derepressed in certain tumours, causing humoral hypercalcaemia of malignancy.

The consequences of most disturbances of calcium metabolism can be predicted from a knowledge of the actions of PTH on bone and on renal tubular cells, and from plasma concentrations of calcium and phosphate. A low plasma free-ionized calcium concentration normally stimulates PTH secretion which results in phosphaturia; the loss of urinary phosphate overrides the tendency to hyperphosphataemia due to the action of PTH on bone. Consequently the plasma phosphate

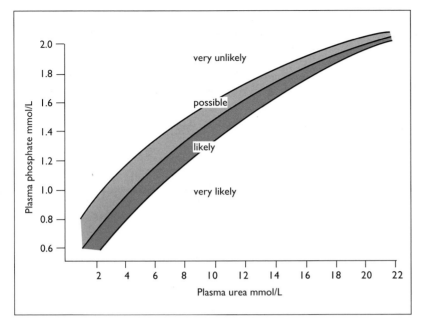

Fig. 9.2 The relation between plasma phosphate and urea concentrations in the differential diagnosis of proven hypercalcaemia. The lower the plasma phosphate with respect to the plasma urea concentration, the greater the probability that hypercalcaemia is caused by inappropriate PTH or PTHRP secretion. If the diagnosis is not obvious on clinical grounds these two conditions can often be differentiated by measuring the plasma PTH concentration.

concentration is usually low normal or low when the plasma PTH concentration is increased. Conversely, a high plasma free-ionized calcium concentration, unless due to inappropriate excess of PTH, inhibits PTH secretion and causes a high plasma phosphate concentration (p.**180**). Therefore, plasma calcium and phosphate concentrations vary in the same direction unless:

- there is inappropriate excess or deficiency of PTH, due to a primary disorder of the parathyroid gland or to secretion of PTHRP; in such cases calcium and phosphate vary in opposite directions;
- renal glomerular dysfunction is severe enough to impair the phosphaturic, and therefore hypophosphataemic, effect of PTH or PTHRP (Fig. 9.2).

Metabolism and Action of Vitamin D

Vitamin D is derived from:

- *cholecalciferol* (vitamin D_3), formed in the skin by the action of ultraviolet light on 7-*dehydrocholesterol* (Fig. 9.3); this is the form found in animal tissues, especially the liver;

- *ergocalciferol* (vitamin D_2), obtained from plants after irradiation.

In normal adults much more cholecalciferol is derived from the action of sunlight on skin than from food. Dietary sources are important when requirements are high, such as during growth or pregnancy, or in those elderly or chronically sick individuals who are confined indoors and not exposed to the sun.

Vitamin D is transported in plasma bound to specific carrier proteins. Vitamin D is inactive until metabolized.

In the liver cholecalciferol is hydroxylated to 25-hydroxycholecalciferol (25-OHD$_3$) by the enzyme 25-hydroxylase. The rate of formation of 25-OHD$_3$ is affected by the supply of substrate in the form of calciferol, whether derived from the skin or from the diet. 25-OHD$_3$ is the main circulating form and store of the vitamin.

In the proximal renal tubular cells of the kidney 25-OHD$_3$ undergoes a second hydroxylation, catalysed by the enzyme *1α-hydroxylase* to form the active metabolite, 1,25-dihydroxycholecalciferol (1,25-(OH)$_2$D$_3$). Other hydroxylated metabolites are formed in the kidney but their biological functions are not known at the time of writing.

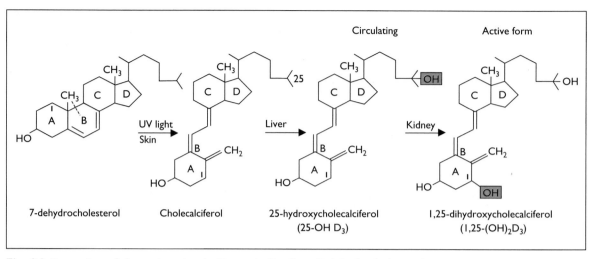

Fig. 9.3 Formation of the active vitamin D metabolite from 7-dehydrocholesterol.

1α-hydroxylase activity, and hence the production of 1,25-(OH)$_2$D$_3$, may be *stimulated* by:

- a low plasma phosphate concentration;
- an increase in plasma PTH concentration, possibly because of its phosphate lowering effect;
- oestrogens, prolactin and growth hormone, which increase 1,25-(OH)$_2$D$_3$ production and which therefore increase calcium absorption during pregnancy, lactation and growth.

It may be *inhibited* by:

- hyperphosphataemia;
- free-ionized hypercalcaemia.

The kidney is thus an endocrine organ, synthesizing and releasing the hormone 1,25-(OH)$_2$D$_3$; impairment of the final hydroxylation probably explains the hypocalcaemia of renal disease.

1,25-(OH)$_2$D$_3$ increases calcium absorption by intestinal mucosal cells. In conjunction with PTH it stimulates osteoclastic activity releasing calcium from bone.

Relation Between PTH and 1,25-(OH)$_2$D$_3$

The action of PTH on bone is impaired in the absence of 1,25-(OH)$_2$D$_3$. A fall in plasma free-ionized calcium concentrations stimulates PTH secretion. PTH enhances 1α-hydroxylase activity and therefore stimulates 1,25-(OH)$_2$D$_3$ synthesis. The two hormones act synergistically on the osteoclasts of bone, releasing calcium into the circulation. 1,25-(OH)$_2$D$_3$ also increases calcium absorption from the intestinal lumen. In the short term, the homeostatic mechanisms involving the effects on bone are the more important; if hypocalcaemia is prolonged more efficient absorption becomes important. As soon as the plasma free-ionized calcium concentration is corrected both PTH and 1,25-(OH)$_2$D$_3$ secretion are suppressed.

Calcium homeostasis follows the general rule that extracellular concentrations are controlled rather than the total body content. The effectiveness of this control depends on:

- normal functioning of the:
  parathyroid glands;
  kidneys;
  intestine.
- an adequate supply of:
  calcium;
  vitamin D.

If any one of these factors is impaired calcium leaves bone by passive physico-chemical diffusion and plasma concentrations may be maintained at the expense of bone calcification.

Action of Thyroid Hormone on Bone

Thyroid hormone excess may be associated with the histological appearance of osteoporosis and with increased faecal and urinary excretion of calcium, probably following its release from bone. Hypercalcaemia is a very rare complication of severe hyperthyroidism. Unless there is gross excess of thyroid hormone, the effects on plasma calcium are overridden by homeostatic reduction of PTH secretion and by urinary loss.

Disorders of Calcium Metabolism

The plasma phosphate concentration, *interpreted with the plasma urea concentration*, usually indicates whether either hyper- or hypocalcaemia is caused by an excess of PTH or PTH-like activity (PTHRP) or some other cause. Consequently the measurement of PTH is rarely necessary in order to make an initial diagnosis.

Hypercalcaemia

CLINICAL EFFECTS OF AN INCREASED FREE-IONIZED CALCIUM CONCENTRATION

Effects on the kidneys.

- *Renal damage* is the most serious clinical consequence of prolonged hypercalcaemia. Because of the high plasma free-ionized calcium concentration the solubility of calcium phosphate may be exceeded and precipitate in extraosseous sites of which the kidneys are the most clinically important.
- *Polyuria*, characteristic of chronic hypercalcaemia, may result from impairment of renal concentrating ability due to calcification of the tubular cells; acute hypercalcaemia may cause reversible inhibition of the tubular response to antidiuretic hormone rather than to cell damage.

- *Hypokalaemia*, often with a metabolic alkalosis, is a common finding in association with hypercalcaemia. Calcium may directly inhibit potassium reabsorption from the tubular lumen.
- *Renal calculi*, without significant parenchymal damage, may be caused by precipitation of calcium salts in the urine if the free-ionized calcium concentration is high in the glomerular filtrate due to hypercalcaemia. Any patient with radio-opaque calcium-containing renal stones should have plasma calcium concentrations estimated at regular intervals.

Effects on neuromuscular excitability. High extracellular free-ionized calcium concentrations depress neuromuscular excitability in both voluntary and involuntary muscle. The patient may complain of *constipation and abdominal pain*. There may also be muscular hypotonia.

Effects on the central nervous system. Depression is a common complaint, even in patients with only mild hypercalcaemia. *Depression, anorexia, nausea and vomiting*, associated with high plasma calcium concentrations, are probably caused by an effect on the central nervous system.

Effects on the stomach. Calcium stimulates gastrin, and therefore gastric acid, secretion (p.**248**). There is an association between chronic hypercalcaemia and *peptic ulceration*.

Effects on blood pressure. Some patients with hypercalcaemia may be *hypertensive.* If renal damage is not severe the hypertension may respond to reducing the plasma calcium concentration.

Effects on the heart. Severe hypercalcaemia causes characteristic changes in the electrocardiogram with shortening of the Q–T interval and broadening of the T waves. If plasma concentrations exceed about 3.75 mmol/L (15 mg/dl), there is a risk of sudden *cardiac arrest or ventricular arrhythmias.* For this reason marked hypercalcaemia should be treated as a matter of urgency.

Table 9.1 The possible effects of prolonged excess PTH secretion on bone in the presence of vitamin D. *Note that these changes are rarely found nowadays as diagnosis is made earlier*

Clinical
　　bone pain
　　bony swellings
Radiological
　　generalized decalcification
　　subperiosteal erosions and/or bone cysts
Histological
　　increasesd number of osteoclasts
Plasma
　　raised free-ionized calcium concentration
　　low phosphate concentration in relation to urea
　　normal or slightly raised alkaline phosphatase activity
　　(*only raised in advanced, prolonged cases*)

Causes of Hypercalcaemia

HYPERCALCAEMIA WITH HYPOPHOSPHATAEMIA RELATIVE TO THE GFR

True free-ionized hypercalcaemia with hypophosphataemia is caused by inappropriate secretion of PTH or PTHRP. The term 'inappropriate secretion' is used in this book to indicate that the release of hormone into the circulation is not adequately inhibited by negative feedback control. Inappropriate PTH secretion occurs in the following clinical situations.

- **PTH production** by the parathyroid glands due to:
　　primary hyperparathyroidism;
　　tertiary hyperparathyroidism.
- **PTHRP production** by non-parathyroid tissue.

If renal glomerular function is adequate the high circulating PTH or PTHRP concentrations cause hypercalcaemia, which is associated with a low normal or low plasma phosphate concentration in relation to GFR (p.**175**), and to phosphaturia. If glomerular damage develops due to hypercalcaemia, the kidneys cannot respond normally to the phosphaturic effect of PTH and, because of impaired hydroxylation of 25-OHD$_3$, plasma calcium concentrations may fall towards or within the reference range as renal failure progresses. Because plasma phosphate concentrations tend to rise, diagnosis may be difficult at this stage.

The *clinical features* of PTH- or PTHRP-induced hypercalcaemia are due to:

- excess circulating concentration of free-ionized calcium which is the direct consequence of increased osteoclastic activity and release of calcium from bone, and enhanced absorption of calcium from the intestinal lumen by vitamin D; PTH increases the formation of 1,25-(OH)$_2$D$_3$.
- the effects of persistent PTH or PTHRP activity on bone in the presence of a normal supply of Vitamin D and calcium, are shown in Table 9.1.

The differences between the clinical presentations, associated with inappropriately high plasma PTH concentrations, depend on the duration of the disease. *The following effects on bone only become evident in long-standing cases.* Prolonged decalcification of bone causes a secondary increase in osteoblastic activity. Alkaline phosphatase-rich osteoblasts release the enzyme into the circulation and if the number of cells is greatly increased *plasma alkaline phosphatase activity rises.*

Primary hyperparathyroidism is caused by inappropriate secretion of PTH by the parathyroid glands, causing hypercalcaemia. It is usually due to one or more parathyroid adenomas, but occasionally to hyperplasia of all four parathyroid glands or to carcinoma of one of the glands. Ectopic parathyroid tumours do occur. Primary hyperparathyroidism may be associated with other multiple endocrine neoplasias (MEN), such as pituitary and pancreatic adenomas (MEN Type I), or with phaeochromocytomas and medullary carcinoma of the thyroid (MEN Type II) (p.**397**).

The incidence of primary hyperparathyroidism increases with age, being commonest in elderly females. It may be found in young people and occasionally in children in whom the sex incidence seems to be equal.

The majority of cases of primary hyperthyroidism are diagnosed after the chance finding of high plasma calcium with low plasma phosphate concentrations. *Clinical symptoms and signs* at presentation are due to a high plasma free-ionized calcium concentration and include:

- *generalized ill health*, depression, nausea, anorexia and abdominal pain and polyuria;
- *renal calculi*. About 10 per cent of patients who present with renal calculi have primary hyperparathyroidism;
- *bone pain*. In most patients *subperiosteal bone erosions* or cysts may be seen on X-ray of the terminal phalanges. However, extensive, severe bone disease, osteitis fibrosa cystica, is now a rare presenting feature as patients are usually diagnosed before the disorder is extensive and consequently *plasma alkaline phosphatase activity is usually normal or only slightly increased;*
- *medical emergency*. Occasionally the patient is admitted as an emergency with abdominal pain, vomiting and constipation. Severe hypercalcaemia is a recognized cause of acute pancreatitis and should be considered as one cause of an 'acute abdomen'.

Tertiary hyperparathyroidism may occur if the parathyroid glands have been subjected to long-standing and sustained positive feedback by low plasma free-ionized calcium concentrations of secondary hyperparathyroidism (p.**181**), which has been subsequently corrected. The parathyroid glands hypertrophy; PTH secretion becomes partly autonomous and is not suppressed by negative feedback by the hypercalcaemia. The diagnosis is usually made when the cause of the original hypocalcaemia is removed, for example by renal transplantation or correction of long standing calcium or vitamin D deficiency. A history of previous hypocalcaemia and the finding of a very high plasma alkaline phosphatase activity due to the prolonged osteomalacia distinguish it from primary hyperparathyroidism. In some cases, the glandular hypertrophy gradually regresses and the plasma calcium concentration returns to normal.

Humoral hypercalcaemia of malignancy. PTHRP is synthesized by some malignant tumours of nonendocrine tissues and is not subject to normal feedback control by the high plasma free-ionized calcium concentration. Initially the biochemical findings are identical to those of primary hyperparathyroidism. Bony lesions due to circulating PTHRP are not normally present because the underlying disease is usually either fatal or successfully treated in a relatively short time. However, the plasma alkaline phosphatase activity may be raised because of secondary deposits in bone, the liver or both. In humoral hypercalcaemia of malignancy, the plasma calcium concentration may rise from normal to a dangerously high concentration very rapidly, in contrast with primary hyperparathyroidism. Ectopic hormone production is discussed more fully in Chapter 21.

Familial hypocalciuric hypercalcaemia. Hypercalcaemia, with an inappropriately high plasma PTH concentration in the presence of hypocalciuria, has been reported in families, in none of whom was a parathyroid adenoma found at operation. The condition is inherited as an autosomal dominant trait. The aetiology of the condition is not known and is extremely rare.

HYPERCALCAEMIA WITH HYPERPHOSPHATAEMIA RELATIVE TO THE GFR

Hypercalcaemia, not caused by inappropriate PTH secretion, suppresses the release of the hormone, and is associated with a rise of the plasma phosphate concentration, from its basal level.

Hypercalcaemia with hyperphosphataemia relative to GFR, may be due to:

- *vitamin D excess;*
- *sarcoidosis;*
- rare causes, such as:
    prolonged immobilization, for example in patients with Paget's disease;
    idiopathic hypercalcaemia of infancy;
    severe hyperthyroidism;
    some cases of extensive secondary malignant deposits in bone and possibly myelomatosis.

The clinical picture in these conditions may be caused by the high plasma free-ionized calcium concentration (p.**172**). Generalized decalcification of bone is rare in this group, and is only associated with thyrotoxicosis, sarcoidosis, and sometimes with myelomatosis or bony deposits. The plasma alkaline phosphatase activity is usually normal in myelomatosis (p.**329**) and in those conditions not involving bone.

Vitamin D excess may be caused by overvigorous treatment of hypocalcaemia. Increased intestinal calcium absorption may cause dangerous hypercalcaemia. Vitamin D therapy, with either ergocalciferol or the active metabolite, 1,25-dihydroxyvitamin D, should always be monitored by frequent estimation of plasma calcium concentrations and, if there is osteomalacia, by measuring plasma alkaline phosphatase activity. If the cause of hypercalcaemia is obscure a careful drug history should be taken. Occasionally patients overdose themselves with vitamin D, which is available in most countries without prescription.

PTH secretion is suppressed by negative feedback inhibition and therefore the plasma phosphate concentrations are usually normal or high.

Abnormal vitamin D metabolism, as a cause of hypercalcaemia, may be associated with:

- *sarcoidosis.* Hypercalcaemia is a rare complication. $1,25\text{-}(OH)_2D_3$ is synthesized in the granuloma tissue and increases calcium absorption from the intestinal tract. *Chronic beryllium poisoning* produces a granulomatous reaction very similar to that of sarcoidosis and may also be associated with hypercalcaemia;
- *idiopathic hypercalcaemia of infancy* which includes a number of conditions that cause hypercalcaemia during the first year of life. Excessive vitamin D supplementation of cow's milk is now a very uncommon cause. Williams' syndrome is a rare familial disorder asscoiated with increased intestinal calcium absorption and hypercalcaemia. Clinical features include growth retardation, mental deficiency and characteristic 'elfin' facies. Congenital heart disease may also be present.

Malignant disease of bone. The production of PTHRP by malignant tumours has been discussed (p.**174**). A different syndrome may occur in some patients with multiple bony metastases or with myelomatosis in whom the parallel rise of plasma phosphate, with plasma calcium, concentration suggests that the hypercalcaemia is caused by direct bone breakdown due to the local action of malignant deposits, rather than to PTHRP. The paraproteins of myelomatosis very rarely bind calcium to any significant extent and are unlikely to account for hypercalcaemia in this condition. Malignant deposits in bone stimulate a local osteoblastic reaction and hence a rise in plasma alkaline phosphatase activity (p.**306**). This osteoblastic reaction does not occur in bone eroded by the marrow expansion of myelomatosis. Therefore in the latter condition the plasma concentration of alkaline phosphatase of bony origin is normal, despite extensive bone involvment.

Hypercalcaemia of hyperthyroidism. Prolonged excess of thyroid hormone in severe hyperthyroidism may be associated with the histological appearance of osteoporosis and a consequent increase in urinary calcium excretion. Hypercalcaemia is a very rare complication. Unless there is a marked excess of thyroid hormone the effects on plasma calcium are overridden by a reduction of PTH secretion by negative feedback and the increase in urinary calcium loss. If the plasma calcium concentration fails to fall when the hyperthyroidism is controlled, and especially if there is hypophosphataemia, the possibility of coexistent hyperparathyroidism should be considered; these may be part of the syndrome of multiple endocrine neoplasia (p.**397**).

Hypocalcaemia

CLINICAL EFFECTS OF A REDUCED FREE-IONIZED CALCIUM CONCENTRATION

Low plasma free-ionized calcium concentrations, including those associated with a normal total calcium concentration of alkalosis (p.**173**), cause increased neuromuscular activity eventually leading to *tetany*.

Prolonged hypocalcaemia, even when mild, interferes with the metabolism of the lens in the eye and may cause cataracts. Because of this, asymptomatic hypocalcaemia should be sought when there has been a known risk of parathyroid damage, such as after partial or total thyroidectomy and, if found, treated. Hypocalcaemia may also cause *depression and other psychiatric symptoms*.

HYPOCALCAEMIA WITH HYPOPHOSPHATAEMIA RELATIVE TO THE GFR

High plasma PTH concentrations cause phosphaturia with hypophosphataemia if glomerular function is normal.

Secondary hyperparathyroidism ('appropriate' secretion of PTH) occurs in response to a low plasma free-ionized calcium concentration. The parathyroid glands respond with appropriate secretion of PTH. If the response is effective, the plasma calcium concentration returns to normal, the stimulus to secretion is removed and hormone production is then inhibited by negative feedback. Preservation of plasma calcium concentrations occurs at the expense of bone mineralization and therefore decalcification may result. PTH cannot act effectively on bone in the absence of 1,25-$(OH)_2D_3$. In cases of vitamin D deficiency with hypocalcaemia, plasma PTH concentrations may be very high but the effects on bone differ from those with inappropriate PTH secretion due to primary hyperparathyroidism. Without an adequate supply of calcium and phosphate osteoid cannot be calcified despite marked osteoblastic proliferation. The histological finding of uncalcified osteoid is characteristic of osteomalacia in adults or rickets in children. *Osteomalacia, before fusion of the epiphyses,* may present with a slightly different clinical, radiological and histological picture and *is called rickets.* Plasma alkaline phosphatase activity is increased because of osteoblastic proliferation. The effects on bone of a high plasma PTH concentration in prolonged vitamin D and calcium deficiency are shown in Table 9.2. Disorders of bone disease, associated with secondary hyperparathyroidism, may present with:

- *osteomalacia in adults, or rickets in children,* presenting before fusion of the epiphyses is due to long-standing deficiency of calcium, phosphate and vitamin D. Predisposing factors include:
  reduced dietary intake of vitamin D, calcium and phosphate in malnutrition;
  impaired absorption of vitamin D in steatorrhoea after gastrectomy;
  impaired metabolism of vitamin D to 1,25-$(OH)_2D_3$ due to renal disease;
  increased inactivation of vitamin D due to anticonvulsant therapy (p.**183**);
  renal tubular disorders of phosphate reabsorption (p.**184**).

Table 9.2 The possible effects of prolonged excess PTH secretion with deficiency of vitamin D (secondary hyperparathyroidism)

Clinical
  bone pain
  rarely bony swelling
Radiological
  generalized decalcification
  sometimes pseudofractures (cortical fractures; Looser's zones)
  rarely subperiosteal erosions or bone cysts
Histological
  Uncalcified osteoid and wide osteoid seams
  osteoblastic proliferation
  occasionally an increased number of osteoclasts
Plasma
  low free-ionized calcium concentration
  low phosphate concentration in relation to urea
  raised alkaline phosphatase activity

- *without osteomalacia or rickets.* If PTH action is inadequate to correct the abnormality, the plasma calcium concentration remains low and bone disorders are not present. Predisposing factors include:
    early calcium and vitamin D deficiency, most cases of the *very rare* pseudohypoparathyroidism (p.**183**).

In secondary hyperparathyroidism the plasma calcium concentration is never high and usually both the plasma calcium and phosphate concentrations tend to be low. High normal or high plasma calcium concentrations in renal glomerular dysfunction suggest that either primary hyperparathyroidism has caused the renal disease, or that prolonged calcium deficiency has led to the development of tertiary hyperparathyroidism.

Reduced intake and absorption of calcium and vitamin D. $1,25\text{-}(OH)_2D_3$ is essential for normal intestinal absorption of calcium. Vitamin D can only be absorbed from the intestinal lumen if it is dissolved in fat (p.**268**). In steatorrhoea fat, and therefore vitamin D, absorption is impaired; this malabsorption may be aggravated if calcium combines with unabsorbed fatty acids to form insoluble soaps in the lumen. Deficiency due to malnutrition is more commonly caused by deficiency of vitamin D than of calcium.

In relatively affluent countries, *malabsorption is the commonest cause of calcium and vitamin D deficiencies.* However, in the world as a whole, dietary deficiency is important. The following groups are at risk of developing osteomalacia or rickets:

- *children and pregnant women*, in whom increased needs may not be met by the normal supply from the skin;
- subjects, such as the *elderly and chronically sick*, who are not exposed to sunlight because they are confined indoors.

There is a relatively high incidence of osteomalacia and rickets amongst the Asian community in Western countries, most common in those not fully integrated into the community. The causes are unclear but probably include dietary habits, lack of sunlight and possibly genetic factors.

Malnutrition, with protein deficiency, may reduce the plasma concentration of protein bound calcium. In this group the plasma free-ionized concentration may not, therefore, be as low as the plasma total calcium concentration would suggest.

Impaired metabolism of vitamin D. *Renal disease* causes relative resistance to vitamin D because of:

- the direct effect of the disease on the functioning renal tubular cells and therefore on 1α-hydroxylation of 25-OHD$_3$;
- inhibition of 1α-hydroxylation by hyperphosphataemia associated with the low GFR of renal glomerular dysfunction.

Hypocalcaemia may develop within a few days of the onset of renal damage. Low plasma protein concentrations often contribute to the reduction in the total calcium concentration. Tetany is rare in renal disease, probably because the accompanying acidosis increases the plasma free-ionized calcium concentration above tetanic concentrations. Treatment of the metabolic acidosis with bicarbonate is usually contraindicated because a rise in blood pH may cause precipitation of calcium phosphate in extraosseous sites. In the kidney it may aggravate renal dysfunction.

Chronic liver disease may occasionally be associated with mild osteomalacia, especially if there is cholestasis causing malabsorption due, for example, to primary biliary cirrhosis (p.**286**). However, it is unlikely that significant impairment of vitamin D hydroxylation is the cause.

Prolonged anticonvulsant therapy, especially if both barbiturates and phenytoin are taken, may be associated with hypocalcaemia and even osteomalacia. These drugs probably induce the synthesis of hepatic enzymes which catalyse the conversion of vitamin D to inactive metabolites.

In all these conditions, the low plasma free-ionized calcium concentration stimulates PTH secretion; the plasma phosphate concentration tends to be low *relative to the GFR*. However, if there is renal glomerular dysfunction the plasma phosphate concentration may be increased but tends to be lower than in those cases with the same concentration of plasma urea but normal plasma PTH concentrations. In chronic cases a rising plasma alkaline phosphatase activity indicates the onset of the bone changes of osteomalacia or rickets.

HYPOCALCAEMIA WITH HYPERPHOSPHATAEMIA RELATIVE TO THE GFR

A low concentration of circulating PTH is associated with hyperphosphataemia.

Primary Hypoparathyroidism

Surgical causes. Hypoparathyroidism is most commonly caused *by surgical damage* to the parathyroid glands, either directly or indirectly by impairment of their blood supply during partial *thyroidectomy*. Total thyroidectomy or *laryngectomy* is almost inevitably associated with removal of the parathyroid glands. Post-thyroidectomy hypocalcaemia is not always due to damage to the glands. Most, even minor, operations cause temporary hypoalbuminaemia (p.**318**) with a consequent fall in plasma total but not free-ionized calcium concentration.

Parathyroidectomy, carried out to treat primary or tertiary hyperparathyroidism, also carries a slight risk of damage to the remaining parathyroid tissue. However, there are several causes of temporary hypocalcaemia, which usually need no treatment:

- apparent hypocalcaemia may be due to postoperative hypoalbuminaemia;
- in rare cases of primary hyperparathyroidism with overt bone disease, rapid entry of calcium into bone, when plasma PTH concentrations fall, may cause true, but temporary, postoperative hypocalcaemia;
- if the hypercalcaemia has been severe and prolonged, the remaining parathyroid tissue may have been suppressed by negative feedback for so long that there may be true hypoparathyroidism evidenced by a rising plasma phosphate concentration, which usually recovers within a few days. Unless persistent it should be treated only if there is tetany. Mild hypocalcaemia stimulates the remaining parathyroid tissue to regenerate.

Evidence for asymptomatic hypocalcaemia should always be sought after partial thyroidectomy or parathyroidectomy. Although early postoperative parathyroid insufficiency may recover, a low plasma calcium concentration persisting for more than a few weeks should be treated because of the danger of cataract formation (p.**181**). Even with highly skilled surgery there is always a danger of parathyroid damage.

Idiopathic hypoparathyroidism is rare. It may occur as:

- *a familial disorder*, presenting either during childhood or in adults;
- *an autoimmune disorder* with antibodies against parathyroid tissue.

Congenital absence of the parathyroid glands, associated with impaired cellular immunity, a characteristic facial appearance and cardiac abnormalities is known as the DiGeorge syndrome. It is very uncommon.

Pseudohypoparathyroidism. A very rare inborn error is associated with an impaired response of both kidneys and bone to PTH.

Plasma calcium concentrations are low despite increased PTH secretion because of the impaired action of PTH on renal 1α-hydroxylase activity. The biochemical changes of hypoparathyroidism, not hyperparathyroidism, are therefore present.

HYPOCALCAEMIA OF 'SHOCK'

Any cause of the 'shock' syndrome, including minor surgery, may cause a temporary fall in the plasma albumin concentration with a consequent fall in total calcium. Although plasma free-ionized calcium concentrations very occasionally fall, they are almost always normal even in acute pancreatitis. Calcium should only be given if there are clinical symptoms of hypocalcaemia.

Disorders of Bone not Affecting the Plasma Calcium Concentration

Some disorders of bone rarely alter plasma calcium concentrations but are important in the differential diagnosis of changes in mineral metabolism.

Osteoporosis is *not* a primary disorder of calcium metabolism. The reduction of bone mass is due to thinning of the protein on which the calcium is usually deposited. A slight increase in urinary calcium loss is secondary to this. Disorders associated with an increased incidence include:

- *low plasma oestrogen concentrations*, such as after the menopause, the most common cause and prolonged amenorrhoea;
- *endocrine disorders*:
    hypercortisolism;
- *elderly subjects* in whom there may also be mild osteomalacia because of impaired renal function (p.**182**).

Clinically and radiologically it may resemble osteomalacia, but plasma calcium and phosphate concentrations do not fall and, because there is no increase in osteoblastic activity, the plasma alkaline phosphatase activity does not rise. These findings are invaluable in distinguishing between osteomalacia and osteoporosis.

Paget's disease of bone is caused by disorganized osteoclastic and osteoblastic function and occurs with increasing frequency in the elderly. It may be asymptomatic or may present with *bone pain* and high output cardiac failure due to increased vascularity within the bone. Plasma calcium and phosphate concentrations are rarely affected unless the patient is immobilized; the plasma calcium concentrations may then rise. *Plasma alkaline phosphatase activity is typically very high.* A small minority of patients may develop *osteosarcomas* and this complication may be associated with a rapidly rising plasma alkaline phosphatase activity.

Rickets or osteomalacia caused by renal tubular disorders of phosphate reabsorption. In a group of inborn errors of renal tubular function *less phosphate than normal is reabsorbed* from the glomerular filtrate. The consequent rickets or osteomalacia, unlike the usual form, responds poorly to vitamin D therapy. The syndrome has therefore been called 'resistant rickets'. *Familial hypophosphataemia* is an X-linked dominant trait; the syndrome may also be part of a more generalized reabsorption defect in the Fanconi syndrome (p.**356**).

In these disorders failure to calcify bone is probably due to phosphate deficiency, although impaired vitamin D metabolism may also be present. Plasma phosphate concentrations are usually very low and fail to rise when vitamin D is given; there is phosphaturia inappropriate to the plasma concentration. The high plasma alkaline phosphatase activity reflects increased osteoblastic activity. The usually normal plasma calcium concentrations differ from the findings in the 'classical' syndrome. Because the free-ionized calcium concentration is normal the parathyroid glands are not overstimulated and therefore evidence in the bone of high PTH concentrations is rare. The conditions respond to large doses of oral phosphate and to a small dose of the active metabolite of vitamin D.

Tests for Diagnosis of Disorders of Calcium Metabolism

If careful attention is paid to the history and clinical examination, the concentration of plasma calcium in relation to albumin, phosphate *in relation to that of urea* (Fig. 9.2; p.**175**) and alkaline phosphatase activity, together with haematological and radiological findings, other biochemical tests are usually unnecessary.

The non-invasive techniques of isotope subtraction scanning or ultrasonography of the neck may help to localize a parathyroid adenoma before operation and so help the surgeon. Photon absorptiometry may occasionally be useful to measure bone density in those individuals at risk of developing osteoporosis before the onset of symptoms.

Plasma parathyroid hormone assay. If the negative feedback mechanism for PTH release is functioning normally a rise in free-ionized hypercalcaemia should reduce secretion of PTH. Detectable plasma PTH, even if the concentration is within the reference range, is inappropriate in the presence of free-ionized hypercalcaemia and is consistent with primary, or more rarely tertiary, hyperparathyroidism. Undetectable plasma PTH concentrations do not always exclude the diagnosis of primary hyperparathyroidism, nor high ones necessarily confirm it, as some proven parathyroid adenomas secrete biologically active hormone, which fails to react in some assays.

The measurement of plasma PTH concentration may help if the exceedingly rare

pseudohypoparathyroidism is suspected as a cause of hypocalcaemia (p.**183**). If it is very high despite hypocalcaemia and hyperphosphataemia, it suggests that the feedback mechanism is intact, but that there is end-organ unresponsiveness to circulating PTH.

At the time of writing, there is no routine clinical indication to measure plasma PTHRP concentrations.

Urinary calcium and phosphate estimation. Estimation of urinary calcium excretion is almost never of diagnostic value in the differential diagnosis of hypercalcaemia. If glomerular function is normal hypercalcaemia, unless due to familial hypocalciuric hypercalcaemia, increases the calcium load on the glomeruli and causes hypercalciuria. Excess PTH, by increasing tubular reabsorption, might be expected to reduce calcium excretion below that appropriate for the plasma concentration but the 'normal' response is too variable for the test to be helpful. If renal glomerular function is impaired calcium excretion is low even if there is hypercalcaemia.

Hypercalciuria, in the absence of hypercalcaemia, occurs in:

- *idiopathic hypercalciuria* and may predispose to the formation of renal stones (p.**22**);
- some cases of *osteoporosis* in which calcium cannot be deposited in normal amounts because the bone matrix is reduced;
- *acidosis*, in which the release of free-ionized calcium from bone is increased.

Urinary phosphate excretion falls as the plasma phosphate, and therefore glomerular filtrate, concentrations decrease in response to reduced dietary phosphate intake. The measurement of urinary phosphate concentration may occasionally be useful to distinguish hypophosphataemia due to true depletion (low urinary phosphate) and the increased urinary phosphate excretion found in renal tubular disorders, such as familial hypophosphataemic rickets.

Plasma Vitamin D assay. 25-OHD$_3$ is the circulating, inactive form of vitamin D and plasma concentrations fall in deficiency states. In most cases the diagnosis of vitamin D deficiency is evident after clinical examination and simple investigations. The measurement of the biologically active metabolite, 1,25-(OH)$_2$D$_3$, which circulates in plasma in very low concentrations, is never indicated as it does not reflect body stores but disordered metabolism.

Biochemical Basis of Treatment

HYPERCALCAEMIA

Mild to moderate hypercalcaemia. Protein-bound hypercalcaemia due to hyperalbuminaemia should *never* be treated.

If the plasma calcium concentration is below about 3.75 mmol/L (15 mg/dl), and if there are no significant electrocardiographic changes attributable to hypercalcaemia, there is no need for rapidly-acting treatment. However, treatment should be started as soon as the abnormality is found and preliminary investigations performed because of the danger of renal damage. If possible, the primary cause should also be diagnosed and treated.

The patient should be volume repleted. The plasma total calcium concentration will almost certainly fall as the plasma albumin concentration is diluted, but the plasma free-ionized calcium concentration is probably little affected. Correcting haemoconcentration enables a more realistic assessment of the degree of true hypercalcaemia to be made.

Bisphosphonates have largely replaced the use of oral sodium phosphate, calcitonin and mithramycin in the medical management of hypercalcaemia.

- *Bisphosphonates* are structurally similar to pyrophosphate. They bind to hydroxyapatite in bone, thus inhibiting bone turnover and the mobilization of calcium. They are poorly absorbed from the intestinal tract and may have to be given intravenously to patients with severe hypercalcaemia. Cyclical administration may prevent the long-term complication of osteomalacia.
- *Oral sodium phosphate*, by forming calcium phosphate, prevents the absorption of dietary calcium and the reabsorption of calcium entering the gut lumen in intestinal secretions: it therefore removes calcium from the body. This treatment is effective, safe and cheap. The tendency to develop osmotic diarrhoea is minimized if the phosphate is dissolved in enough water to make it isosmolar. It may be used in conjunction with steroids to treat intractable hypercalcaemia due to extensive malignancy.
- *Calcitonin* is expensive and relatively ineffective; it should only be used if bisphosphonates are contraindicated and oral phosphate treatment is not possible, for example because the patient is vomiting.
- *Mithramycin* may be used to treat intractable hypercalcaemia of malignancy. It inhibits calcium mobilization from bone; the effect lasts for several days. It is a bone marrow suppressant and should only be used at low dosage and for a short time.
- *Steroids* lower the plasma calcium concentration in some cases, particularly if the hypercalcaemia is caused by malignancy, sarcoidosis or vitamin D intoxication.

The management of apparently asymptomatic mild hypercalcaemia due to primary hyperparathyroidism is controversial. It has been suggested that prolonged hypercalcaemia does not always cause obvious renal dysfunction and that the risk of parathyroidectomy is greater than that of mild hypercalcaemia. Nevertheless, almost all patients volunteer the information that a successful operation has improved their feeling of well-being and has made them aware of previous vague ill health. In the hands of an experienced surgeon the morbidity of the procedure is minimal and short-lived. The decision as to whether to operate must be made on clinical grounds; of particular importance are the fitness of the patient for operation if other disease is present and age.

Symptomatic hypercalcaemia in a patient unfit for operation must be treated medically.

Severe hypercalcaemia. The plasma concentration at which urgent treatment is indicated varies in different subjects, but, because of the danger of cardiac arrest, it is usually necessary if it exceeds about 3.75 mmol/L (15 mg/dl). If in doubt, abnormalities associated with hypercalcaemia should be sought on the electrocardiogram. Oral phosphate, steroids and calcitonin have no significant effect for about 24 hours.

- *Rehydration.* The patient should be volume repleted, intravenously if vomiting. Frusemide may be given in an attempt to increase urinary calcium clearance. Because there is an inverse relation between plasma calcium and potassium concentrations, many patients are hypokalaemic and need potassium supplementation.
- *Bisphosphonates.* After rehydration and correction of any electrolyte abnormalities, bisphosphonates are the treatment of choice. They are probably the most effective and have the least toxic side effects. A single infusion restores normocalcaemia in about 80 per cent of patients and the response lasts for up to 20 days.
- *Intravenous sodium, sometimes with potassium, phosphate* lowers the plasma calcium concentration within a few hours. The response depends, at least in part, on precipitation of insoluble calcium salts. Because some of this precipitation may occur in the kidney the treatment carries a slight risk of initiating or aggravating renal dysfunction; this is rarely a problem in practice, probably because little precipitation is needed to reduce the plasma calcium concentration quickly.
- *Steroids* may sometimes lower the plasma calcium concentration in malignancy and almost always in cases of sarcoidosis and vitamin D intoxication.
- *Calcitonin* is sometimes used to treat severe hypercalcaemia. The effect lasts

about three days; repeated doses are often less successful in maintaining a 'normal' plasma calcium concentration.

As with most other extracellular constituents, rapid changes in plasma calcium concentration may be dangerous because time is not allowed for equilibration across cell membranes. The aim of emergency treatment should be to lower the plasma concentration to one that is not immediately dangerous, while initiating treatment for mild hypercalcaemia as outlined above. *Too rapid a reduction, even to only normal or slightly raised concentrations, may cause tetany or, more seriously, hypotension.*

HYPOCALCAEMIA

Postoperative hypocalcaemia. Hypocalcaemia, during the first week after a thyroidectomy or parathyroidectomy, should only be treated if there is severe tetany, and then only with calcium supplements which, unlike calciferol, have a rapid effect and a short half-life. Mild hypocalcaemia is of no immediate danger and helps to stimulate recovery of suppressed parathyroid tissue; some of the fall in the plasma total calcium concentration may be due to postoperative haemodilution. Persistent hypocalcaemia may indicate that the glands are permanently damaged and that long-standing, or even life-long, calciferol treatment is necessary.

Asymptomatic hypocalcaemia. Apparent hypocalcaemia, due to low plasma albumin concentrations, should not be treated.

Asymptomatic true hypocalcaemia, or that causing only mild clinical symptoms, can usually be treated effectively with oral vitamin D supplements. It is difficult to give enough oral calcium by itself to make a lasting and significant difference to plasma calcium concentrations. If a normal diet is being taken, vitamin D, by increasing absorption of calcium from the intestine, is usually adequate without calcium supplements; *management using one drug is simpler than with two.*

Because of the danger of ectopic calcification by precipitation of calcium phosphate, hypocalcaemia with hyperphosphataemia in renal disease should be treated cautiously and only if there are signs of osteomalacia, such as a raised plasma alkaline phosphatase activity. The plasma phosphate concentration should first be lowered by giving oral aluminium hydroxide which binds phosphate in the intestinal lumen. $1,25-(OH)_2D_3$ or 1α-hydroxycalciferol, the active vitamin D metabolites, have been used.

Hypocalcaemia with severe tetany. If there is severe tetany shown to be due to hypocalcaemia, intravenous calcium, usually as calcium gluconate, should be given at once.

Phosphate Metabolism

Factors that affect the absorption, metabolisn and excretion of phosphate have been discussed (p.179).

Abnormalities of Plasma Phosphatase Concentration

Hypophosphataemia, associated with disturbances of calcium metabolism is usually due to high circulating PTH concentrations. In such conditions, and in renal tubular disorders of phosphate reabsorption (p.184), phosphate is lost from the body in urine. Hypophosphataemia may also be caused by severe and prolonged dietary deficiency; urinary phosphate excretion is then usually significantly reduced.

Phosphate, like potassium, enters cells from the extracellular fluid if the rate of glucose metabolism is increased. This may be associated with *glucose infusion* during, for example, the treatment of diabetic coma with insulin. The redistribution of phosphate is a common cause of hypophosphataemia in patients receiving parenteral nutrition with insulin and glucose. Long-term parenteral feeding, without phosphate supplementation, may cause true phosphate depletion. Hypophosphataemia in such circumstances, whether due to deficiency or redistribution, may cause neurological abnormalities such as *convulsions*.

Hyperphosphataemia. Normal plasma phosphate concentrations are higher in infants and children than in adults. The commonest cause of hyperphosphataemia is renal glomerular dysfunction; it is important not to correct hypocalcaemia until this abnormality has been corrected. Less common causes include hypoparathyroidism and acromegaly.

Magnesium Metabolism

Bone mineral contains magnesium as well as calcium and the two ions tend to move in and out of bone together. Cells contain magnesium at a much higher concentration than the extracellular fluid and magnesium, potassium and phosphate usually enter and leave cells under the same circumstances.

Large amounts of magnesium can be lost in faeces in diarrhoea, or in fluid lost through intestinal fistulae.

Plasma Magnesium and its Control

About 35 per cent of plasma magnesium is protein bound. Less is known about the importance of this binding than that of calcium.

The mechanism of control is poorly understood. Aldosterone increases its renal excretion. PTH may affect its absorption and excretion in a similar way to that of calcium.

CLINICAL EFFECTS OF ABNORMAL PLASMA MAGNESIUM CONCENTRATIONS

Hypomagnesaemia. The symptoms of hypomagnesaemia are very similar to those of hypocalcaemia. If the plasma calcium concentrations, allowing for that of albumin, and blood pH are normal in a patient with tetany, the plasma magnesium concentration should be assayed. If the deficiency is severe, magnesium may be given intravenously but in less severe cases oral treatment is adequate.

Hypermagnesaemia causes muscular hypotonia but, as it is rarely found without other abnormalities such as hypercalcaemia

or those due to renal failure, it is not always easy to distinguish those signs and symptoms specifically due to hypermagnesaemia.

CAUSES OF ABNORMAL PLASMA MAGNESIUM CONCENTRATIONS

Hypomagnesaemia is uncommon and is rarely associated with clinical problems. Causes include:

- *excess loss of magnesium.* This is by far the most important cause, often serious enough to warrant treatment. It may be due to losses either in *severe, prolonged diarrhoea*, or through *intestinal fistulae.* Loss in urine due to renal tubular dysfunction is usually less severe. Cytotoxic drugs, such as cisplatin, may cause hypomagnesaemia by impairing renal tubular reabsorption;

- *hypomagnesaemia accompanied by hypocalcaemia.* This may occur in hypoparathyroidism, or following a parathyroidectomy which is associated with the fall of plasma calcium concentrations. Prolonged magnesium deficiency may impair PTH secretion from the parathyroid glands and cause hypocalcaemia by altering the normal feedback control mechanism;

- *hypomagnesaemia accompanied by hypokalaemia.* Since magnesium moves in and out of cells with potassium, hypomagnesaemia tends to occur with hypokalaemia, for example during diuretic therapy, or due to primary hyperaldosteronism. Such hypomagnesaemia is rarely of clinical importance. The low plasma magnesium concentration due to renal tubular dysfunction may also be associated with hypokalaemia. Hypomagnesaemia can also occur following chronic alcohol ingestion and may sometimes cause symptoms.

Hypermagnesaemia. The commonest cause of hypermagnesaemia is renal glomerular dysfunction. It rarely needs specific treatment and responds to measures to treat the underlying condition. Magnesium salts should never be given to patients with renal glomerular failure.

Summary

Calcium Metabolism

1. About half the plasma calcium is protein-bound and half in the free-ionized form.
2. The free-ionized calcium is the physiologically active fraction. Plasma total calcium concentrations should be interpreted together with albumin concentrations.
3. The plasma calcium concentration is controlled by PTH and vitamin D in the form of $1,25\text{-}(OH)_2D_3$. PTH secretion is increased if the plasma free-ionized calcium concentration is reduced.
4. PTH acts on:

   - *bone*, stimulating osteoclastic activity and so releasing calcium and phosphate into the plasma; if prolonged, this action increases the number of osteoblasts and the plasma alkaline phosphatase activity;
   - *kidneys*, stimulating calcium and inhibiting phosphate reabsorption, and so lowers the plasma phosphate concentration. It may also increase the rate of 1α-hydroxylation of $25\text{-}OHD_3$.
5. Signs and symptoms and laboratory findings of altered calcium metabolism can be related to the plasma concentrations of free-ionized calcium and PTH, and to renal function.
6. If the parathyroid glands are functioning normally appropriately high concentrations of PTH are present if plasma free-ionized calcium concentration falls.
7. Inappropriately high plasma PTH concentrations are present in primary and tertiary hyperparathyroidism. In these circumstances the plasma free-ionized calcium concentration is high.
8. Plasma PTH concentrations are appropriately low if hypercalcaemia is caused by a condition other than primary or tertiary hyperparathyroidism. They are inappropriately low if hypocalcaemia is due to hypoparathyroidism.

Magnesium Metabolism

1. Hypomagnesaemia may cause tetany in the absence of hypocalcaemia.
2. The commonest cause of significant hypomagnesaemia is severe diarrhoea.
3. Magnesium tends to move in and out of bone with calcium and in and out of cells with potassium.

INVESTIGATION OF DISORDERS OF CALCIUM METABOLISM

The concentration of plasma calcium should never be interpreted without those of albumin and phosphate; the latter can only be interpreted if the urea concentration is known.

Differential Diagnosis of Hypercalcaemia

Three groups of causes must be differentiated:

- raised protein-bound, with normal free-ionized calcium;
- raised free-ionized calcium due to inappropriately high PTH;
- raised free-ionized calcium due to other causes and associated with low PTH concentrations.

The following procedure outlines a simple and reliable sequence of investigations to elucidate the cause of hypercalcaemia. The diagnosis is usually obvious before all the steps have been followed.

Is the high plasma total calcium concentration due only to a high protein-bound fraction?

1. What is the plasma albumin concentration?
2. If the total calcium concentration is less than about 2.80 mmol/L (11.2 mg/dl), *in vivo* or artefactual haemoconcentration may be the cause. If the plasma calcium concentration is much higher than this, true hypercalcaemia is likely.

   - Following rehydration, take a specimen without venous stasis to eliminate artefactual haemoconcentration (p.**424**) and repeat the plasma calcium and albumin assays. If true hypercalcaemia is confirmed a cause for a high plasma free-ionized calcium must be sought.

   - If the plasma calcium concentration is at the upper end of the reference range repeat the assay at about three monthly intervals, to exclude developing hypercalcaemia.

3. Is the plasma albumin concentration low? If so, plasma calcium concentrations at the upper end of the reference range may indicate a high plasma free-ionized fraction. Many formulae have been proposed in an attempt to 'correct' the plasma total calcium for abnormal plasma protein concentrations. Unfortunately the relation between the plasma albumin concentration and calcium binding is not simple, and results of such calculations are often misleading.

What is the cause of a raised plasma free-ionized calcium concentration?

The commonest causes of hypercalcaemia are primary hyperparathyroidism and malignancy; the latter is usually obvious following clinical examination and radiological, haematological and simple biochemical investigations.

1. Take a careful history, with special reference to the drug history, such as vitamin D containing preparations and thiazide duretics.
2. Is the plasma phosphate concentration low *in relation to the plasma urea concentration?*

   If so the most important differential diagnosis is now between primary hyperparathyroidism and malignancy.

   - Repeat the clinical examination, paying special attention to palpation of the breasts and pelvic examination. Seek evidence of carcinoma of the bronchus.

     A very *high plasma alkaline phosphatase activity* is unlikely to be due to uncomplicated primary hyperparathyroidism; a normal activity is the rule, although it may be slightly raised if there is radiological evidence of bone involvement. If it is very high it suggests either malignancy, or some concurrent disease such as Paget's disease.

If myeloma is suspected perform serum and urine protein electrophoresis.

If all the findings are negative, if the blood haemoglobin concentration and ESR are normal, and especially if there is a history of, for example peptic ulceration or renal calculi, this suggests chronic hypercalcaemia. Primary hyperparathyroidism is by far the most likely cause, and other investigations are rarely necessary. Of course either of these complications may occur without hypercalcaemia. Isotope subtraction scanning or ultrasound of the neck may help to localize the adenoma.

- PTH assay may help make a diagnosis but remember that the results can only be interpreted if there is concomitant hypercalcaemia; a high concentration may be appropriate in its absence.

3. If the plasma phosphate concentration is normal or high, is the urea concentration high? Both phosphate and urea are retained if there is glomerular dysfunction. If there is hypercalcaemia Figure 9.2 (p.**175**) gives a rough guide to the significance of the plasma phosphate concentration at different urea concentrations.

   - By far the commonest cause is ingestion of vitamin D alone or in multivitamin preparations, in which case the patient may not know that he has taken vitamin D. Some people seem to be sensitive to diets high in calcium and vitamin D. A fall in both plasma calcium and phosphate during a supervized stay in hospital suggests vitamin D as a cause.
     Look for evidence of sarcoidosis.
     Is there severe thyrotoxicosis?
     In infants consider 'idiopathic' hypercalcaemia.

   In all these conditions the plasma calcium concentration falls following administration of steroids.

STEROID SUPPRESSION TEST

A steroid suppression test is rarely necessary to identify the cause of hypercalcaemia. However it is included here for completeness as it may occasionally be useful if the cause of severe hypercalcaemia remains obscure. The test differentiates primary and tertiary hyperparathyroidism from any other cause.

Procedure. All specimens should be taken without venous stasis.

- At least two specimens for plasma calcium and albumin assay should be taken on two different days before starting the test.
- The patient takes 40 mg of hydrocortisone orally eight hourly for 10 days.
- Blood is taken for plasma calcium and albumin estimation on the fifth, eighth and 10th days after starting the hydrocortisone.

Interpretation. If the plasma calcium concentration remains elevated and does not fall to within the reference range by the end of the test the diagnosis of primary hyperparathyroidism is very probable.

Significant fluid retention during high-dose steroid administration may dilute the protein-bound calcium. This effect must be allowed for when interpreting the results.

Differential Diagnosis of Hypocalcaemia

As in the case of hypercalcaemia, the causes of hypocalcaemia fall into three groups:

- reduced protein-bound, with normal free-ionized calcium concentration;
- reduced free-ionized calcium concentration due to primary PTH deficiency;
- reduced free-ionized calcium concentration due to other causes and associated with appropriately high PTH concentrations.

Is the fall in plasma total calcium concentration due only to a low protein-bound fraction?

- Patients with a low albumin concentration should not be given calcium or vitamin D unless there is clinical evidence of an associated free-ionized calcium concentration.

What is the cause of the low plasma free-ionized calcium concentration?

1. Is the plasma phosphate concentration low? If so, calcium deficiency with normal secretion of PTH in response to feedback is likely.

   - Is the plasma alkaline phosphatase activity high? This finding would suggest prolonged secondary hyperparathyroidism due to calcium deficiency.
   - Do bone X-rays show signs of osteomalacia? This confirms very prolonged calcium deficiency.

   - Look for causes of malnutrition, especially malabsorption.

2. Is the plasma phosphate concentration high? If the plasma urea concentration is high glomerular dysfunction is the likely cause. If the plasma urea concentration is also normal hypoparathyroidism is the most likely cause.

   - Is there a history of an operation on the neck? Hypoparathyroidism may be of autoimmune origin. This may be distinguished from the even more rare 'pseudohypoparathyroidism' by measuring plasma PTH concentrations. Concentrations will be low in true hypoparathyroidism but very high if there is the end organ unresponsiveness of pseudohypoparathyroidism.

Carbohydrate Metabolism

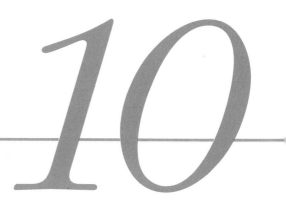

In most of the world carbohydrate is the major source of energy intake. Under normal circumstances starch is the main dietary carbohydrate; disaccharides contribute significantly and monosaccharides are a minor component.

CHEMISTRY

The principal monosaccharide hexoses are all reducing sugars; they therefore reduce copper compounds, such as those incorporated in Clinitest tablets (Ames Division, Miles Laboratories), to produce a colour change (Table 10.1).

Naturally occurring polysaccharides are long-chain carbohydrates composed of glucose subunits:

- *glycogen*, found in animal tissue, is a highly branched polysaccharide;
- *starch*, found in plants, is a mixture of amylose (straight chains) and amylopectin (branched chains).

Table 10.1 Common reducing and non-reducing sugars

	Reducing sugars	Non-reducing sugars
Monosaccharides	Glucose Fructose Galactose	
Disaccharides	Lactose (galactose + glucose) Maltose (glucose + glucose)	Sucrose (fructose + glucose)

PHYSIOLOGY

The Importance of Extracellular Glucose Concentrations

Brain cells are very dependent on the extracellular glucose concentration for their energy supply; *hypoglycaemia is likely to impair cerebral function*. This is because they cannot:

- *store glucose in significant amounts*;
- *synthesize glucose*;
- *metabolize substrates other than glucose and ketones*. Plasma ketone concentrations are usually very low and are of little importance as an energy source under physiological conditions;

- *extract enough glucose from the extracellular fluid at low concentrations for their metabolic needs*, because entry into brain cells is not facilitated by insulin.

Hyperglycaemia, especially of rapid onset, can also cause cerebral dysfunction by increasing extracellular osmolality, resulting in a shift of fluid out of the cells (p.35).

Normally the plasma glucose concentration remains between about 4.5 and 11 mmol/L (about 80 and 200 mg/dl) despite the intermittent load entering the body from the gastrointestinal tract. The maintenance of plasma glucose concentrations below about 11 mmol/L minimizes loss from the body as well as providing the optimal supply to the brain. Renal tubular cells reabsorb almost all the glucose filtered by the glomeruli and urinary glucose concentration is normally too low to be detected by the usual tests, even after a carbohydrate meal. Significant glycosuria only occurs if the plasma glucose concentration exceeds about 11 mmol/L – the '*renal threshold*'.

Maintenance of Extracellular Glucose Concentrations

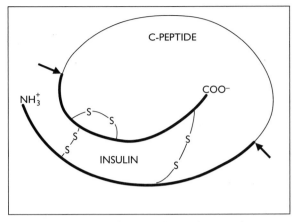

Fig. 10.1 Structure of proinsulin, indicating the cleavage sites at which insulin and C-peptide are produced.

HORMONES CONCERNED WITH GLUCOSE HOMEOSTASIS

Some of the more important effects of hormones on glucose homeostasis are summarized in Table 10.2.

Insulin is the most important hormone controlling plasma glucose concentrations, which it, in turn, controls. The β-cells of the pancreatic islets produce proinsulin which incorporates the 51-amino acid polypeptide insulin, and a linking peptide (C-peptide) (Fig. 10.1). Splitting the peptide bonds releases equimolar amounts of insulin and C-peptide into the extracellular fluid.

Insulin binds to specific cell-surface receptors on adipose tissue and muscle and enhances the rate of glucose entry into these cells. The intracellular glucose concentration is kept low by insulin-induced activation of enzymes which stimulate its incorporation into glycogen synthesis (*glycogenesis*) in liver and muscle. Insulin also inhibits the production of glucose (*gluconeogenesis*) from fats and amino acids partly by reducing these substrates by inhibiting fat and protein breakdown (*lipolysis* and *proteolysis*).

The transport of glucose into liver cells is insulin independent but, by reducing the intracellular glucose concentration, insulin does indirectly promote the passive diffusion of glucose into them. Insulin also directly increases transport of amino acids, potassium and phosphate into cells, especially muscle; these processes are independent of glucose transport.

The normal response to hyperglycaemia therefore depends on:

- adequate insulin secretion;
- normal insulin receptors;
- normal intracellular reaction to receptor binding of insulin ('postreceptor events').

Circulating C-peptide is probably of little physiological importance but its measurement may help in the differential diagnosis of hypoglycaemia (p.**213**).

Glucagon is a single-chain polypeptide synthesized by the α-cells of the pancreatic islets. Its secretion is stimulated by hypoglycaemia. Glucagon enhances hepatic glycogenolysis and gluconeogenesis.

When plasma insulin concentrations are low, for example during fasting, the hyperglycaemic actions of other hormones, such as growth hormone (GH), glucocorticoids, adrenaline and glucagon, become apparent, even if there is no increase in secretion rates. Secretion of these hormones may increase during stress and in patients with acromegaly (GH) (p.**111**), Cushing's syndrome (glucocorticoids) (p.**122**) or phaeochromocytoma (adrenaline and noradrenaline) (p.**395**) and thus oppose the normal action of insulin.

Table 10.2 Action of hormones that affect intermediary metabolism

	Insulin	Glucagon	Growth Hormone	Glucocorticoids	Adrenaline
Carbohydrate metabolism					
In liver					
• glycolysis	+				
• glycogenesis	+				
• glycogenolysis		+			+
• gluconeogenesis	−	+		+	
In muscle					
• glucose uptake	+		−	−	
• glycogenesis	+				
• glycogenolysis					+
Protein metabolism					
• synthesis	+		+		
• breakdown	−			+	
Lipid metabolism					
• synthesis	+				
• lipolysis	−		+	+	+
Secretion					
• stimulated by	Hyperglycaemia Amino acids Glucagon Gut hormones	Hypoglycaemia Amino acids Fasting	Hypoglycaemia Stress Sleep	Hypoglycaemia Stress	Stress
• inhibited by	Adrenaline Fasting	Insulin			
Results	Uses and stores available glucose	Provides glucose	Spares glucose	Provides glucose	
			Provide FFA as alternative fuel		
Plasma FFA levels	Fall			Rise	
Plasma glucose levels	Fall			Rise	

+ = stimulates, − = inhibits.

CONTROL OF PLASMA GLUCOSE CONCENTRATION

During normal metabolism little glucose is lost unchanged from the body. Maintenance of plasma glucose concentrations within a relatively narrow range, between about 4.5 to 11 mmol/L, despite the widely varying input from the gastrointestinal tract, depends on the balance between the glucose entering cells from the extracellular fluid or leaving them into this compartment. In order to understand the pathological disturbances of carbohydrate metabolism, including ketosis and lactic acidosis, we must first consider the metabolic interactions between tissues and how these affect plasma glucose control.

THE LIVER

The liver is the most important organ maintaining a constant energy supply for other tissues, including the brain, under a wide variety of conditions. It is also of importance in controlling the postprandial plasma glucose concentration. It is well adapted to these roles for many reasons.

- Portal venous blood leaving the absorptive area of the intestinal wall reaches the liver first and consequently the hepatic cells are in a key position to buffer the hyperglycaemic effect of a high carbohydrate meal (Fig. 10.2).
- The entry of glucose into liver and cerebral cells is not directly affected by insulin, but

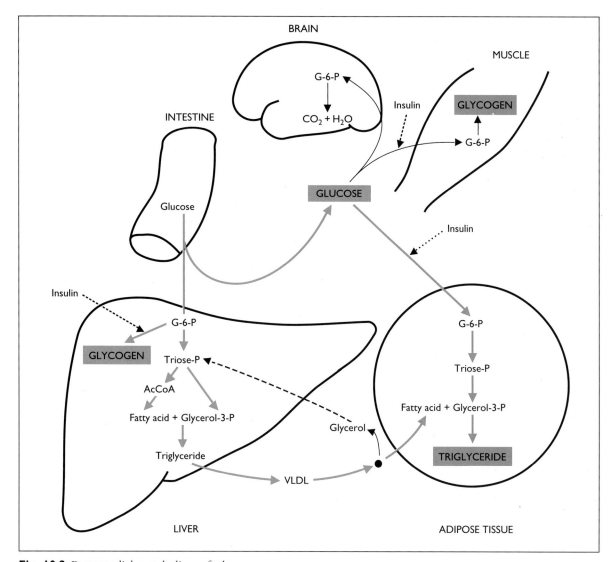

Fig. 10.2 Postprandial metabolism of glucose.

depends on the extracellular glucose concentration. The conversion of glucose to glucose-6-phosphate (G-6-P), the first step in glucose metabolism in all cells, is catalysed in the liver by the enzyme glucokinase, which has a low affinity for glucose compared with that of hexokinase found in most other tissues. Glucokinase activity is induced by insulin. Therefore, proportionally less glucose is extracted by hepatic cells during fasting, when concentrations in portal venous plasma are low, than after carbohydrate ingestion. This helps to maintain a fasting supply of glucose to vulnerable tissues such as the brain.

- The liver cells can store some of the excess glucose as glycogen. The rate of glycogen synthesis (*glycogenesis*) from G-6-P may be increased by insulin secreted by the β-cells of the pancreas in response to systemic hyperglycaemia.
- The liver can convert some of the excess glucose to fatty acids, which are ultimately transported as triglyceride in very low density lipoprotein (VLDL) and stored in adipose tissue.

- Under normal aerobic conditions the liver can synthesize glucose by *gluconeogenesis* using the metabolic products from other tissues, such as glycerol, lactate or the carbon chains resulting from deamination of certain amino acids (mainly alanine) (Table 10.3).
- The liver contains the enzyme glucose-6-phosphatase, which, by hydrolysing G-6-P derived from either glycogen breakdown (*glycogenolysis*) or gluconeogenesis, releases glucose and helps to maintain extracellular fasting concentrations. Hepatic glycogenolysis is stimulated by the hormone glucagon, secreted by the α-cells of the pancreas in response to a fall in the plasma glucose concentration, and by catecholamines such as adrenaline (epinephrine) or noradrenaline (norepinephrine).
- *During fasting* the liver converts fatty acids, released from adipose tissue as a consequence of low insulin activity, to ketones. The carbon chains of some amino acids may also be converted to ketones (Table 10.3). Ketones can be used by other tissues, including the brain, as an energy source when plasma glucose concentrations are low.

This combination of properties is unique to the liver. The renal cortex is the only other tissue capable of gluconeogenesis, and of converting G-6-P to glucose. The gluconeogenic capacity of the kidney is probably mainly of importance in hydrogen ion homeostasis (p.**88**) and during prolonged fasting.

Other tissues, such as muscle, can store glycogen to a greater or lesser extent, but, because they do not contain glucose-6-phosphatase, they cannot release glucose from cells and so can only use it locally; this glycogen plays no part in maintaining the plasma glucose concentration.

SYSTEMIC EFFECTS OF A GLUCOSE LOAD (FIG. 10.2)

As discussed, the liver modifies the potential hyperglycaemic effect of a high carbohydrate meal by extracting relatively more glucose than in the fasting state from the portal plasma. However, some glucose does pass through the liver and the rise in the systemic concentration stimulates the β-cells of the pancreas to secrete insulin. Insulin may further enhance hepatic and muscle glycogenesis. More importantly, *entry of glucose into adipose tissue and muscle cells*, unlike that into liver and brain, is *stimulated by insulin* and under physiological conditions the plasma glucose concentration falls to near fasting levels. Conversion of intracellular glucose to G-6-P in adipose and muscle cells is catalysed by the enzyme *hexokinase which, because its affinity for glucose is greater than that of hepatic glucokinase*, ensures that glucose enters the metabolic pathways in these tissues at lower extracellular concentrations than those in the liver. The relatively high insulin activity after a meal also *inhibits* the breakdown of triglyceride (*lipolysis*) and protein (*proteolysis*). If there is relative or absolute insulin deficiency, as in diabetes mellitus, these actions are impaired.

Both muscle and adipose tissue store the excess postprandial glucose, but the mode of storage and the function of the two types of cell is very different. By examining the metabolic relations of each of these tissues with the liver, many of the disturbances of carbohydrate metabolism can be explained.

Table 10.3 Metabolism of the carbon skeleton of some amino acids to either carbohydrate (glycogenic) or fat (ketogenic)

Glycogenic	Glycogenic and ketogenic	Ketogenic
Alanine	Isoleucine	Leucine
Arginine	Lysine	
Glycine	Phenylalanine	
Histidine	Tyrosine	
Methionine		
Serine		
Valine		

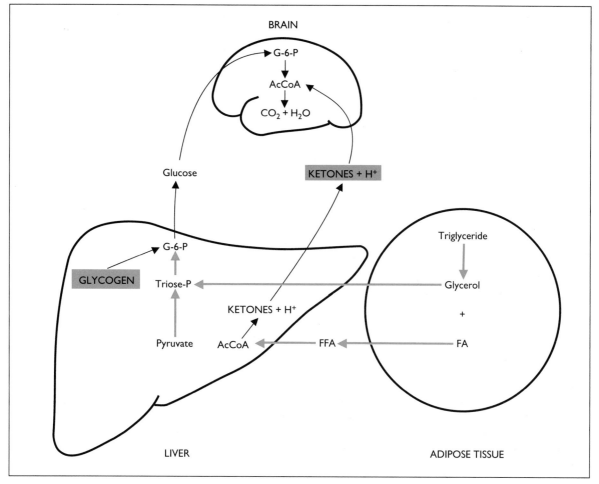

Fig. 10.3 Intermediary metabolism during fasting: ketosis.

Ketosis

ADIPOSE TISSUE AND THE LIVER

Adipose tissue triglyceride is the most important long-term energy store in the body. Greatly increased use of fat stores, for example during prolonged fasting, is associated with ketosis.

Adipose tissue cells, acting in conjunction with the liver, convert excess glucose to triglyceride and stores it in this form rather than as glycogen. The components are both derived from glucose, fatty acids from that entering hepatic cells and glycerol from glucose entering adipose tissue cells.

In the liver triglycerides are formed from:

- glycerol-3-phosphate (from triose phosphate);
- fatty acids (from acetyl CoA).

The triglycerides are transported to adipose tissue cells incorporated in VLDL, where they are hydrolysed by lipoprotein lipase (p.**229**). The released fatty acids, of hepatic origin, are re-esterified within these cells with glycerol-3-phosphate, derived from glucose, which has entered this tissue under the influence of insulin. The resultant triglyceride is stored. Far more energy can be stored as triglyceride than as glycogen.

During fasting, when exogenous glucose is unavailable and the plasma insulin concentration is therefore low, endogenous triglycerides are reconverted to free fatty acids (FFA) and glycerol by *lipolysis* (Fig. 10.3). Both are transported to the liver in plasma, the FFA being protein bound predominantly to albumin. Glycerol enters the hepatic gluconeogenic pathway at the triose phosphate stage; the glucose synthesized can be released from these cells, thus minimizing the fall in glucose concentrations. Most tissues, other than the brain, can oxidize fatty acids to acetyl CoA, which can then be used in the tricarboxylic acid (TCA) cycle as an energy source. When the rate of synthesis exceeds its use the hepatic cells produce *acetoacetic acid* by enzymatic condensation of two molecules of acetyl CoA; acetoacetic acid can be reduced to *β-hydroxybutyric acid* and decarboxylated to *acetone*. These ketones can be used as an energy source by brain and other tissues at a time when glucose is in relatively short supply.

Therefore *ketosis* occurs when *fat stores are the main energy source* and may result from fasting, or from reduced nutrient absorption, for example, due to vomiting. Mild ketosis may occur after as little as 12 hours fasting. Its presence should not be misinterpreted as being caused by diabetic ketoacidosis. After short fasts metabolic acidosis is not usually detectable, but after longer periods more hydrogen ions may be produced than can be dealt with by homeostatic buffering mechanisms, depleting the plasma bicarbonate concentration, which therefore falls. The plasma glucose concentration is maintained, principally by hepatic gluconeogenesis, but during prolonged starvation, such as that in anorexia nervosa or during childhood (p.**214**), *ketotic hypoglycaemia* may occur. The brain may tolerate ketotic hypoglycaemia better than the same degree of insulin-induced hypoglycaemia; in the former the brain adapts to ketone metabolism, while in the latter ketone concentrations are low, thus depriving the brain of its only non-glucose energy source.

During starvation low extracellular glucose concentration reduces the supply to cells and therefore reduces adipose tissue glycolysis and fat synthesis (*lipogenesis*); this tendency inhibits insulin secretion and therefore the rate of lipolysis and fatty acid, and hence ketone, production are increased (Table 10.2).

Diabetic ketoacidosis is differentiated from that of fasting by hyperglycaemia and is usually more severe. Despite the differences in plasma glucose concentrations, the ketone production in both cases is due to intracellular glucose deficiency. *In diabetic ketosis this is due to low insulin activity.*

Ketosis always reflects excessive use of fat as an energy source due to:

- intracellular glucose deficiency;
- low insulin activity.

The low insulin activity increases the rate of production of gluconeogenic substrates by glycolysis and proteolysis, and the rate of hepatic gluconeogenesis. The resultant increased rate of glucose released into the ECF is appropriate in starvation, but aggravates the hyperglycaemia in diabetes mellitus.

Lactate Production and Lactic Acidosis

STRIATED MUSCLE AND THE LIVER

Glucose enters muscle postprandially under the influence of insulin and is stored as glycogen. This glycogen cannot be reconverted to glucose because of the absence of glucose-6-phosphatase and can only supply local needs. Quantitatively, muscle glycogen stores are second only to those in the liver.

Muscular contraction (Fig. 10.4). During muscular activity glycogenolysis is stimulated by adrenaline (epinephrine), and the resultant G-6-P is metabolized by glycolysis and in the TCA cycle to supply energy. The rate of glycolysis may exceed the availability of

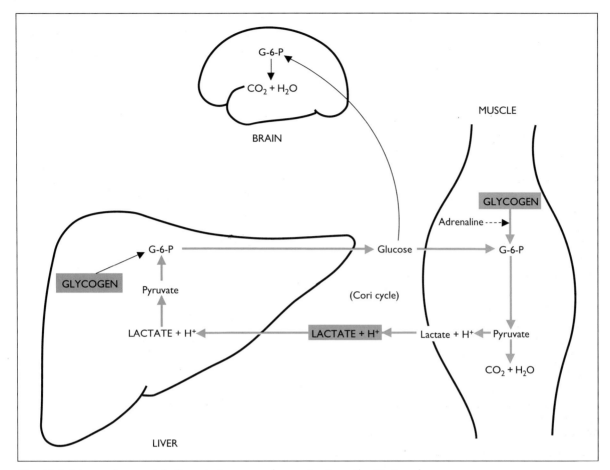

Fig. 10.4 Intermediary metabolism during muscular contraction: the Cori cycle.

oxygen needed in the TCA cycle and glycolytic products may then accumulate.

The overall reaction for anaerobic glycolysis is:

$$Glucose \longrightarrow 2\ Lactate^- + 2H^+$$

The lactate is transported in the blood to the liver where it can be used for gluconeogenesis, providing further glucose for the muscle (Cori cycle). During gluconeogenesis hydrogen ions are reused. *Under aerobic conditions the liver consumes much more lactate than it produces.*

The physiological accumulation of lactic acid during muscular contraction is a temporary phenomenon and rapidly disappears at rest, when slowing of glycolysis allows aerobic processes to 'catch up'.

PATHOLOGICAL LACTIC ACIDOSIS

Lactic acid, produced by anaerobic glycolysis, may be oxidized either to CO_2 and water in the TCA cycle or be reconverted to glucose by gluconeogenesis in the liver. Both the TCA cycle and gluconeogenesis need oxygen; *anaerobic glycolysis is the only non-oxygen-requiring pathway.* Pathological accumulation of lactate may occur because:

- *production is increased* by an increased rate of anaerobic glycolysis;
- *use is decreased* by:
   impairment of the TCA cycle;
   impairment of gluconeogenesis.

The *clinical syndromes* associated with lactic acidosis are usually associated with more than one of these factors.

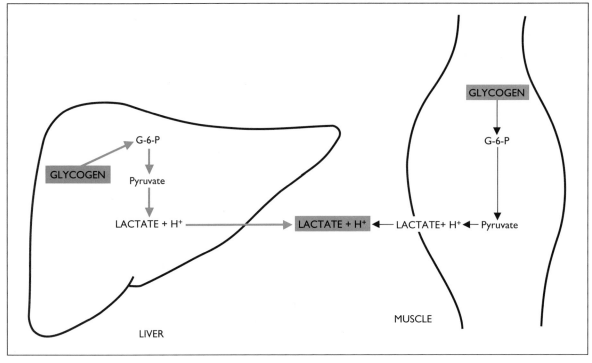

Fig. 10.5 Metabolic pathways during tissue hypoxia.

Tissue hypoxia (Fig. 10.5) due to the poor tissue perfusion of the 'shock' syndrome is the *commonest cause of lactic acidosis.* Such hypoxia increases plasma lactate concentrations because:

- the TCA cycle cannot function anaerobically and oxidation of pyruvate and lactate to CO_2 and water is impaired;
- hepatic and renal gluconeogenesis from lactate cannot occur anaerobically;
- anaerobic glycolysis is stimulated because the falling ATP levels cannot be regenerated by the TCA cycle under anaerobic conditions.

The combination of impaired gluconeogenesis and increased anaerobic glycolysis converts the liver from a lactate and H^+ consuming organ to one generating large amounts of lactic acid.

Severe hypoxia, for example following a cardiac arrest, causes marked lactic acidosis. If diabetic ketoacidosis is associated with significant volume depletion this hypoxic syndrome may aggravate the acidosis. Other causes of lactic acidosis include:

- *severe illnesses,* such as leukaemias and lymphomas. A variety of factors, including poor tissue perfusion and increased anaerobic glycolysis by malignant tissue, may contribute to the lactic acidosis;
- *biguanides,* such as metformin or phenformin. These drugs, which inhibit both the TCA cycle and gluconeogenesis, are rarely used now to treat diabetes mellitus because they can cause lactic acidosis;
- *glucose-6-phosphatase deficiency* (von Gierke's disease; glycogen storage disease (GSD) Type I, p.**214**). The rate of glycolysis increases if G-6-P cannot be converted to glucose by the liver and kidney.

The treatment of lactic acidosis depends on the cause and on the degree of acidosis. *Measurement of plasma lactate concentrations is rarely necessary, because it is the acidosis that is dangerous: lactate itself is harmless.* Lactic acidosis may be suspected if the plasma bicarbonate concentration is very low in the absence of another obvious cause of metabolic acidosis. The plasma anion gap is increased (p.**91**).

Urinary Glucose

Glycosuria is defined as a concentration of urinary glucose detectable using relatively insensitive, but specific, screening tests. These tests depend on the action of the enzyme, glucose oxidase, incorporated into a diagnostic strip (p.**221**). Usually most of the glucose in the glomerular filtrate is reabsorbed by the proximal tubular cells. Although very low urinary glucose concentrations may be detectable by more sensitive methods even in normal subjects, glycosuria, as defined above, occurs only when the plasma, and therefore glomerular filtrate concentrations, exceed the tubular reabsorptive capacity. This may be because:

- the plasma and glomerular filtrate concentrations are more than about 11 mmol/L, and therefore the normal tubular reabsorptive capacity is significantly exceeded;
- the tubular reabsorptive capacity is reduced, as for example during pregnancy, so that glycosuria occurs at a lower filtrate concentration ('renal glycosuria'). This is usually a harmless condition

Very rarely, if the GFR is much reduced, there may be no glycosuria despite plasma glucose concentrations above 11 mmol/L. If the volume of glomerular filtrate is very low the *total amount* of glucose delivered to tubular cells may be less than normal, even if the concentration is high. In such rare cases urine

Table 10.4 Reducing substances in urine that may give a positive reaction with Clinitest tablets

Reducing substance	Comment
Glucose Glucuronates	Common
Lactose	Common in pregnancy
Galactose Fructose Pentoses Homogentisic acid	Rare
Urate Creatinine	Weakly positive at high concentrations

testing cannot be used to monitor diabetic control.

Glycosuria should be sought in a urine specimen produced *by the kidneys*, collected about an hour after a meal, when peak plasma concentrations are reached by the *double void technique* (p.**217**). This ensures that the specimen being tested reflects the plasma glucose concentration at the same time and has not been stored in the bladder for some time, prior to collection. Specimens collected after a period of fasting will yield positive results only when fasting plasma glucose concentrations are above about 11 mmol/L (diabetes mellitus, or during infusion of glucose), or if there is gross renal glycosuria.

Reducing substances in the urine (including glucose) can be detected using copper-containing reagents such as those incorporated in Clinitest tablets (Table 10.4). In the neonatal period, the finding of other reducing substances may suggest an inborn error of metabolism, such as galactosaemia (p.**290**). It is therefore important to use this test in such cases rather than one specific for glucose.

Hyperglycaemia and Diabetes Mellitus

Hyperglycaemia may be due to:

- diabetes mellitus;
- intravenous infusion of glucose-containing fluids;
- severe stress (temporary effect) such as cerebrovascular accidents.

DIABETES MELLITUS

Diabetes mellitus is caused by an absolute or relative insulin deficiency. It has been defined by the World Health Organization (WHO), on the basis of laboratory findings, as a fasting venous plasma glucose concentration greater than 7.8 mmol/L (140 mg/dl) or greater than 11.1 mmol/L (200 mg/dl) two hours after a carbohydrate meal or two hours after the oral ingestion of the equivalent of 75 g of glucose, even if the fasting concentration is normal (p.**217**). Severe cases have persistent hyperglycaemia. Diabetes mellitus is classified into the following categories.

Insulin-dependent diabetes mellitus (IDDM, Type 1) is the term used to describe the condition in patients for whom insulin therapy is essential because they are prone to develop ketoacidosis. It usually presents during childhood. It has been suggested that many cases follow a viral infection, which has destroyed the β-cells of the pancreatic islets. Subjects most at risk are those with HLA-types DR3 and DR4 of the major histocompatibility complex.

Non-insulin-dependent diabetes mellitus (NIDDM, Type 2) is the commonest variety. Patients are much less likely to develop ketoacidosis than those with IDDM and although insulin may sometimes be needed, it is not essential for survival. Onset is most usual during adult life. Although no genetic markers have been found, there is a familial tendency. A variety of inherited disorders

may be responsible for the syndrome, either by reducing insulin secretion, or by causing relative insulin deficiency because of resistance to its action or of postreceptor defects, despite high plasma insulin concentrations. Factors increasing the risk of developing NIDDM include obesity, sustained stress and a sedentary life style.

Diabetes mellitus associated with other conditions includes:

- *absolute insulin deficiency*, due to pancreatic disease (chronic pancreatitis, haemochromatosis, cystic fibrosis);
- *relative insulin deficiency*, due to excessive growth hormone (acromegaly), glucocorticoid secretion (Cushing's syndrome), or increased plasma glucocorticoid concentrations due to administration of steroids;
- *drugs, such as thiazide diuretics.*

IMPAIRED GLUCOSE TOLERANCE

The WHO definition of impaired glucose tolerance is a finding of a fasting venous plasma glucose concentration between 5.5 and 7.8 mmol/L (100 and 140 mg/dl) and/or a plasma glucose concentration between 7.8 and 11.1 mmol/L (140 and 200 mg/dl) two hours after taking a standard glucose load (glucose tolerance test). Only a small proportion of subjects with such mild impaired glucose tolerance develop diabetes mellitus later. Because it is not possible to predict the outcome at the time of presentation subjects must not be diagnosed as having diabetes mellitus merely on the basis of impaired glucose tolerance, because of the serious psychological, social and economic implications. However, because of the increased risk of vascular complications, secondary causes of impaired glucose tolerance should be sought and dietary advice given if necessary.

SUBJECTS AT RISK OF DEVELOPING DIABETES MELLITUS

A strong family history of diabetes mellitus or the birth of an abnormally large baby may suggest that an individual is at risk of developing diabetes mellitus despite normal plasma glucose concentrations and a normal response to a glucose load at that time. These subjects should be given dietary advice and, if overweight, advised to lose weight.

Clinical and Metabolic Features of Insulin-dependent Diabetes Mellitus

Most of the metabolic changes of diabetes mellitus are a consequence of insulin deficiency.

Hyperglycaemia is, by definition, an invariable finding. If plasma glucose concentrations exceed about 11 mmol/L and renal function is normal, there will be *glycosuria*. High urinary glucose concentrations produce an osmotic diuresis and therefore *polyuria*. Cerebral cellular dehydration due to hyperosmolality, secondary to hyperglycaemia, causes thirst (*polydipsia*) (p.**35**). A prolonged osmotic diuresis may cause excessive urinary electrolyte loss. *These 'classical' symptoms of diabetes mellitus are only present in advanced cases.*

Abnormalities in lipid metabolism may be secondary to insulin deficiency. Lipolysis is enhanced and plasma free fatty acid (FFA) concentrations rise. In the liver FFA are converted to acetyl CoA and ketones, or are re-esterified to form endogenous triglycerides and incorporated into VLDL; the latter accumulate in plasma because lipoprotein lipase, which is necessary for VLDL catabolism, requires insulin for optimal activity. If insulin deficiency is very severe there may also be chylomicronaemia. The rate of cholesterol synthesis is also increased, with an associated increase in plasma LDL concentrations.

Increased breakdown of protein may cause muscle wasting.

LONG-TERM EFFECTS

Vascular disease is a common complication of diabetes mellitus.

- *Macrovascular disease*, due to abnormalities of large vessels, may present as coronary artery, cerebrovascular or peripheral vascular insufficiency. The condition is probably related to alterations in lipid metabolism.
- *Microvascular disease*, due to abnormalities of small blood vessels, particularly affects the retina (*diabetic retinopathy*) and the kidney; the incidence of both may be related to inadequate glucose control.

Kidney disease is associated with several abnormalities, including proteinuria and progressive renal failure. Diffuse nodular glomerulosclerosis (*Kimmelstiel-Wilson lesions*) may cause the nephrotic syndrome. The presence of small amounts of albumin in the urine (microalbuminuria) is associated with an increased risk of developing progressive renal disease (p.**330**) which may sometimes be prevented by more stringent plasma glucose and blood pressure control. The renal complications may partly be due to the increased glycation of structural proteins in the arterial walls supplying the glomerular basement membrane; similar vascular changes in the retina may account for the high incidence of diabetic retinopathy. Glycation of protein in the lens may cause cataracts.

Glycation of haemoglobin and plasma proteins may also occur, and may be assayed to assess, *retrospectively*, long-term diabetic control. Glycated haemoglobin (HbA$_{1c}$) is most commonly measured for this purpose. Glucose bound to plasma proteins undergoes a rearrangement to form fructosamine, and this sugar amine has also been estimated.

Infections are common in diabetic patients and may aggravate renal and peripheral vascular disease. Infants born to women with poorly controlled diabetes mellitus tend to be large at birth and to have an increased incidence of fetal abnormalities.

Principles of Management of Diabetes Mellitus

The management of diabetes mellitus will be considered briefly.

Insulin requirements vary in patients with IDDM. For example, the dose may need to be increased during any illness or during pregnancy. In patients with NIDDM, plasma glucose concentrations can often be controlled by diet, associated with weight reduction, but insulin may be required during periods of stress. In this group insulin secretion can be stimulated by the sulphonylurea drugs, such as tolbutamide or glibenclamide. Biguanides, (metformin and phenformin), have been used but they are now rarely prescribed because of the danger of lactic acidosis (p.**204**).

Blood glucose concentrations may be measured by the patients themselves using glucose oxidase-containing reagent strips. The colour change of the strip can be quantitated visually or by using a portable reflectance meter. It is *essential that reflectance meters are checked regularly by laboratory staff.* Although the measurement of blood glucose concentrations involves the discomfort of several skin punctures, many motivated patients are able to adjust their insulin dose more accurately, based on these results than on those obtained by testing their urine. If urine testing is used, the renal threshold for glucose must first be established by a glucose tolerance test and the patients must be instructed how to collect urine by the double void technique (p.**217**). All diabetic patients must remain under regular medical supervision.

Glycated haemoglobin (HbA$_{1c}$) expressed as a percentage of total blood haemoglobin concentration gives a retrospective assessment of the mean plasma glucose concentration during the preceding six to eight weeks, the higher the percentage the poorer the mean diabetic control. HbA$_{1c}$ is formed by nonenzymatic glycation of haemoglobin and is dependent on the mean plasma glucose concentrations and on the lifespan of the red cell; falsely low values may be found in patients with haemolytic disease. *Measurement of blood HbA$_{1c}$ is an adjunct to, not a replacement for, serial plasma glucose estimations*, which are necessary to reveal potentially dangerous short-term swings. It does not detect hypoglycaemic episodes.

The measurement of plasma *fructosamine* concentrations may be used to assess glucose control over a shorter time course than that of HbA$_{1c}$ (about two to four weeks), but the assay has methodological limitations.

Acute Metabolic Complications of Diabetes Mellitus

Patients with diabetes mellitus may develop one of several metabolic complications needing emergency treatment. These include:

- diabetic ketoacidosis;
- hyperosmolal non-ketotic coma;
- hypoglycaemia caused by excess insulin or sulphonylurea administration (p.**212**).

DIABETIC KETOACIDOSIS

Diabetic ketoacidosis is a more severe form of the metabolic events outlined in p.**219**. It may be precipitated by infection or by vomiting. Insulin may be mistakenly withheld by the patient, who reasons 'no food, therefore no insulin'. In the absence of insulin, there is increased lipid and protein breakdown, enhanced hepatic gluconeogenesis and impaired glucose entry into cells.

The clinical consequences of diabetic ketoacidosis are due to:

- *hyperglycaemia causing plasma hyperosmolality;*
- *metabolic acidosis;*
- *glycosuria.*

Plasma glucose concentrations are usually in the range 20 to 40 mmol/L (about 350 to 700 mg/dl) but may be considerably higher. Hyperglycaemia causes *glycosuria* and hence an *osmotic diuresis.* Water and electrolyte loss due to vomiting, common in this syndrome, increases fluid depletion. There may be haemoconcentration and reduction of the GFR enough to cause uraemia due to renal circulatory insufficiency. The extracellular *hyperosmolality* causes a shift of water out of the cellular compartment and severe cellular dehydration occurs. Loss of water from cerebral cells is probably the reason for the confusion and coma. Thus, there is both cellular and extracellular volume depletion.

The rate of *lipolysis is increased* because of decreased insulin activity; more FFA are produced than can be metabolized by peripheral tissues. They are either converted to *ketones* by the liver or, of less immediate clinical importance, incorporated as endogenous triglycerides into VLDL, sometimes causing *hyperlipidaemia.* Hydrogen ions, produced with ketones other than acetone, are buffered by plasma bicarbonate. However, when their rate of production exceeds the rate of bicarbonate generation the plasma bicarbonate falls. Hydrogen ion secretion causes a fall in urinary pH.

The deep, sighing respiration (*Kussmaul respiration*) and the odour of acetone on the breath are classical features of diabetic ketoacidosis.

Plasma potassium concentrations may be raised, secondarily to the metabolic acidosis before treatment is started, because of failure of glucose entry into cells in the absence of insulin and because of the low GFR. Despite hyperkalaemia, there is a *total body deficit* due to increased urinary potassium loss in the presence of an osmotic diuresis. During treatment plasma potassium concentrations may fall as potassium re-enters cells, sometimes causing severe hypokalaemia unless potassium is prescribed.

Plasma sodium concentrations may be low or low normal at presentation, partly because of the osmotic effect of the high extracellular glucose concentration which draws water from the cells and dilutes the sodium. In the presence of a very high plasma glucose concentration, a normal or raised plasma sodium concentration is suggestive of significant water depletion. If there is severe hyperlipidaemia the possibility of *pseudohyponatraemia* must be considered (p.**38**). When insulin is given gluconeogenesis is inhibited, glucose enters cells and sodium-free water follows along the osmotic gradient. If plasma sodium concentrations rise rapidly the patient may remain confused or even comatose as long as the plasma osmolality remains significantly raised, despite a satisfactory fall in plasma glucose concentration. This may also occur if isosmolar or stronger saline solutions are given inappropriately.

A summary of the usual clinical and biochemical findings in a patient presenting with diabetic ketoacidosis are shown in Table

Table 10.5 Clinical and biochemical findings in a patient presenting with diabetic ketoacidosis

Findings	Underlying cause/abnornality
Clinical	
confusion and later coma	Hyperosmolality
hyperventilation (Kussmaul respiration)	Acidosis
signs of volume depletion	Osmotic diuresis
Biochemical	
Plasma:	
hyperglycaemia	
bicarbonate concentration (metabolic acidosis)	Low
potassium concentration	High normal or high
mild uraemia	Decreased GFR
Urine:	
glycosuria	If GFR is adequate
ketonuria	
low pH	Unless there is renal impairment

10.5. Associated biochemical findings may include:

- *hypophosphataemia* as plasma phosphate concentrations parallel those of potassium. This may persist for several days after recovery from diabetic coma;
- plasma and urinary *amylase* activities may be markedly elevated and, even in the presence of abdominal pain mimicking an 'acute abdomen', do not necessarily indicate acute pancreatitis. In some patients the amylase is of salivary rather than of pancreatic origin.

HYPEROSMOLAL NON-KETOTIC COMA

In diabetic ketoacidosis there is always plasma hyperosmolality due to the hyperglycaemia and many of the symptoms, including those of confusion and coma, are related to it. However, the term 'hyperosmolal' coma or 'precoma' is usually confined to a condition in which there is marked hyperglycaemia but *no detectable ketoacidosis*. The reason for these different presentations is not clear. It has been suggested that *insulin activity is sufficient to suppress lipolysis* but insufficient to suppress hepatic gluconeogenesis or to facilitate glucose transport into cells. This does not explain why the plasma glucose concentration is often higher in non-ketotic coma than in ketoacidosis.

Hyperosmolal non-ketotic coma may be of sudden onset. It is commoner in older patients. Plasma glucose concentrations may exceed 50 mmol/L (900 mg/dl). The effects of glycosuria are as those described above, but hypernatraemia due to predominant water loss is more commonly found than in ketoacidosis and aggravates the plasma hyperosmolality. Cerebral cellular dehydration, which contributes to the coma, may also cause hyperventilation; the consequent respiratory alkalosis may cause a slight fall in the plasma bicarbonate concentration. This should not be confused with that due to metabolic acidosis.

OTHER CAUSES OF COMA IN PATIENTS WITH DIABETES MELLITUS

In addition to the metabolic complications described above, a patient with diabetes mellitus may present in coma, or in a confused state (precoma), due to hypoglycaemia, a cerebrovascular accident or to an unrelated cause. The onset of coma due to these causes is often more sudden than that due to hyperglycaemia.

- *Hypoglycaemia* is most commonly caused by accidental over-administration of insulin or sulphonylureas. The patient may not eat normally, or may take excessive exercise after the usual dose of insulin or oral hypoglycaemic drugs.
- *Cerebrovascular accidents* are relatively common in diabetic patients because of the increased incidence of vascular disease. Such an event may be associated with hyperglycaemia and glycosuria. Stimulation of the respiratory centre may cause hyperventilation and consequent respiratory alkalosis, with a low plasma bicarbonate concentration.

The assessment of a diabetic patient presenting in coma or precoma is considered on p.217.

Principles of Treatment of Diabetic Coma

Only the outline of treatment will be discussed. For details of management the reader should consult a textbook of endocrinology. The treatment of hypoglycaemia is considered on p.215.

Diabetic ketoacidosis. *Repletion of fluid and electrolytes should be vigorous.* If the plasma sodium concentration is low normal or low, isosmolal saline should be given initially. The plasma sodium concentration should be monitored frequently and when the concentration returns to within the reference range, hypo-osmolal saline solutions should be used. If the metabolic acidosis is very severe (pH below 7.00) bicarbonate may be infused, but only until the blood pH rises to between about 7.15 and 7.20. It is unnecessary and often dangerous to correct the plasma bicarbonate concentration completely; it rapidly returns to normal following adequate fluid and insulin therapy. 8.4 per cent sodium bicarbonate is grossly hyperosmolar (Table 2.7, p.**54**) and may cause hypernatraemia and aggravate hyperosmolality. A rapid rise in the blood pH may aggravate the hypokalaemia associated with treatment.

The plasma potassium concentration should be measured before insulin is given. It is almost always raised at presentation due to the metabolic acidosis and reduced GFR, although total body potassium may be decreased. The plasma potassium concentration *may fall rapidly* once treatment is started and therefore it should be monitored frequently and potassium given as soon as the plasma concentration starts to fall.

Urinary volume should be monitored; if it fails to rise despite adequate rehydration further fluid and potassium should only be given if clinically indicated, and then with care.

Insulin is given either by continuous intra-venous infusion or by intermittent intramuscular injections, as soon as the plasma glucose and potassium concentrations are known. The insulin dose should be 'titrated' against the plasma glucose concentration.

Another clinical condition such as infection may have precipitated the coma and should be sought and treated.

Frequent monitoring of plasma glucose, potassium and sodium concentrations is essential to assess progress and to detect developing hypoglycaemia, hypokalaemia or hypernatraemia.

Hyperosmolal nonketotic coma. Treatment of hyperosmolal coma is similar to that of ketoacidosis; a sudden reduction of extracellular osmolality may do more harm than good (p.**35**), and it is especially important to give *small doses of insulin* to reduce plasma glucose concentrations slowly. These patients are often very sensitive to the action of insulin. Hypo-osmolal solutions should be used to correct volume depletion, but these too should be given slowly.

Hypoglycaemia

By definition *hypoglycaemia is present if the plasma glucose concentration is less than 2.5 mmol/L* (45 mg/dl) in a specimen collected into a tube containing an inhibitor of glycolysis; blood cells continue to metabolize glucose *in vitro* and low concentrations, found in a specimen collected without such an inhibitor, can be dangerously misleading. Symptoms of hypoglycaemia may develop at higher concentrations if there has been a rapid fall from a previously raised value, when adrenaline secretion is stimulated and causes sweating, tachycardia and agitation. Symptoms may not occur even at concentrations below 2.5 mmol/L, especially if the fall has been gradual, or if the autonomic nervous system is unresponsive to stress because the patient is taking β-blocking agents or has a severe peripheral neuropathy; the latter is a complication of diabetes mellitus. As discussed earlier, cerebral metabolism depends on an adequate supply of glucose from extracellular fluid and the symptoms of hypoglycaemia may resemble those of cerebral hypoxia. Faintness, dizziness or lethargy may progress rapidly to coma and, if untreated, permanent cerebral damage or death may occur. Existing cerebral or cerebrovascular disease may aggravate the clinical picture.

There is no completely satisfactory classification of the causes of hypoglycaemia as there is overlap between the different groups. A practical approach to diagnosis is based on the history. Attention should be paid to the relation of symptoms to meals and to particular food and drugs. The patient can usually be allocated to one of the two main groups:

- *Fasting hypoglycaemia.* Symptoms occur typically at night or in the early morning, or may be precipitated by a prolonged fast or strenuous exercise. This pattern suggests excessive utilization of glucose or an abnormality of the glucose-sparing or glucose-forming mechanisms (p.**198**) (Table 10.6).
- *Non-fasting hypoglycaemia.* Symptoms typically occur within five or six hours after a meal and may be related to ingestion of a particular type of food, or be associated with medication. Substances that may provoke hypoglycaemia are summarized in Table 10.7. Reactive and drug-induced hypoglycaemia are the commonest causes in adults. Fructose or leucine ingestion are important causes in infants.

On the basis of the history alone, it is not always possible to distinguish between early fasting and provoked hypoglycaemia.

Table 10.6   Principal causes of fasting hypoglycaemia in adults

Inappropriately high insulin concentrations due to:
  pancreatic tumour
  hyperplasia of the pancreatic islet cells
Glucocorticoid deficiency
Severe liver disease
Some nonpancreatic tumours

Table 10.7   Substances that may provoke hypoglycaemia

Drugs:
  insulin
  sulphonylureas
Alcohol
Glucose   (reactive hypoglycaemia)
Fructose   (in sucrose-containing foods)
Leucine   (an amino acid in casein, a protein in milk)

Hypoglycaemia, Particularly in Adults

Symptoms can only be attributed to hypoglycaemia if hypoglycaemia has been documented. This statement may seem superfluous, but it is not unknown for a patient to be submitted to multiple tests for the differential diagnosis of hypoglycaemia that does not exist, or worse, to be treated for it. Once demonstrated the following main causes must be considered.

Insulin- or other drug-induced hypoglycaemia. These are probably the commonest causes. It is most important to take a careful drug history. Unless the facts are deliberately concealed by the patient the offending drug should be easily identifiable. Hypoglycaemia in a diabetic patient may be caused by accidental insulin overdosage, by changing insulin requirements, or by failure to eat after insulin has been given. Self-administration for suicidal purposes or to gain attention is not unknown, and homicidal use is a remote possibility. Sulphonylureas may also induce hypoglycaemia, especially in the elderly; it may be a complication of salicylate poisoning. Other drugs, such as antihistamines, have been suspected but not proven as a cause.

Hypoglycaemia due to exogenous insulin suppresses insulin and C-peptide secretion. Measurement of plasma C-peptide concentrations may help to differentiate exogenous insulin administration, when the peptide secretion is inhibited, from endogenous insulin secretion together with C-peptide, whether it is from an insulinoma or following pancreatic stimulation by sulphonylurea drugs. Some very rare nonpancreatic tumours secret an insulin-like growth factor, which may cause hypoglycaemia but in these cases plasma insulin and C-peptide concentrations are low (Table 10.8).

Insulinoma. An insulinoma is usually a small histologically benign primary tumour of the islet cells of the pancreas. It may present at any age. Multiple tumours may occur and it may be part of the syndrome of multiple

Table 10.8 Results of plasma insulin and C-peptide estimations during hypoglycaemia (spontaneous or after a prolonged fast)

Hypoglycaemia caused by:	Plasma insulin	Plasma C-peptide
Insulin administration	} Inappropriately high	Low
Insulinoma or ectopic insulin secretion		} High
Sulphonylurea administration		
Alcohol	} Appropriately low	
Non-pancreatic non-insulin-secreting tumour (IGF)		} Low
Pituitary or adrenal failure		

endocrine neoplasia (p.**397**). As with other functioning endocrine tumours, hormone secretion is inappropriate and usually excessive. C-peptide is released in parallel with insulin and plasma concentrations are therefore inappropriately high in the presence of hypoglycaemia.

Attacks of hypoglycaemia occur typically at night and before breakfast, and may be precipitated by strenuous exercise. Personality or behavioural changes may be the first feature; some patients present initially to psychiatrists.

Alcohol-induced hypoglycaemia. Hypoglycaemia may develop between two and 10 hours after ingestion of large amounts of alcohol. It is found most often in malnourished subjects and chronic alcoholics but may occur in young subjects when they first drink alcohol. Hypoglycaemia is probably caused by suppression of gluconeogenesis during metabolism of alcohol. Differentiation of hypoglycaemia from alcoholic stupor may be impossible unless the plasma glucose concentration is estimated. It may be necessary to infuse glucose frequently during treatment, until glycogen stores are repleted and plasma glucose concentrations are stable.

During prolonged fasting, when glycogen stores are depleted, gluconeogenesis is the main source of plasma glucose, and hypoglycaemia is potentially severe.

Non-pancreatic tumours. Although carcinomas, especially of the liver, and sarcomas have been reported to cause hypoglycaemia, it occurs most commonly in association with retroperitoneal tumours of mesenchymal origin. The tumours are slow-growing but may become very large. Hypoglycaemia may be the presenting feature; the mechanism is not always clear, but may sometimes be due to the secretion of an insulin-like growth factor (p.**110**).

Reactive (functional) hypoglycaemia. Some people develop symptomatic hypoglycaemia between two and four hours after a meal or a glucose load. Loss of consciousness is very rare. Similar symptoms may follow a gastrectomy, when rapid passage of glucose into the intestine, and rapid absorption, may stimulate excessive insulin secretion ('late dumping syndrome', p.**249**). Reactive hypoglycaemia is uncommon except after gastrectomy; it is diagnosed too often.

Endocrine causes. Hypoglycaemia may occur in pituitary or adrenal insufficiency (Chapters 5 and 6). It is rarely the presenting manifestation of these conditions.

Impaired liver function. The functional reserve of the liver is so great that, despite its central role in the maintenance of plasma glucose concentrations, hypoglycaemia is a rare complication of liver disease. It may complicate very severe hepatitis, hypoxic liver disease associated with congestive cardiac failure or liver necrosis if the whole liver is affected. This is less a problem of the differential diagnosis of hypoglycaemia than of the awareness that it may occur and need treatment.

Hypoglycaemia in Infants and Children

Hypoglycaemia is not uncommon in infancy. It may cause permanent brain damage, especially during the first few months of life.

Table 10.9 Principal causes of hypoglycaemia in infants and children

Neonatal period
  'Small for dates' infants
  Hypoxia at birth
  Infants of diabetic mothers
  Erythroblastosis fetalis (rare)

Early infancy
  Endocrine causes
    hypopituitarism
    adrenal insufficiency
  Inborn errors of metabolism
    glycogen storage disease, such as von Gierke's disease
    hereditary fructose intolerance

Late infancy
  Ketotic hypoglycaemia of infancy
  Nesidioblastosis (islet cell hyperplasia)
  Leucine sensitivity

Causes of hypoglycaemia are shown in Table 10.9 but only the principal ones will be outlined in more detail.

NEONATAL PERIOD

There may be no obvious clinical signs of hypoglycaemia even if the plasma glucose concentration is as low as 1.7 mmol/L (about 30 mg/dl) during the first 72 hours of life, or 2.2 mmol/L (about 40 mg/dl) in the later neonatal period. Clinical signs may be absent in very premature infants weighing less than 2.5 kg (5.5 lb) even at concentrations as low as 1.1 mmol/L (about 20 mg/dl). However, impaired neurological development has been reported in some infants who have had repeated episodes of asymptomatic hypoglycaemia and it is now recommended that the plasma glucose concentration should be maintained above 2.2 mmol/L (40 mg/dl).

Clinical signs of hypoglycaemia include convulsions, tremors and attacks of apnoea with cyanosis; the need for treatment is urgent because of the danger of permanent brain damage. Neonatal hypoglycaemia occurs particularly in:

- *infants born to diabetic mothers.* If the fetus is exposed to hyperglycaemia during pregnancy, fetal islet-cell hyperplasia may occur. The consequent hyperinsulinism may cause hypoglycaemia when the high glucose supply from the mother is removed after parturition. Asymptomatic hypoglycaemia occurs in about 50 per cent of such infants;

- *'small for dates' infants* suffering from intrauterine malnutrition, for example, infants of mothers with toxaemia of pregnancy, or the smaller of twins. These infants may develop hypoglycaemia during the first week of life. Prematurity is an aggravating factor, because most of the liver glycogen is laid down after 36 weeks of gestation. Low fat stores also limit the availability of ketones as an alternative energy source for brain cells;

- *erythroblastosis fetalis*, which may also be associated with islet-cell hyperplasia.

EARLY INFANCY

Soon after birth, or after the introduction of milk to the diet, hypoglycaemia may be due to one of the following causes.

Glycogenoses. A deficiency of one of the enzymes involved in glycogenesis or glycogenolysis results in the accumulation of normal or abnormal glycogen with *hepatomegaly*. In von Gierke's disease, the least rare glycogen storage disorder, there is a deficiency of *glucose-6-phosphatase. Fasting hypoglycaemia* occurs because the enzyme is essential for the conversion of glucose-6-phosphate (G-6-P) to glucose. There may also be *ketosis* and *endogenous hypertriglyceridaemia* due to excessive lipolysis caused by low insulin activity, lactic acidosis due to excessive anaerobic glycolysis, and hyperuricaemia (p.**370**).

Diagnosis is made either directly by demonstrating the absence of the enzyme in a liver biopsy specimen, or indirectly by demonstrating failure of plasma glucose concentrations to rise after giving glucagon to stimulate glycogenolysis. Infusion of galactose or fructose, which are normally converted to glucose via G-6-P, also fails to increase plasma glucose concentrations because G-6-P cannot be converted to glucose.

Treatment. Frequent meals should be given to maintain normal plasma glucose levels and so prevent cerebral damage.

Hereditary fructose intolerance is a rare cause of hypoglycaemia. It is due to deficiency of *fructose-1-phosphate aldolase*. The accumulation of *fructose-1-phosphate* in several tissues causes many of the clinical features; hypoglycaemia may be due to inhibition of glycogenolysis and gluconeogenesis. Symptoms only present after sucrose (fructose and glucose) and fructose-containing fruit or fruit drinks have been introduced into the diet. Hypoglycaemia, with nausea, vomiting and abdominal pain, and fructosuria follow about 30 minutes after fructose ingestion or intravenous infusion; this can be used as a diagnostic test. The infant fails to thrive. Liver deposits of fructose-1-phosphate cause hepatomegaly with jaundice; this may progress to cirrhosis with ascites.

LATER INFANCY

Idiopathic hypoglycaemia of infancy. The diagnosis of this condition is made by excluding other causes. Symptoms usually develop after fasting or a febrile illness. There is a high incidence of brain damage. In some cases there is excessive insulin secretion and it may not be possible to differentiate this condition from an insulinoma. Islet cell hyperplasia (*nesidioblastosis*) is a difficult diagnosis to make and is an uncommon cause of hypoglycaemia occurring before the age of three.

During the second year of life hypoglycaemia associated with ketosis may also develop after fasting or a febrile illness. It is the most common cause of hypoglycaemia in this age group. These children were usually 'small for dates' at birth.

Adult causes of hypoglycaemia, including insulinoma, must always be considered in the differential diagnosis.

Leucine sensitivity. There is often a familial incidence of leucine sensitivity. During the first six months of life casein, present in milk, may cause severe hypoglycaemia, due to its high leucine content. Leucine sensitivity is probably due to stimulation of insulin secretion by the amino acid. The condition appears to be self-limiting and does not usually persist beyond the age of six years. The diagnosis is confirmed by demonstrating hypoglycaemia within 30 minutes after an oral dose of leucine or casein. Normal subjects do not respond to leucine with a significant fall in plasma glucose concentration, but a number of patients with insulinoma are leucine sensitive.

Treatment. The diet should be low in leucine containing food.

Treatment of Hypoglycaemia

Hypoglycaemia should be treated by urgent intravenous administration of 10 to 20 ml of at least 10 per cent, and in adults 50 per cent, glucose solution *after* withdrawal of a blood sample for glucose and insulin assays (p.**220**). Some cases may need to be maintained on a glucose infusion until the cause has been established and treated.

An insulinoma should be removed surgically. If this is contraindicated for clinical reasons a combination of diazoxide and chlorothiazide may maintain normoglycaemia.

Summary

1. Glucose is the main product of dietary carbohydrate metabolism.
2. After a carbohydrate-containing meal excess glucose is:

   - stored as glycogen in liver and muscle;
   - converted to fat and stored in adipose tissue

   Insulin stimulates these processes. The brain is almost entirely dependent on extracellular glucose as an energy source. Maintenance of plasma glucose concentrations is important for normal cerebral function.
3. During fasting:

   - glycogen breakdown in the liver and, to a lesser extent, in the kidneys releases glucose into the plasma;
   - triglyceride breakdown in adipose tissue releases glycerol, which can be converted to glucose, and fatty acids which can be metabolized by most tissues other than the brain.

   The liver converts excess fatty acids to ketones which can be used as an energy source by the brain and other tissues.
   If ketoacid formation exceeds the capacity of homeostatic mechanisms ketoacidosis may develop.
4. Anaerobic glycolysis produces lactic acid:

   - lactic acid production occurs temporarily in contracting muscles;
   - lactic acid is produced by hypoxic tissues. The hypoxic liver becomes a major lactic acid-producing rather than a lactic acid-consuming organ, and lactic acidosis results. Other factors may also cause lactic acidosis by increasing glycolysis or by reducing the utilization of lactic acid.
5. Diabetes mellitus is caused by relative or absolute insulin deficiency. It is characterized by hyperglycaemia which may be intermittent. In severe diabetes mellitus excessive lipolysis may cause ketosis and later acidosis. Confusion and coma are probably due to hyperosmolality. There is severe water and electrolyte depletion in both ketoacidosis and non-ketotic hyperosmolal coma.
6. Hypoglycaemia may occur during fasting, or be provoked by drugs or by some foods.

   - In adults, insulinoma is the most important cause of fasting hypoglycaemia; it is diagnosed by demonstrating high plasma insulin and C-peptide concentrations despite hypoglycaemia. In diabetic patients insulin administration is the commonest cause.
   - In childhood factors causing hypoglycaemia vary with age. Many inborn errors of carbohydrate metabolism may cause hypoglycaemia.

INVESTIGATION OF DISORDERS OF CARBOHYDRATE METABOLISM

ESTIMATION OF PLASMA OR BLOOD GLUCOSE

Glucose is measured in the laboratory by specific enzymatic methods. The supply of glucose to cells depends on extracellular (*plasma*) concentrations. The measurement of plasma glucose concentrations is preferable to that of whole blood. Blood cells, with very low glucose concentrations, 'dilute' glucose, giving results 10 to 15 per cent lower than in plasma, the actual amount depending on the haematocrit. Capillary blood from a finger prick is used for home glucose monitoring and results on such samples usually fall between those of venous whole blood and venous plasma.

Unless plasma is separated from the blood cells within about a hour of collection, the whole blood sample must be mixed with an inhibitor of glycolysis, such as fluoride or iodoacetate, to prevent an *in vitro* fall in the plasma glucose concentration as glycolysis continues.

COLLECTION OF URINE SAMPLE FOR GLUCOSE ESTIMATION

Double void technique. Glycosuria should be sought on a urine specimen produced by the kidneys at that time. The double void technique ensures that the specimen being tested reflects the plasma glucose at the same time and has not been stored in the bladder for some time, before collection. The patient should empty the bladder and discard the specimen; a further specimen passed 10 to 15 minutes later is collected and tested.

Investigation of Suspected Diabetes Mellitus

Diabetes mellitus should not be diagnosed unless unequivocally high plasma glucose concentrations have been found in specimens taken on at least *two different occasions*. If the plasma glucose concentrations are not within the normal reference range and are not above that defined as diabetic, the patient is said to have *impaired glucose tolerance*.

INITIAL INVESTIGATIONS

Blood for plasma glucose estimation should be taken if a patient presents with symptoms of diabetes mellitus, glycosuria, or if it is desirable to exclude the diagnosis because, for example, of a strong family history.

Blood samples may be taken:

- at least 10 hours after a fast;
- two hours after a meal;
- at random;
- as part of a glucose load test.

Diabetes mellitus is confirmed if one of the following is present:

- a fasting plasma concentration of 7.8 mmol/L (140 mg/dl) or more on two occasions;
- a random plasma concentration of 11.1 mmol/L (200 mg/dl) or more on two occasions;
- both a fasting concentration of more than 7.8 mmol/L and a random concentration of more than 11.1 mmol/L.

Diabetes mellitus is usually excluded if:

- a fasting plasma glucose concentration is less than 5.5 mmol/L (100 mg/dl) on two occasions. Samples taken at random times

Table 10.10 Interpretation of fasting and random plasma glucose concentrations.

	Venous plasma glucose mmol/L (mg/dl)	
	Fasting	Random
Diabetes unlikely		5.5 (100) or less
Diabetic	7.8 (140) or more	11.1 (200) or more

Table 10.11 Frequency of sampling and duration of test, depending on the suspected diagnosis or indication for performing a glucose tolerance test

Diagnosis	Frequency sampling (minutes)	Duration of of test (hours)
Diabetes mellitus	120	2
Renal threshold for glucose	60	2
Reactive hypoglycaemia	30	5
Excess growth hormone	30	2

after meals are less reliable for excluding than for confirming the diagnosis

These findings are summarized in Table 10.10. Indications for performing an oral glucose load test are rare. They include:

- fasting plasma glucose concentrations between 5.5 and 7.8 mmol/L;
- random plasma concentration between 7.8 and 11.1 mmol/L;
- a high index of clinical suspicion.

A patient without symptoms may be suspected of having diabetes mellitus because of the chance finding of glycosuria or hyperglycaemia. If the plasma glucose concentration is more than 11.1 mmol/L two hours after a standard glucose load the finding should be confirmed before a definitive diagnosis is made. If the glucose concentration is measured in whole blood the results will be approximately 1.0 mmol/L (18 mg/dl) lower (see above).

ORAL GLUCOSE TOLERANCE TEST (GTT)

Before starting this test contact your laboratory; local details may vary.

Procedure. The patient should be resting and should not smoke during the test.

- The patient fasts overnight (for at least 10, but not more than 16 hours). Water, but no other beverage, is allowed.
- A venous sample is withdrawn for plasma glucose estimation. A urine specimen is collected using the double void technique (p.**217**).

Table 10.12 Interpretation of oral glucose tolerance test

	Venous plasma glucose mmol/L (mg/dl)	
	Fasting	Two hours
Diabetes unlikely	5.5 (100) or less	7.8 (140) or less
Impaired glucose tolerance	5.5–7.8	7.8–11.1
Diabetic	7.8 (140) or more	11.1 (200) or more

- a solution containing 75 g of glucose in 300 ml of water is hyperosmolar, and may not only cause nausea and occasionally vomiting and diarrhoea, but because of delayed absorption, may affect the results of the test. It is therefore more usual to give a solution of a mixture of glucose and its oligosaccharides, because fewer molecules per unit volume have less osmotic effect than the equivalent amount of monosaccharide; the oligosaccharides are all hydrolysed at the brush border, and the glucose immediately enters the cells. Solutions which contain the equivalent of 75 g of hydrated glucose include:

  113 ml of 'Fortical' (Cow and Gate Ltd) made up to approximately 300 ml with water;

  353 ml of 'Lucozade' (SmithKline Beecham Ltd).

  These solutions should be drunk slowly over about four minutes.
- Further blood and urine samples are taken at two hours after the ingestion of glucose. The frequency of blood sampling depends

on the indication for performing the investigation. Examples are shown in Table 10.11.

The plasma glucose concentrations are measured and the urine samples tested for glucose and ketones.

Interpretation of the oral glucose tolerance test is shown in Table 10.12. It is the same for pregnant and nonpregnant women. Because of the increased risks of congenital malformations in offspring of diabetic women, optimal glycaemic control should be achieved. Therefore, it is recommended that the two hour plasma glucose concentration should be less than 7.8 mmol/L.

The following factors may affect the result of the test:

- *Previous diet.* No special restrictions are necessary if the patient has been on a normal diet for three to four days. However, if the test is performed after a period of carbohydrate restriction, perhaps as part of a reducing diet, this may cause abnormal glucose tolerance, probably because metabolism is adjusted to the 'fasted state' and so favours gluconeogenesis.
- *Time of day.* Most glucose tolerance tests are performed in the morning and the reference values quoted are for this time of day. There is evidence that tests performed in the afternoon yield higher plasma glucose concentrations and that the

accepted 'reference values' may not be applicable. This may be due to a circadian variation in islet cell responsiveness.
- *Drugs*, such as steroids, oral contraceptives and thiazide and loop diuretics may impair glucose tolerance.

INITIAL INVESTIGATION OF A DIABETIC PATIENT PRESENTING IN COMA

A diabetic patient may be in coma due to hyperglycaemia, hypoglycaemia or any of the causes shown in Table 10.13. After a thorough clinical assessment proceed as follows.

- *Notify* the laboratory that specimens are being taken and ensure that they are delivered *promptly*. This minimizes delays.
- Take blood *immediately* for estimation of plasma:
  - glucose
  - sodium and potassium
  - urea and/or creatinine
  - bicarbonate and/or arterial blood pH and P_{CO_2}

Repeated arterial puncture is undesirable and often unnecessary. If arterial pH is measured initially, plasma T_{CO_2} (bicarbonate) concentration may be estimated if monitoring of acid–base balance is needed.

Table 10.13   Clinical and biochemical features of a diabetic patient presenting in coma

Diagnosis	Clinical features	Laboratory findings			
		Plasma		Urine	
		glucose	bicarbonate	glucose	ketones
Ketoacidosis	Volume depletion Hyperventilating	High	Low	+++	+++
Hyperosmolar coma	Volume depletion May be hyperventilating	Very high	N or slightly reduced	+++	Neg
Hypoglycaemia	Non-specific	Low	N	Neg	Neg
Cerebrovascular accident	Neurological May be hyperventilating	May be raised	May be low	May be +	Usually absent

N = normal.

- Test a urine sample for glucose and ketones. *Urine testing alone must never be used to diagnose hyperglycaemia.* The urine may have been in the bladder for some time and may reflect earlier and very different plasma glucose concentrations.
- A rapid assessment of blood glucose concentration may be obtained using a reagent strip; results may be dangerously wrong if:

    reagent strips are outdated or improperly stored;

    the manufacturers' instructions are not followed;

    the skin is contaminated with glucose for any reason.

    Results should always be checked with results obtained from the laboratory.
- If hypoglycaemia is suspected on clinical grounds or because of the results obtained using reagent strips, glucose should be given *immediately* while waiting for the laboratory results. It is less dangerous to give glucose to a patient with hyperglycaemia than to give insulin to a patient with hypoglycaemia.

Blood samples must be sent to the laboratory immediately after the blood has been taken; the plasma potassium concentration should be measured before insulin is given but rehydration should never be delayed. Results of side-room tests must be interpreted with caution.

Investigation of Hypoglycaemia

The most important test in a patient with proven hypoglycaemia is to measure the plasma insulin concentration when that of glucose is low. This should differentiate exogenous insulin administration or endogenous insulin production, for example from an insulinoma, from other causes of hypoglycaemia. If the plasma insulin concentration is inappropriately high for that of glucose, and if doubt remains about the cause, plasma C-peptide concentrations should be assayed. If high, it suggests endogenous insulin secretion, causes of which include pancreatic stimulation by sulphonylureas. An undetectable plasma concentration suggests exogenous insulin administration.

If a patient is seen during an episode of hypoglycaemia, before giving glucose take blood for plasma glucose, insulin and C-peptide assays. Plasma for the last two assays should be separated from cells immediately and the plasma stored at $-20°C$ until hypoglycaemia has been proven. This may considerably shorten the time needed for further investigation.

However, more commonly the patient has been referred for investigation of previously documented hypoglycaemia or with a history strongly suggestive of hypoglycaemic attacks. A full assessment should be made, paying special attention to:

- the time of attacks in relation to meals (reactive hypoglycaemia);
- drug (especially hypoglycaemic drugs) or alcohol ingestion. This information may not be freely given and a negative history does not exclude it;
- possible hypopituitarism or adrenocortical hypofunction. If either of these diagnoses is considered likely, investigate as outlined on p.**147**;
- possible non-pancreatic tumour (p.**213**).

If no cause is identified, it may be possible to induce hypoglycaemia by fasting for up to 72 hours, accompanied by exercise *under close supervision*. Blood should be taken every six hours for plasma glucose and insulin estimations and, if symptoms occur, should be assayed for glucose immediately. The test can be stopped if hypoglycaemia is demonstrated. If hypoglycaemia is not induced by prolonged fasting, endogenous hyperinsulinism is unlikely to be the cause of the symptoms.

Insulin should be measured in a sample taken at the time of proven hypoglycaemia. If insulin administration is suspected, C-peptide should also be assayed. The interpretation of results is summarized in Table 10.8 (p.**213**).

If results of fasting plasma glucose and insulin assays are equivocal, an insulin suppression test can be performed. Hypoglycaemia induced by intravenous injection of insulin should suppress endogenous insulin and C-peptide secretion. Failure of C-peptide concentrations to fall confirms autonomous insulin secretion, usually due to an insulinoma.

INSULIN SUPPRESSION TEST

The precautions outlined on p.148 must be observed.

Procedure:

- The patient must fast overnight for 10 to 16 hours but is allowed small amounts of water.
- Insert an indwelling intravenous cannula (p.**147**) and keep it patent with either sodium citrate solution or heparinized saline.
- Take fasting samples for glucose and C-peptide estimation.
- Give soluble insulin (0.15 U/kg body weight) intravenously.
- After the insulin injection, take further samples for glucose and C-peptide assay after 30, 60, 90, 120 and 150 minutes. If clinically indicated, cortisol may also be measured to assess hypothalamic–pituitary–adrenal function (p.**148**).

Interpretation. In normal subjects plasma C-peptide concentrations fall by more than 50 per cent of the initial value. In most cases of insulinoma this degree of fall does not occur.

GLYCOSURIA

Glycosuria is best detected by enzyme reagent strips. Directions for use are supplied with the strips. Glycosuria may be due to:

- diabetes mellitus;
- glucose infusion;
- renal glycosuria, which may be inherited as an autosomal dominant trait;
- pregnancy.

False negative results may occur:

- if the urine contains large amounts of ascorbic acid, after ingestion of therapeutic doses;
- after injection of tetracyclines, which contain ascorbic acid as a preservative.

False positive results may occur if the urine container is contaminated with detergent.

Reducing substances

The reagents in Clinitest tablets react with reducing substances and are caustic so they should be handled carefully. Clinitest tablets must be used as directed. They should be used rather than glucose specific reagent strips to screen the urine in newborn infants or children because of the diagnostic importance of non-glucose reducing substances, such as galactose, in these age groups.

Causes of a positive result with Clinitest are shown in Table 10.4 (p.**205**). Nonglucose reducing substances are identified by chromatography and specific tests. In adults a positive reaction with Clinitest is usually due to glucose and can be confirmed using glucose oxidase impregnated reagent strips. The significance of a positive result varies with the substance.

Glucose (see p.**205**).

Glucuronates are relatively common urinary reducing substances. A large number of drugs, such as salicylates and their metabolites, are excreted in the urine after conjugation with glucuronate in the liver (p.**282**).

Galactose is found in the urine in galactosaemia (p.**290**).

Fructose may appear in the urine after very large oral doses of sucrose, or after excessive fruit ingestion, but usually fructosuria is due to one of two rare inborn errors of metabolism, both transmitted as autosomal recessive disorders.

- Essential fructosuria is a harmless condition.

- Hereditary fructose intolerance (p.**205**) is a serious disease characterized by hypoglycaemia that may lead to death in infancy.

Lactose. Lactosuria may occur in:

- late pregnancy and during lactation;
- lactase deficiency (p.**255**).

Pentoses. Pentosuria is very rare. It may occur in:

- alimentary pentosuria after excessive ingestion of fruits such as cherries and grapes. The pentoses are arabinose and xylose;
- essential pentosuria, a rare recessive disorder due to a block in glucuronate metabolism characterized by the excretion of xylose. It is harmless.

Homogentisic acid appears in the urine in the rare inborn error alkaptonuria (p.**358**). It is usually recognizable because it forms a blackish precipitate in urine on standing.

KETONURIA

Most simple urine tests for ketones are more sensitive for detecting acetoacetate than acetone; β-hydroxybutyrate does not react in these tests. Ketonuria may be detected after the patient has fasted for several hours. Occasional colour reactions resembling, but not identical with, that of acetoacetate may be given by phthalein compounds when used as a laxative.

Ketostix and Acetest are strips and tablets respectively, impregnated with ammonium sulphate and sodium nitroprusside.

Plasma Lipids and Lipoproteins

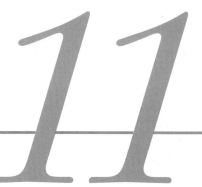

11

An understanding of the pathophysiology of plasma lipid metabolism is based on the concept of lipoproteins, the form in which lipids circulate in plasma. The first part of this chapter will describe the classifications used and show how terminologies are related.

TERMINOLOGY

Plasma Lipids

The chemical structures of the four forms of lipid present in plasma are illustrated in Fig. 11.1.

Fatty acids are straight-chain carbon compounds of varying lengths. They may be *saturated*, containing no double bonds, *monounsaturated* with one, or *polyunsaturated* with more than one, double bond (Table 11.1). Fatty acids may be esterified with glycerol to form triglycerides, or be *nonesterified* or *free* (NEFA or FFA). Plasma FFA liberated from adipose tissue are transported, mainly bound to albumin, to the liver and muscle where they are metabolized. They provide a significant proportion of the energy requirements of the body. This aspect of fat metabolism is considered further on p.**201**.

Triglycerides are fatty acid esters of glycerol, each containing three different fatty acids. They are transported from the intestine and the liver to various tissues, such as adipose tissue, as lipoproteins. Following hydrolysis, fatty acids are taken up, re-esterified and

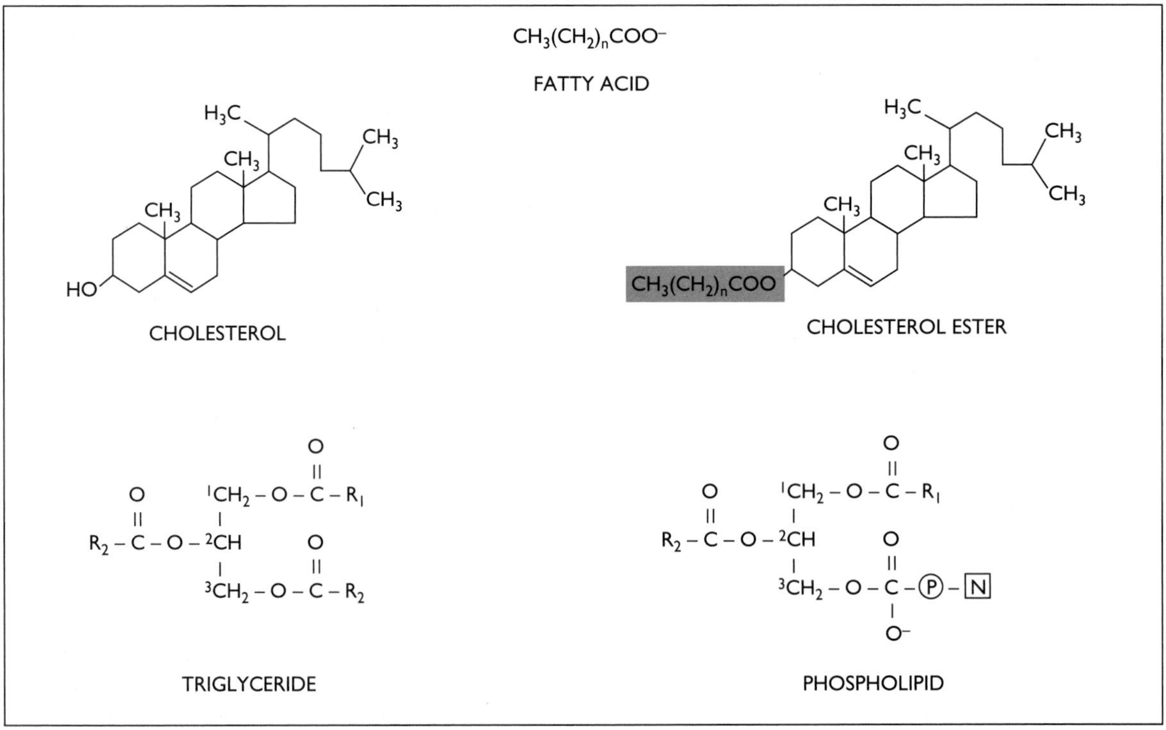

Fig. 11.1 Chemical structure of lipids present in plasma. $\textcircled{P}$ = phosphate, $\boxed{N}$ = nitrogenous base, R = fatty acid.

Table 11.1 Fatty acids present in plasma

	Name	Chain length	Source
Saturated	Myristic acid	C_{14}	Coconut oil
	Palmitic acid	C_{16}	Animal/plant fat
	Stearic acid	C_{18}	Animal/plant fat
Monounsaturated	Palmitoleic acid	C_{16}	Fat
	Oleic acid	C_{18}	Natural fat
Polyunsaturated	Linoleic acid	C_{18}	Plant oils
	Linolenic acid	C_{18}	Plant oils
	Arachidonic acid	C_{20}	Plant oils
	Eicosapentaenoic acid	C_{20}	Fish oils

stored as triglycerides. Plasma triglyceride concentrations rise after a fatty meal and remain increased for several hours.

Phospholipids are complex lipids, resembling triglycerides, but containing phosphate and a nitrogenous base in place of one of the fatty acids. They are important components of cell membranes and lipoproteins, maintaining the solubility of non-polar lipids and cholesterol.

Cholesterol, a steroid, is a precursor to many physiologically important steroids, such as bile acids and steroid hormones (Fig. 6.1; p.**119**). Cholesterol synthesis initially involves the conversion of acetate to mevalonic acid. The rate-limiting step is catalysed by the enzyme β-hydroxy-β-methyl glutaryl coenzyme A reductase (HMGCoA reductase), the activity of which is controlled by negative feedback by the intracellular cholesterol concentration. About two-thirds of the plasma cholesterol is esterified with fatty acids to form cholesterol esters. Assays in routine use measure the plasma total cholesterol concentrations and do not distinguish between the unesterified and esterified forms. *Unlike that of triglyceride, plasma concentration of cholesterol does not rise after a fatty meal.*

Lipoproteins

Plasma lipids are derived from food (exogenous) or are synthesized in the body (endoge-

nous). Lipids are relatively insoluble in water; they are carried in body fluids as soluble protein complexes known as lipoproteins. The core of insoluble (nonpolar) cholesterol esters and triglycerides is surrounded by proteins, phospholipids and free cholesterol with their water-soluble (polar) groups facing outwards.

Lipoproteins are classified by their density which, in turn, reflects size. The greater the lipid/protein ratio in the complex, the larger it is and the lower its density. There are five main classes of lipoproteins. *Triglyceride-rich* particles include:

- *chylomicrons*, which transport exogenous lipid from the intestine to all cells;
- *VLDL (very low density lipoproteins)*, which transport endogenous lipid from the liver to cells;
- *IDL (intermediate density lipoproteins)*, which are usually undetectable in normal plasma. It is normally a transient intermediate lipoprotein formed during the conversion of VLDL to LDL. It contains both cholesterol and endogenous triglycerides. IDL is undetectable in normal plasma.

Because of their large size these particles reflect light and plasma containing a high concentration appears turbid or milky (lipaemia). If a turbid plasma sample is left standing for 18 hours at 4°C the larger chylomicrons, because of their low density, rise to form a creamy layer on the surface. The smaller, denser VLDL and IDL particles

Table 11.2   The composition and electrophoretic mobility of the main lipoprotein particles

| Lipoprotein | Source | Composition (% mass) | | | | Apolipoproteins | Electrophoretic mobility |
		Prot.	Chol.	TG.	PL.		
Chylomicrons	Intestine	1	4	90	5	A, B, (C), (E)	Origin
VLDL	Liver	8	25	55	12	B, C, E	pre-β
LDL	VLDL (via IDL)	20	55	5	20	B	β
HDL	Liver, intestine	50	20	5	25	A, C, E	α

Prot. = apolipoprotein. Chol. = cholesterol. TG. = triglyceride. PL. = phospholipid. The apolipoproteins in brackets are acquired after secretion.

do not rise and the sample remains diffusely turbid. If hyperlipidaemia is gross the distribution may be less easy to distinguish.

Two smaller lipoproteins contain mostly *cholesterol*:

- *LDL (low density lipoproteins)*, formed from VLDL, transport cholesterol to cells;
- *HDL (high density lipoproteins)* are involved in the transport of cholesterol from the cells to the liver.

Another lipoprotein $Lp_{(a)}$ is similar in composition to LDL but has a higher protein content; it contains a portion which is structurally similar to one of the clotting factors. Unlike LDL, it is synthesized in the liver. $Lp_{(a)}$ is normally present in low plasma concentrations.

Lipoproteins of smaller size do not scatter light; even very high concentrations in plasma do not produce lipaemia.

Although the classification of lipoproteins is based on their densities determined by ultracentrifugation, the lipoprotein composition of plasma can usually be inferred from simple lipid assays. Plasma taken from a fasting subject contains only LDL, VLDL and HDL in normal individuals and in many cases of hyperlipidaemia (p.**232**). Because 70 per cent of the plasma cholesterol is incorporated in LDL and only 20 per cent in HDL, the measured plasma total cholesterol concentration primarily reflects LDL concentrations and the plasma triglyceride concentration those of VLDL. The cholesterol content in HDL can be quantitated by precipitation techniques and LDL calculated if the plasma triglyceride

Table 11.3   WHO (Fredrickson) classification of hyperlipidaemia, based on the electrophoretic pattern of the lipoproteins. However, an individual with primary hyperlipidaemia may have different patterns at different times

Type	Electrophoretic pattern	Lipoprotein increased
I	Increased chylomicrons	Chylomicrons
IIa	Increased β-lipoproteins	LDL
IIb	Increased pre-β and β lipoproteins	VLDL and LDL
III	'Broad β' band	IDL
IV	Increased pre-β lipoprotein	VLDL
V	Increased pre-β lipoprotein and chylomicrons	VLDL and Chylomicrons

concentration is less than about 5.0 mmol/L (425 mg/dl). If the plasma triglyceride concentration is increased, the cholesterol content within either chylomicron or VLDL particles makes the calculation inaccurate.

The nomenclature and composition of the main lipoprotein classes are summarized in Table 11.2.

In some cases of hyperlipidaemia the lipoprotein pattern may be defined according to its electrophoretic mobility (Table 11.3). This classification is less frequently used now than formerly but is included here because it still appears in the medical literature. The technique separates the particles by electrical charge into four principal bands, named according to their relative positions by protein electrophoresis, as α, pre-β and β, which correspond to HDL, VLDL, and LDL respectively and chylomicron fractions. IDL excess may produce a broad β band.

METABOLISM OF LIPOPROTEINS

Lipoproteins are synthesized in the liver or intestine. After secretion they are modified by enzyme-catalysed reactions and the remnants are taken up by receptors on cells surfaces. These processes are regulated by the protein component of the particle, the apolipoproteins.

Apolipoproteins are classified into several groups, such as apoA and apoB. Some are incorporated into the lipoprotein structure, but others, such as apoC and apoE, interchange freely between lipoproteins. The apolipoproteins have several functions. They are involved in normal lipid secretion by cells; apoA-I and apoC-II activate enzymes concerned with lipid metabolism and others, such as apoB and apoE, recognize receptors involved in cellular uptake of the lipoprotein particle. These functions are described in the text and summarized in Table 11.4.

Exogenous Lipid Pathways (Fig. 11.2)

Fatty acids and cholesterol, released by digestion of dietary fat together with cholesterol from the bile, are absorbed into intestinal mucosal cells where they are re-esterified to form triglycerides and cholesterol esters.

These, together with phospholipids, apoA and apoB, are secreted from cells into the lymphatic system as chylomicrons. This secretion depends on the presence of apoB. Chylomicrons enter the systemic circulation by the thoracic duct. ApoC and apoE, both derived from HDL, are added to them in both lymph and plasma.

CHYLOMICRON METABOLISM

Chylomicrons are metabolized in adipose tissue and muscle. The enzyme, *lipoprotein lipase*, located on capillary walls, is activated by apoC-II and hydrolyses triglyceride to glycerol and fatty acids. The fatty acids are either taken up by adipose or muscle cells or are bound to albumin in the plasma. The glycerol enters the hepatic glycolytic pathway. As the chylomicron shrinks, surface material containing apoA and some apoC and phospholipid is released and incorporated into HDL.

The small chylomicron remnants are composed mainly of cholesterol, apoB and apoE. They rapidly bind to hepatic chylomicron-remnant receptors, which recognize the constituent apoE. The remnants then enter the liver cells where the protein is catabolized and the cholesterol released. The uptake of chylomicron remnants, unlike that of LDL (p.**229**), is not influenced by the amount of cholesterol in hepatic cells.

Table 11.4 The main apolipoproteins and their known functions

Apolipoprotein	Occurrence	Known functions
A	Chylomicrons, HDL	Cofactor for LCAT (A-I)
B	Chylomicrons, VLDL, IDL, LDL	Secretion of chylomicrons and VLDL Binding of LDL to receptors
C	HDL, VLDL, IDL, chylomicrons (from HDL)	Cofactor for lipoprotein lipase (C-II)
E	HDL, VLDL, IDL, chylomicrons (from HDL)	Binding of IDL and remnant particles to receptors

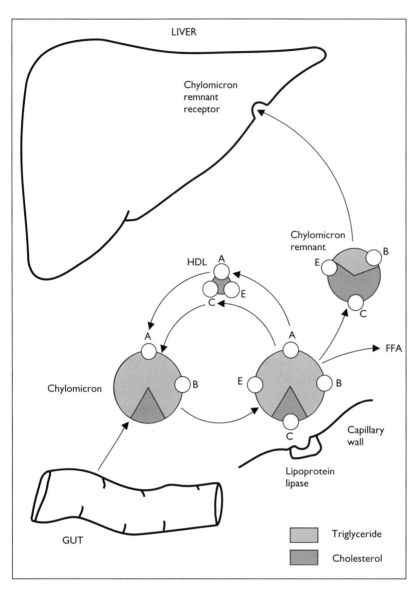

Fig. 11.2 Exogenous pathway of lipid metabolism.

At the end of this pathway dietary triglycerides have been delivered to adipose tissue and muscle, and cholesterol to the liver.

Endogenous Lipid Pathways (Fig. 11.3)

The liver is the main source of endogenous lipids. Triglycerides are synthesized from glycerol and fatty acids, which may reach the liver from the fat stores or from glucose. Hepatic cholesterol may be synthesized locally or be derived from lipoproteins, such as chylomicron remnants, after they have been taken up by liver cells. These lipids are transported from the liver in VLDL.

VLDL METABOLISM

VLDL is a large triglyceride-rich particle incorporating apoB, apoC and apoE. After secretion it incorporates more apoC from HDL. In

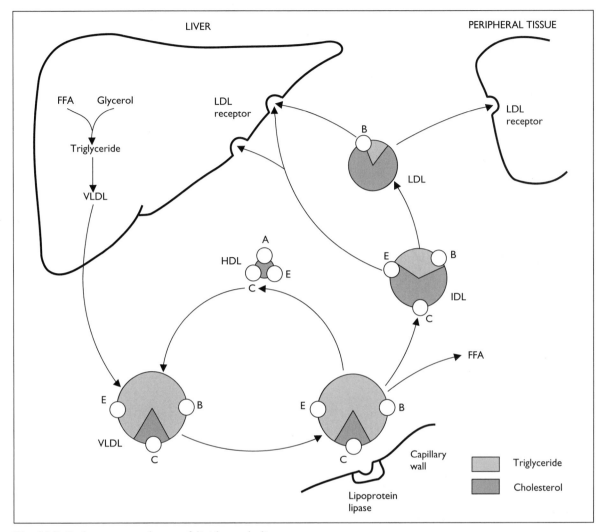

Fig. 11.3 Endogenous pathway of lipid metabolism.

peripheral tissues triglycerides are removed after hydrolysis by *lipoprotein lipase*. Up to this stage the metabolism of VLDL is similar to that of chylomicrons, although it occurs more slowly. However, the disposal of the resulting remnant particle differs.

The 'VLDL remnant', or IDL, which contains both triglycerides and cholesterol, as well as apoB and apoE, is either rapidly taken up by the liver or loses the remaining triglycerides and apoE to become LDL. The mechanism and site of this conversion is unknown.

LDL METABOLISM

LDL is a small cholesterol-rich lipoprotein containing only apoB. It has a longer life than its precursors, VLDL and IDL, and accounts for about 70 per cent of the total cholesterol in plasma. It is taken up by specific receptors located on cell surfaces (LDL receptors or apoB/E receptors). Although these are present on all cells, they are most abundant in the liver. They recognize apoB and apoE and so can take up either LDL or IDL. After entering cells LDL particles are broken down by lysosomes; much of the released cholesterol

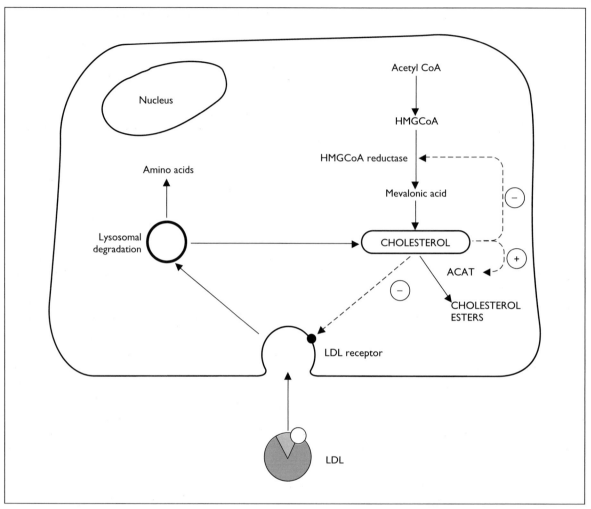

Fig. 11.4 The relation between the cellular uptake of LDL and the endogenous synthesis of cholesterol.
+ = stimulation; − = suppression

contributes to membrane formation or, in the adrenal cortex and gonads, to steroid synthesis. Most cells can synthesize cholesterol but several feedback mechanisms prevent its intracellular accumulation. Cholesterol, taken up by receptors, inhibits intracellular cholesterol synthesis and prevents further uptake by reducing the rate of synthesis of LDL receptors (Fig. 11.4).

Most of the plasma LDL is removed by LDL receptors. If plasma concentrations are high some may also enter cells by a passive, unregulated route. Because of their small size LDL particles can infiltrate tissues, such as those of the arterial wall, and cause damage.

FACTORS INFLUENCING PLASMA LDL CONCENTRATIONS

The plasma LDL concentration, and therefore the measured plasma cholesterol concentration, is determined mainly by the rate of uptake by LDL receptors. The liver has a central role in cholesterol metabolism because it:

- contains most of the LDL receptors;
- synthesizes most of the endogenous cholesterol;
- receives cholesterol from the diet and from lipoproteins;
- is the only organ that can excrete cholesterol from the body in bile.

The concentration of LDL receptors on hepatic cell surfaces depends on the amount of cholesterol in cells. As intracellular cholesterol accumulates the number of receptors is reduced. Factors that lead to cholesterol accumulation in the liver will, by reducing receptor numbers, increase plasma LDL concentrations. One of these factors is the amount of cholesterol reaching the liver from the intestine.

Between 30 and 60 per cent of cholesterol entering the intestinal lumen from the diet and in bile is absorbed. The rate of absorption increases if the diet is rich in saturated fat, possibly because of more efficient micelle formation (p.**246**). In affluent societies dietary cholesterol is derived mainly from egg yolk (the richest source), dairy products and red meat; the daily intake is about 1.5 to 2.0 mmol (600 to 800 mg). Absorbed cholesterol is transported to the liver in chylomicron remnant particles which are taken up by chylomicron-remnant receptors.

Inhibition of hepatic cholesterol synthesis, *by suppression of the enzyme HMGCoA reductase*, may not prevent intracellular accumulation if dietary intake is excessive. As in all other cells, intracellular cholesterol accumulation leads to a reduction in LDL receptor activity. LDL entry into cells therefore falls and plasma concentrations rise.

Cholesterol may be secreted into plasma, incorporated into VLDL, with no net loss to the body, or may be excreted from the body in bile either as cholesterol or after conversion to bile acids. Some bile acids are reabsorbed from the intestinal lumen and returned to the liver via the *enterohepatic circulation* (p.**246**); they then control further

bile acid synthesis. Any interruption to the enterohepatic circulation, for example by combination with bile salt sequestrants (p.**237**), results in an increased conversion of cholesterol to bile acids, reduction in hepatic cholesterol stores and an increase in the number of LDL receptors. The rate of hepatic LDL receptor synthesis is also increased by oestrogens and by thyroid hormones.

ROLE OF HIGH DENSITY LIPOPROTEIN (HDL)

Cholesterol synthesized in cells would accumulate there if not removed. The only excretory route is in the bile. The transport of cholesterol from non-hepatic cells to liver involves HDL.

HDL is synthesized in hepatic and intestinal cells and secreted from them as small particles containing phospholipid, free cholesterol and apoA and apoE ('nascent' HDL). It may also be formed from the surface coat of the large triglyceride-rich lipoproteins, VLDL and chylomicrons (p.**226**). HDL synthesis is increased by oestrogen; consequently plasma concentrations are higher in menstruating women than in women after the menopause or in men.

Esterification of free cholesterol, derived from cells and from other lipoproteins, is catalysed by the enzyme *lecithin-cholesterol acyltransferase (LCAT)*, which is part of the HDL particle and which is activated by apoA-I. Most of the esterified cholesterol is transferred to LDL, VLDL and chylomicron remnants and so reaches the liver. A small amount is stored in the core of the now spherical HDL particle. Some cholesterol-rich HDL may be taken up directly by the liver.

When plasma VLDL or chylomicron concentrations are low, most of the apoC in plasma is carried in HDL. As the plasma concentrations of the triglyceride-rich lipoproteins rise, these particles take up apoC-II from HDL. The role of apoC-II in activating lipoprotein lipase has been mentioned. After the triglyceride has been hydrolysed, the apoprotein returns to the HDL particle.

Disorders of Lipid Metabolism

Most common disorders of lipid metabolism are associated with hyperlipidaemia. Very rare inherited disorders may be associated with accumulation of lipid in tissues and not in plasma.

Clinical Manifestation of Hyperlipidaemia

The accumulation of lipid in tissues is usually, but not always, the result of severe and prolonged hyperlipidaemia and causes cell damage. Lipid accumulations, for example under skin or mucous membranes, may be visible. Lipid may accumulate in:

- **arterial walls**. *This is by far the commonest and most important manifestation of lipid disorders.* Cholesterol accumulation and associated cellular proliferation and fibrous tissue formation produce atheromatous plaques. *Atherosclerosis* is due to distortion and obstruction of the artery which may result from calcification and ulceration of plaques. The small lipoproteins LDL and IDL are atherogenic;
- **subcutaneous tissue**, causing *xanthomatosis*. The nature of the lipid fraction most affected usually determines the clinical appearance:
  eruptive xanthomata are crops of small, itchy, yellow nodules. They are associated with *very high plasma VLDL or chylomicron (triglyceride) concentrations*, which disappear if plasma lipid concentrations fall to normal;
  tuberous xanthomata are yellow plaques found mainly over the elbows

and knees, and can be large and disfiguring. These, and raised linear lipid deposits in the palmar creases, are associated with high plasma concentrations of IDL, which contain both triglyceride and cholesterol;
  xanthelasma are lipid deposits under the periorbital skin and may be associated with high plasma LDL-cholesterol concentrations.
- **tendons**. *Xanthomata*, usually on the Achilles tendons or the extensor tendons of the hands, occur in familial hypercholesterolaemia;
- **cornea**. *Corneal arcus* in subjects under the age of about 40 may be caused by deposition of lipid and associated with high plasma LDL-cholesterol concentrations. A corneal arcus must be distinguished from an arcus senilis, which presents in older subjects.

Tendinous xanthomata, and corneal arcus have a poor prognosis.

Hypertriglyceridaemia whether due to chylomicrons, VLDL, or both, causes *plasma turbidity*. Sustained and very high plasma concentrations of chylomicrons are associated with *abdominal pain* and even *acute pancreatitis*, as well as eruptive xanthomata. However, many cases of hypertriglyceridaemia are symptom free. These large lipoproteins are unlikely to cause atheroma *per se*. However, many patients with increased concentrations of VLDL-triglyceride have a reduced concentration of plasma HDL and increased plasma concentration of LDL or IDL, which contain cholesterol. The slightly increased risk of atheroma which has been attributed to hypertriglyceridaemia may be explained by the secondary effects on cholesterol metabolism.

Lipid and Cardiovascular Disease

There is a positive correlation between the risk of developing ischaemic heart disease and a raised plasma total and LDL-cholesterol concentrations and a negative one with plasma HDL-cholesterol. Lowering high plasma LDL-cholesterol concentrations reduces the risk of cardiovascular disease. Hypercholesterolaemia is just one of the major risk factors of cardiovascular disease; others include smoking and hypertension.

Most of our knowledge of the clinical effects is based on plasma total, or on LDL or HDL, cholesterol concentrations. As methods for estimating plasma apoA and apoB concentrations become more generally available they may prove better indicators of cardiovascular risk but, at the time of writing, lipoprotein disorders are usually diagnosed by measuring plasma lipid patterns rather than their plasma concentrations directly. Therefore these disorders will be considered under three headings:

- predominant hypercholesterolaemia;
- predominant hypertriglyceridaemia;
- mixed hyperlipidaemia.

Predominant Hypercholesterolaemia

WHAT IS HYPERCHOLESTEROLAEMIA?

Plasma cholesterol concentrations at birth (cord blood) are usually below 2.5 mmol/L (about 100 mg/dl). They increase slowly, mostly during the first year of life, but do not usually exceed 4.0 mmol/L (about 160 mg/dl) in children. In most affluent populations plasma concentrations increase progressively after the second decade, more in men than in women during the reproductive years. The upper 95 per cent limit of the 'reference range' in many societies is as high as about 8.5 mmol/L (330 mg/dl) in the fifth and sixth decades. This rise with age does not occur in less affluent communities, in which the incidence of ischaemic heart disease is much lower. It is likely that the progressive rise in plasma cholesterol concentration reflects a decreasing concentration of LDL receptors in the liver.

Reference ranges, as usually calculated, are of little significance for plasma cholesterol as they would include many cases not strictly 'normal'. The risk of developing cardiovascular disease increases as the plasma cholesterol concentration rise above about 5.2 mmol/L (200 mg/dl). It is generally accepted that, in the absence of other risk factors of coronary artery disease, it is desirable that plasma cholesterol concentrations be maintained below 6.5 mmol/L (275 mg/dl).

CAUSES OF HYPERCHOLESTEROLAEMIA

Hypercholesterolaemia associated with little or no elevation of plasma triglyceride concentration is almost always due to a raised plasma LDL concentration. The coexistence of an underlying genetic defect, or the development of a disorder that affects plasma LDL concentrations, will cause a greater increase in plasma cholesterol with age than the factors already discussed.

Secondary hypercholesterolaemia. The commonest disorders that may produce a *secondary increase* in plasma total and LDL-cholesterol concentrations are:

- primary hypothyroidism;
- diabetes mellitus;
- nephrotic syndrome;
- cholestasis;
- drugs (Table 11.5).

These disorders must be excluded in any individual presenting with hypercholesterolaemia.

Primary hypercholesterolaemia. The familial incidence of hypercholesterolaemia,

Table 11.5 The effect of some drugs on plasma lipid concentrations

Drug	Cholesterol			Triglyceride
	Total-	**LDL-**	**HDL-**	
Thiazides	↑	↑	↑	↑
Loop diuretics e.g. frusemide	↑	↑	↓	↑
β-blockers	↑	–	↓	↑
ACE inhibitors	–	–	–	–
Calcium antagonists	–	–	–	–
Insulin	–	↓	↑	↓
Sulphonylureas	–	–	↑	↓
Biguanides	↓	–	–	↓

↑ = increased, ↓ = decreased.

often associated with an increased risk of ischaemic heart disease, suggests an inherited disorder, the exact nature of which can only be established by extensive family studies.

In most families in which there is moderate hypercholesterolaemia a graph of the plasma cholesterol concentrations of all individuals in the family shows a continuous distribution. This contrasts with the trimodal distribution found in the *monogenic* pattern of familial hypercholesterolaemia (see below), in which plasma cholesterol concentrations form three distinct peaks. These peaks represent homozygotes with the normal gene, the heterozygotes, and the homozygotes for the abnormal gene. The continuous distribution, with a high mean plasma concentration within a family, is thought to be caused by several gene abnormalities affecting either LDL or cholesterol synthesis and disposal. It is therefore called *polygenic hypercholesterolaemia.* Environmental and dietary factors may determine the expression of the defect. Xanthomata are found relatively rarely. The risk of developing cardiovascular disease is higher than normal, compared with an age- and sex-matched population. In the following two disorders associated with moderate to severe hypercholesterolaemia, the pattern of inheritance is autosomal dominant.

Familial combined hyperlipidaemia, the more common, is associated with excessive hepatic production of apoB, and therefore of LDL, and of VLDL-triglyceride synthesis due to either a primary or secondary disorder.

Family members have a variety of different phenotypes. In one-third there is an increase in plasma LDL-cholesterol concentration. In another third there is an increase in both LDL-cholesterol and VLDL-triglyceride and the remaining third have VLDL-hypertriglyceridaemia. The lipid abnormalities only become apparent after the third decade and the risk of *ischaemic heart disease* in all cases is higher than that for an age and sex matched population. High plasma triglyceride concentrations may cause *eruptive xanthomata.*

Familial (monogenic) hypercholesterolaemia is caused by a LDL receptor defect. In families with this mode of inheritance there is a clear distinction between unaffected, homozygous and heterozygous subjects; this differs from the commoner polygenic disease. In most countries monogenic hypercholesterolaemia *accounts for less than five per cent of all cases of primary hypercholesterolaemia.* There are several variants, all of which are inherited as autosomal dominant traits. The reduced cellular uptake of LDL, particularly by the liver, causes an increase in plasma total- and LDL-cholesterol concentrations. Plasma triglyceride concentrations are either normal or only slightly raised. It is the most lethal of the inherited disorders.

- *In homozygotes* LDL receptors are virtually absent and plasma LDL-cholesterol concentrations are three or four times higher than those in normal subjects; patients rarely survive beyond the age of 20 and usually die from ischaemic heart disease.
- *In heterozygotes* the number of LDL receptors is reduced by about 50 per cent and the plasma cholesterol concentrations are about twice those in normal subjects. They have a 10 to 20-fold higher risk of developing ischaemic heart disease than those with normal plasma concentrations.

Tendinous xanthomata and xanthelasma develop in homozygotes in early childhood but only after the second decade in heterozygotes.

Predominant Hypertriglyceridaemia

Elevated plasma triglyceride concentrations may be due to an increase in plasma VLDL or chylomicrons or both. *Hypertriglyceridaemia is usually secondary to another disorder* (Table 11.6).

Primary hypertriglyceridaemia is less common than primary hypercholesterolaemia.

Familial combined hyperlipidaemia has been discussed above. One-third of affected individuals have raised plasma VLDL concentrations.

Familial endogenous hypertriglyceridaemia is caused by hepatic triglyceride overproduction with increased VLDL secretion. The condition is probably transmitted as an autosomal dominant trait and usually becomes apparent only after the fourth decade. It may be associated with:

- obesity;
- glucose intolerance;
- decrease in plasma HDL-cholesterol concentration;
- hyperuricaemia.

Insulin resistance may be a common factor in the above conditions. Superimposed secondary conditions, such as diabetes mellitus or excessive alcohol intake, may result in very high plasma VLDL concentrations and often chylomicronaemia.

Hyperchylomicronaemia is usually due either to an acquired or inherited deficiency of lipoprotein lipase. Insulin is needed for optimal enzyme activity. Consequently, hyperchylomicronaemia may occur in poorly controlled diabetic patients. It may also be found in those presenting with acute pancreatitis.

Table 11.6 Some important causes of secondary hypertriglyceridaemia.

Obesity and excessive carbohydrate intake
Alcohol
Diabetes mellitus ⎫
Primary hypothyroidism ⎬ with hypercholesterolaemia
Nephrotic syndrome ⎭
Renal glomerular dysfunction
Drugs:
  'the pill' and oestrogens (before and after the menopause)
  β-blockers
  thiazide diuretics
Acute pancreatitis

Inherited lipoprotein lipase deficiency may be due to:

- true deficiency of the enzyme;
- reduced activity of the enzyme because of apoC-II deficiency.

The plasma is very turbid because of the accumulation of chylomicrons. True lipoprotein lipase deficiency usually presents during childhood, with signs and symptoms due to an excess of fat at such sites as:

- skin (eruptive xanthomata);
- liver (hepatomegaly);
- retinal vessels (lipaemia retinalis);
- abdomen (abdominal pain).

Hyperchylomicronaemia due to apoC-II deficiency is most likely to present in adults.

Mixed Hyperlipidaemia

Raised plasma concentrations of both cholesterol and triglycerides are commonest in patients with poorly controlled diabetes mellitus, severe hypothyroidism or the nephrotic syndrome.

The commonest primary cause is familial combined hyperlipidaemia with elevated plasma LDL and VLDL concentrations (p.**234**).

Less commonly, mixed hyperlipidaemia may be caused by the accumulation of IDL and chylomicron remnants, which contain both cholesterol and triglyceride. The patients are homozygous for an uncommon apoE phenotype or variant. The variant does not in itself produce hyperlipidaemia but, if there is another cause for primary or secondary hyperlipidaemia the impaired recognition of the apoE variant by hepatic receptors leads to the accumulation of IDL and chylomicron remnants in plasma (Type III (broad-β) hyperlipidaemia, or dysbetalipoproteinaemia). These patients may present with:

- corneal arcus and xanthelasma;
- tuberous xanthomata on the knees and elbows;
- lipid deposition in the palmar creases;
- a high incidence of vascular disease also involving the peripheral vessels.

Rare Disorders Associated with Lipid Metabolism

A few very rare disorders, which are associated with reduced plasma lipid concentrations but with the accumulation of lipid in tissues, will be discussed.

Inherited disorders of HDL deficiency, associated with premature coronary heart disease, have been described. In *Tangier disease* an abnormal apoA leads to an increased rate of catabolism of HDL. Plasma concentrations are low and cholesterol esters accumulate in the reticuloendothelial system. Characteristically, patients have large yellow tonsils and enlargement of the liver and lymph nodes.

ApoB deficiency (abetalipoproteinaemia; LDL deficiency) results in impaired synthesis of chylomicrons and VLDL, and therefore of LDL. Consequently, lipids cannot be transported from the intestine or liver. The clinical syndrome consists of steatorrhoea, progressive ataxia, retinitis pigmentosa and acanthocytosis ('thorny' red cells).

LCAT deficiency. LCAT is the enzyme needed to catalyse the esterification of free cholesterol (p.**231**) and deficiency results in accumulation of free, mostly unesterified, cholesterol in tissues. This causes premature atherosclerosis, corneal opacities, renal damage and haemolytic anaemia, possibly due to a cell-membrane defect.

*P*RINCIPLES OF TREATMENT OF HYPERLIPIDAEMIA

The decision as to whether to treat a patient with hyperlipidaemia must be based on clinical considerations as well as plasma lipids concentrations. Some forms of treatment carry risks that must be weighed against possible benefits.

General Measures

Secondary causes of hyperlipidaemia and aggravating factors, such as obesity and excessive alcohol consumption (Table 11.6, p.**235**) should be sought and treated.

Whatever the cause of hyperlipidaemia the diet should be regulated and obese patients encouraged to reduce body weight to that appropriate for height. The type of diet indicated depends on the nature of the abnormality but in general it should be low in saturated fats and cholesterol.

HYPERCHOLESTEROLAEMIA

The risk of developing ischaemic heart disease is related to the plasma LDL-cholesterol concentration and lowering the plasma cholesterol concentration reduces that risk. The vigour with which hypercholesterolaemia is treated depends on the clinical circumstances. It is important to understand the nature of the lipid disorder to ensure rational therapy.

Restriction of dietary animal fats, eggs and dairy products reduces the intake of both cholesterol and saturated fatty acids. The proportion of dietary fat as mono- and polyunsaturated triglycerides should be increased (Table 11.1, p.**225**). These dietary measures are not always completely successful in lowering plasma cholesterol concentrations because endogenous cholesterol synthesis may be stimulated by falling plasma concentrations.

Drug treatment includes:

- *bile-salt sequestrants*, such as cholestyramine and colestipol. These are resins that bind bile salts in the intestinal lumen and so prevent their reabsorption and reutilization. Removal of bile acids stimulates hepatic synthesis of cholesterol. A larger amount than normal is used in this process and, despite compensatory stimulation of its synthesis, hepatic cell content is decreased. The consequent increase of hepatic LDL receptors leads to a fall in plasma LDL concentrations (p.**229**). Some patients cannot tolerate bile-salt sequestrants because they may cause constipation or other gastrointestinal symptoms;
- *HMGCoA reductase inhibitors* (Simvastatin or Lovastatin) inhibit the rate-limiting enzyme in the cholesterol synthetic pathway and so reduce endogenous production (p.**230**). As the intracellular concentration of cholesterol falls the rate of synthesis of LDL receptors increases, with a consequent fall in plasma LDL-cholesterol concentration. These drugs are well tolerated; a very few patients develop myositis, particularily if they are also taking fibrates (see below), erythromycin or cyclosporin A. The combination of these inhibitors with bile-salt sequestrants is the most effective treatment available for heterozygous familial hypercholesterolaemia;

- *nicotinic acid* may reduce VLDL secretion and therefore the formation of LDL, but sometimes causes uncomfortable side-effects such as flushing. It also reduces the plasma level of $Lp_{(a)}$.

HYPERTRIGLYCERIDAEMIA

Dietary restriction may be the only treatment needed for hypertriglyceridaemia:

- triglyceride restriction may be effective in lowering plasma chylomicron concentrations;
- carbohydrate restriction reduces endogenous triglyceride synthesis and can be used to treat high VLDL concentrations.

Fibric acid derivitives (gemfibrozil, bezafibrate and fenofibrate) are a group of drugs that activate lipoprotein lipase, and so increase the rates of clearance of VLDL and chylomicrons from the plasma. They also lower LDL-cholesterol by enhancing liver uptake and increase HDL-cholesterol. They are used to treat familial dysbetalipoproteinaemia when dietary measures are ineffective and may also be used in patients with endogenous VLDL-hypertriglyceridaemia if clinically indicated. They may be used with nicotinic acid to lower high VLDL concentrations in combined hyperlipidaemia.

Clofibrate, another fibric acid drug, is rarely used now because it is known to increase the incidence of gall stones. Other side-effects of the fibrates include muscle cramps and rarely, impotence. They potentiate the action of warfarin and should not be given with HMGCoA reductase inhibitors. Plasma alkaline phosphatase and gamma glutamyltransferase activities fall in patients taking these drugs; their measurement may be used to monitor drug compliance. Fenofibrate specifically lowers plasma urate concentrations.

As always, the risks of treatment must be weighed against its possible benefits.

Summary

1. The main plasma lipids are cholesterol, triglycerides, phospholipids and free fatty acids. Of these cholesterol and triglycerides are the most commonly measured.

2. Lipids are transported in plasma incorporated in lipoproteins

   - Exogenous (dietary) lipid is carried in chylomicrons.
   - Endogenous lipid from the liver is carried incorporated in very low density lipoprotein (VLDL), which is metabolized to low density lipoprotein (LDL).
   - High density lipoprotein (HDL) is important for removal of cholesterol from cells.

3. Lipoproteins are modified by enzymes and their remnants are taken up by receptors on cells, mainly in the liver. The metabolism of lipoproteins is controlled by protein components, the apolipoproteins.

4. Plasma LDL concentrations are regulated mainly by hepatic LDL receptor concentrations. The higher the plasma LDL concentration the greater the risk of ischaemic heart disease.

5. Hyperlipidaemia may be primary or secondary to other diseases. The nature of the lipoprotein abnormality can usually be inferred from the plasma cholesterol and triglyceride concentrations. In primary hyperlipidaemia it may be necessary to define the lipoprotein abnormality more fully for the purpose of treatment.

6. Different genetic defects may produce similar lipoprotein abnormalities. Extensive family studies are required to differentiate them. This is rarely practicable, because of the difficulty of tracing family members.

7. Initially hyperlipidaemia should be treated by dietary control. If necessary, drugs may be added.

*I*NVESTIGATION OF LIPID DISORDERS

PLASMA SAMPLING

Plasma lipid concentrations and lipoprotein patterns are labile and affected by eating, smoking, alcohol intake, stress and changes in posture. *It is essential that the samples are taken under standard conditions.* The following points are important.

1. Although plasma cholesterol concentrations are not significantly affected after a fatty meal, plasma triglyceride concentrations are. Therefore, specimens for analysis of both should be taken after the patient has fasted for 12 hours.

   Lipid infusion is a common cause of grossly lipaemic plasma taken from hospital patients. No lipid should be infused for several hours before blood is taken for any such investigation (p.**264**).
2. The patient should be taking a 'normal' diet and his weight should have remained constant for about two weeks before the tests.
3. Unless treatment is being monitored, the patient must not be on any drugs designed to lower plasma lipid concentrations.
4. Lipoprotein concentrations, like those of all large particles, are affected by venous stasis and posture (p.**424** and p.**423**). The plasma cholesterol concentration may be up to 10 per cent higher in the upright than the recumbent position and that of triglyceride may change slightly more than this. A standardized collection procedure is important if serial estimations to assess the effect of treatment are used.
5. Stress may affect plasma lipid concentrations and investigation of hyperlipidaemia should be deferred for three months after a myocardial infarct, a major operation, or any serious illness. However, samples taken within 12 hours of a myocardial infarct seem to reflect 'true' values.

6. The blood sample should not be heparinized and plasma or serum must be separated from cells as soon as possible.

Investigation of Suspected Hyperlipidaemia

There should be a logical progression in the evaluation of a patient suspected of having an abnormality of plasma lipids.

INDICATIONS FOR MEASURING PLASMA LIPIDS

Hyperlipidaemia may be diagnosed because of the lipaemic appearance of the plasma, or for clinical reasons. Plasma total cholesterol and fasting triglyceride concentrations should be measured if there:

- is a clinical indication:
  evidence of arterial disease in a relatively young individual;
  corneal arcus in a patient under about 40;
  xanthelasma or tendinous xanthomata.
- is a family history of arterial disease;
- are risk factors for coronary artery disease such as:
  diabetes mellitus;
  hypertension.

If the plasma total-cholesterol concentration is greater than 6.5 mmol/L (275 mg/dl), or if there are other risk factors for coronary artery disease, measure the plasma HDL-cholesterol concentration. The probable LDL-cholesterol concentration can then be calculated, providing the concentration of cholesterol in VLDL is not too high, that is if the plasma triglyceride concentration is less than about 5.0 mmol/L. The plasma total-cholesterol concentration may be increased because the plasma HDL-cholesterol concentration is increased, not because the plasma LDL-cholesterol is raised.

IS THE CAUSE PRIMARY OR SECONDARY?

Many cases of hyperlipidaemia are secondary to other factors; these secondary causes should be identified and treated before life-long lipid-lowering treatment is prescribed. Common secondary causes (shown in Table 11.6) include:

- *a high fat diet*. The patient should receive dietary advice and should take a diet low in saturated fats and cholesterol for at least three months before the plasma lipid concentrations are measured again;
- *diabetes mellitus*; measure random or fasting plasma glucose concentrations;
- *hypothyroidism*; measure plasma TSH and T_4 concentrations;
- *excessive alcohol intake*; this is a common cause of secondary hypertriglyceridaemia. If this is suspected but denied by the patient measure a random blood alcohol concentration and plasma transaminase and gamma glutamyltransferase (GGT) activities. A raised plasma GGT activity is compatible with excessive alcohol intake, especially if plasma transaminase activities are normal; however, *other causes of raised plasma enzyme activities must be excluded* (p.**308**).

WHAT IS THE NATURE OF THE ABNORMALITY?

If no secondary cause is found and hyper-lipidaemia persists after a three month dietary trial, the hyperlipidaemia should be considered to be a primary abnormality. Selection of appropriate treatment some-times depends on the accurate definition of the basic lipoprotein disturbance. Simple but valuable information may be obtained by

visual inspection of the plasma. If the plasma sample is left standing for 18 hours at 4°C the large, low-density chylomicrons form a creamy layer on the surface. The smaller, denser VLDL particles do not rise and the sample remains diffusely turbid. If hyperlipidaemia is gross the distribution may be less easy to distinguish. On the basis of inspection and the results of simple biochemical tests three main groups can be identified:

- *a predominant increase in plasma LDL-cholesterol concentrations* associated with *clear plasma* possibly due to:
    familial hypercholesterolaemia;
    polygenic hypercholesterolaemia;
    familial combined hyperlipidaemia.
- *a predominant increase in plasma triglyc-eride concentrations* associated with *turbid or even milky plasma* caused by the presence of large lipoproteins, which scatter light. It may be due to:
    familial combined hyperlipidaemia (VLDL);
    familial endogenous hypertriglyceri-daemia (VLDL);
    familial hyperchylomicronaemia.

It is important to determine whether VLDL or chylomicrons are causing the turbidity as the treatment of these conditions differs.

- *an increase in both plasma cholesterol and triglyceride concentrations* in the same proportion, may be due to:
    familial combined hyperlipidaemia (LDL and VLDL);
    familial dysbetalipoproteinaemia (IDL).

In such cases lipoprotein electrophoresis or ultracentrifugation and the identification of the plasma apoE phenotype often help to distinguish the relative contributions from LDL, IDL and VLDL.

FAMILY STUDIES

These are necessary both to identify the disorder and to detect other affected, possibly asymptomatic, individuals.

TREATMENT

The treatment of hyperlipidaemia has been outlined briefly on p.**236**. It is often necessary for life. Initially the patient should be reviewed at regular intervals to ensure that he or she is complying with the diet and drug treatment. Fasting plasma lipids should remain within acceptable limits; this may require adjusting treatment after counselling the patient and identifying any necessary changes in lifestyle.

Intestinal Absorption: Gastric and Pancreatic Function

12

The most important functions of the gastrointestinal tract are the digestion and absorption of nutrients. It also synthesizes some hormones from cells distributed along the tract that act locally (paracrine hormones), so controlling gut motility and the release of digestive enzymes and secretions.

Digestion and absorption depend on food and the products of its digestion being diluted with a large volume of fluid, mostly an ultrafiltrate of extracellular fluid filtered through the 'tight junctions' between epithelial cells, mainly of the duodenum. As in the kidney, energy is expended in reclaiming the bulk of filtered water and electrolytes. Some is reabsorbed in the proximal jejunum, along the osmotic gradient created by reabsorption of the products of digestion; a large amount remains in the lumen to be reclaimed more distally.

A small amount of nutrient from desquamated intestinal cells also enters the lumen; most is reabsorbed, but, for example, almost all the fat in normal faeces is of endogenous origin. This is important when interpreting the results of a faecal fat estimation.

A much smaller volume of fluid enters the lumen by active secretion. As a result the pH and the electrolyte and enzyme concentrations change during passage of fluid through the tract in such a way that conditions for enzyme activity are near optimal for digestion. Adjustment of pH and electrolyte concentrations occurs in the distal ileum and colon (Fig. 4.5, p.**89**); sodium reabsorption, and therefore water reabsorption, is enhanced by aldosterone in the colon. Consequently, the extracellular fluid changes, which would be produced by intestinal secretion, are corrected under physiological conditions.

Disturbances of water, electrolyte and hydrogen ion homeostasis may occur in small intestinal or colonic disease. If there is loss of fluid and electrolytes from the upper intestinal tract because of vomiting or because the function of intestinal cells is so grossly impaired that the amount of fluid and electrolytes entering the distal parts exceeds the reabsorptive capacity, similar changes may occur.

This chapter is primarily concerned with disturbance of digestion and absorption. Water, electrolyte and hydrogen ion disturbances may be marked in diarrhoea but are relatively unimportant in malabsorption syndromes unless gross malabsorption causes severe intestinal hurry.

NORMAL DIGESTION AND CONVERSION OF NUTRIENTS TO ABSORBABLE FORMS

Complex molecules such as protein, polysaccharides and fat are usually acted on by digestive enzymes. This process starts in the mouth where food is mechanically broken down by chewing and is mixed with saliva containing *α-amylase*. In the stomach, acid fluid is added and the low pH initiates protein digestion by pepsin. The stomach also secretes *intrinsic factor*, essential for vitamin B_{12} absorption from the terminal ileum. However, most diges-tion takes place in the duodenum and upper jejunum, where alkaline fluid is added to the now liquid intestinal contents. Pancreatic enzymes digest proteins to amino acids and small peptides, polysaccharides to monosaccharides, disaccharides and oligosaccharides (consisting of a small number of monosaccharide units), and fat to monoglycerides and fatty acids. Severe generalized malabsorption due to failure of digestion is rare.

NORMAL INTESTINAL ABSORPTION

Absorption depends on:

- the integrity and large surface area of absorptive cells;
- the presence of nutrient in an absorbable form (and therefore on normal digestion);
- a normal ratio of the rate of absorption to the rate of passage of contents through the intestinal tract.

The absorptive area of the small intestine is very large. The mucosa forms macroscopically visible folds, increasing the area considerably. Microscopically, these folds are covered with villi lined with absorptive cells (enterocytes), which increase the area about eight-fold. A large number of minute projections (microvilli) cover the surface of each enterocyte, separated by microvillous spaces. These increase the absorptive area about a further 20-fold. The absorptive area is significantly reduced if the villi are flattened, as they are, for example, in gluten-sensitive enteropathy (p.**252**).

Absorption also depends on whether a molecule is:

- lipid-soluble, enabling it to diffuse across the lipid membranes of the enterocytes;
- water-soluble, so that it can be absorbed either by active transport against a physico-chemical gradient or by passive diffusion along gradients.

GUT HORMONES

The release of intestinal secretions and the control of gut motility is, in part, controlled by a series of peptide hormones produced in the mucosa of the gastrointestinal tract. Like other hormones, their release is under feedback control by either the product, or by the physiological response of the target tissue. However, unlike most other hormones, gut peptides are synthesized by cells dispersed throughout the length of the gastrointestinal tract rather than by discrete glands, although the secretory cells are often concentrated in one segment of the tract. Many of these peptides are present in other organs, particularly the brain, where they probably act as neurotransmitters.

The physiological response of some gut peptides is poorly understood whereas others have well-recognized physiological functions.

- **Gastrin** is released from the gastric secreting G-cells in the gastric antrum in response to distension and to protein. It stimulates the contraction of the stomach muscles and secretion of gastric acid. Acid inhibits gastrin release by negative feedback.
- **Cholecystokinin** stimulates contraction of the gall bladder and release of pancreatic digestive enzymes.
- **Secretin** stimulates the release of pancreatic fluid rich in bicarbonate.

Lipid Absorption

Digestion of fats. Triglycerides are the main form of dietary fat. They are esters of glycerol with three, usually different, fatty acids (Fig. 11.1, p.**224**). They are insoluble in water. Cholesterol, in the intestinal lumen, is derived from bile salts and from the diet; only about 30 per cent of the dietary cholesterol is absorbed.

Primary bile acids are synthesized in the liver from cholesterol, conjugated with the amino acids glycine or taurine in the liver, and then enter the intestinal lumen in the bile (p.**293**). In the alkaline duodenal fluid their sodium salts act as detergents, emulsifying and so facilitating the digestion and absorption of fats. Most of the bile salts are actively reabsorbed in the distal ileum. A small proportion enter the colon where they are converted by bacteria to *secondary bile salts*, some of which are absorbed (p.**293**). The absorbed bile salts are recirculated to the liver and resecreted into the bile (the '*entero-hepatic circulation*').

Some bacteria within the gut lumen contain enzymes that catalyse the deconjugation of bile salts; unconjugated bile salts emulsify fat less effectively than conjugated ones and this may contribute to fat malabsorption.

Triglycerides are emulsified by bile salts within the duodenum. They are hydrolysed by pancreatic lipase at the glycerol/fatty acid bond, primarily in positions 1 and 3 (Fig. 11.1, p.**224**). The end products are mainly 2-monoglycerides, some diglycerides and free fatty acids. Colipase, a peptide coenzyme secreted by the pancreas, is essential for lipase activity. It anchors lipase at the fat/water interface, prevents the inhibition of the enzyme by bile salts and reduces its pH optimum from about 8.5 to about 6.5; the latter is the pH in the upper intestinal lumen.

Micelle formation. Monoglycerides and free fatty acids aggregate with bile salts to form water-miscible micelles. The micelles also contain free cholesterol liberated by hydrolysis of cholesterol esters in the lumen and phospholipids, as well as fat-soluble vitamins (A, D, E and K). The diameter of the negatively charged micelles is between 100 and 1000 times smaller than that of the emulsion particles. Both their small size and their charge allow them to pass through the narrow microvillous spaces.

Lipids in the intestinal cells. Within enterocytes, triglycerides are resynthesized from monoglycerides and fatty acids, and cholesterol is re-esterified. Triglycerides, cholesterol esters and phospholipids, together with fat-soluble vitamins, combine with apolipoproteins manufactured in enterocytes to form chylomicrons (p.**247**). These are suspended in water and pass into the lymphatic circulation.

Some short- and medium-chain free fatty acids pass directly through the intestinal cells into the portal blood stream.

The absorption of *lipids and fat-soluble* vitamins depends on:

- the presence of *bile salts*;
- digestion of triglycerides by *lipase* and therefore on normal pancreatic function;
- an adequate *absorptive area of the intestinal* mucosa for chylomicron formation.

Carbohydrate Absorption

Polysaccharides, such as starch, consist either of straight chains of glucose molecules joined by 1:4 linkages, called *amylose*, or of branch chains, in which the branches are joined by 1 : 6 linkages, called *amylopectin*. Salivary and pancreatic α-amylases hydrolyse starch to 1 : 4 disaccharides such as maltose (glucose + glucose). Pancreatic amylase is quantitatively the more important. A few larger branch-chain saccharides (limit dextrans) remain undigested.

Disaccharides (maltose, sucrose (glucose + fructose) and lactose (glucose + galactose)) are hydrolysed to their constituent monosaccharides by the appropriate disaccharidases, β-galactosidases (lactase) and α-glucosidases (maltase, sucrase), located on the surface of enterocytes ('*brush border*'), especially in the proximal jejunum. Sucrase also hydrolyses the 1 : 4, and isomaltase the 1 : 6, linkages of limit dextrans.

Monosaccharides are actively absorbed in the duodenum and proximal jejunum. Glucose and galactose are probably absorbed by a common active process, whereas fructose is absorbed by a different mechanism. Carbohydrate absorption depends on:

- the presence of *amylase,* and therefore on *normal pancreatic function* (polysaccharides only);
- the presence of *disaccharidases* on the luminal membrane of intestinal cells (disaccharides);
- *normal intestinal mucosal cells* with normal active transport mechanisms (monosaccharides).

Polysaccharides can be absorbed only if all three mechanisms are functioning.

Protein Absorption

Protein in the intestinal lumen is derived from the diet, intestinal secretions and desquamated mucosal cells. Dietary protein is broken down by gastric *pepsin* and in the duodenum by *trypsin* and other proteolytic enzymes secreted in pancreatic juice; pancreatic trypsinogen is converted to active trypsin by enterokinase located on the brush border. The products of digestion are small peptides and amino acids. Many peptides are further hydrolysed by peptidases on the brush border.

Amino acids are actively absorbed in the small intestine.

Small peptides are absorbed by an active transport mechanism, independently of amino acids and, with a few exceptions, are hydrolysed intracellularly. Protein absorption depends on:

- the presence of *pancreatic proteolytic enzymes* and therefore on normal pancreatic function;
- *normal intestinal mucosa* with normal active transport mechanisms.

Vitamin B_{12} Absorption

Vitamin B_{12} can be absorbed only when it has formed a complex with *intrinsic factor*, a glycoprotein secreted by the parietal cells of the stomach. This complex is resistant to proteolytic digestion and binds to specific cell receptors in the distal ileum, from where it is absorbed. Some intestinal bacteria need vitamin B_{12} for growth and may prevent its absorption by competing for it with intestinal cells. Intestinal bacterial overgrowth is associated with intestinal strictures, diverticula and 'blind loops'. Vitamin B_{12} absorption therefore depends on normal:

- gastric secretion of *intrinsic factor*;
- intestinal *mucosa in the distal ileum*;
- intestinal *bacterial flora*.

ABSORPTION OF OTHER WATER-SOLUBLE VITAMINS

Most of the other water-soluble vitamins (C and the B group except B_{12}) are absorbed in the upper small intestine, probably by specific transport mechanisms (see Chapter 13). Clinical deficiencies of all but folate are relatively uncommon in the malabsorption syndromes, probably because absorption does not depend on that of fat. *Folate deficiency* may be caused by intestinal malabsorption, inadequate intake or increased use by intestinal bacteria.

Calcium and Magnesium Absorption

Calcium is absorbed mainly from the duodenum and upper jejunum in the free-ionized form; this is enhanced by the vitamin D metabolite, *1,25-dihydroxyvitamin D*, which influences both active transport and passive diffusion (p.**172**). Calcium absorption is impaired by the formation of insoluble salts with free fatty acids and with phosphate. Much of the faecal calcium is endogenous in origin, being derived from intestinal secretions.

Magnesium is also absorbed by an active process that may be shared with calcium.

Calcium and magnesium absorption depend on:

- a *low concentration of fatty acids and phosphate* in the intestinal lumen;
- the absorption and metabolism of *vitamin D* and therefore on normal fat absorption;
- *normal intestinal mucosal cells.*

Iron Absorption

Iron is absorbed in the duodenum and upper jejunum in the ferrous form (Fe^{2+}).

Absorption is increased by anaemia of any kind (p.**377**). Some of the iron absorbed into intestinal cells enters the plasma but some is lost into the lumen with desquamated cells.

GASTRIC FUNCTION

The main components of gastric secretion are *hydrochloric acid, pepsin and intrinsic factor*, all important for normal digestion and absorption. Loss of hydrochloric acid by vomiting, as in pyloric stenosis, may cause a metabolic alkalosis (p.**96**). Gastric secretion may be stimulated by:

- *the vagus nerve*, which, in turn, responds to stimuli from the cerebral cortex, normally resulting from the sight, smell and taste of food. Hypoglycaemia can stimulate gastric secretion and so can be used to assess the completeness of a vagotomy;
- *gastrin*, which is carried by the blood stream to the parietal cells of the stomach; its action is mediated by histamine. Gastrin secretion is inhibited, by negative feedback, by acid in the pylorus. Calcium also stimulates gastrin secretion and this may explain the relatively high incidence of peptic ulceration in patients with chronic hypercalcaemia.

Histamine only stimulates gastric secretion after binding to specific cell-surface receptors of which there are at least two types:

- those for which antihistamines compete with histamine (H_1 receptors). These are found on smooth muscle cells;
- those on which antihistamines have no effect. These H_2 *receptors are found on gastric parietal cells.*

Hypersecretion of gastric juice may cause duodenal ulceration. However, there is overlap between the amount of acid secreted in normal subjects and in those with duodenal ulceration. Estimation of gastric acidity is of very limited diagnostic value.

In the very rare Zollinger-Ellison syndrome, acid secretion is very high due to excessive gastrin production usually by a pancreatic tumour (p.**257**).

Hyposecretion of gastric juice occurs most commonly in association with pernicious anaemia, due to the formation of antibodies to the parietal cells of the gastric mucosa (p.**275**). Extensive carcinoma of the stomach and chronic gastritis may also cause gastric hyposecretion. Plasma gastrin concentrations are raised, because reduced acid secretion causes loss of negative feedback inhibition.

TESTS OF GASTRIC FUNCTION

Tests of gastric function involving measurement of acid secretion have largely been superseded by endoscopic examination of the stomach and duodenum and by histological examination of the biopsy material obtained.

Stimulation of gastric secretion, with the measurement of gastric acidity, may be used to test the completeness of section of the vagus nerve in patients who remain symptomatic after surgery for duodenal ulceration. The stimulus is stress due to insulin-induced hypoglycaemia (compare the use of insulin to stimulate cortisol secretion). If vagotomy is complete, symptomatic hypoglycaemia with a plasma glucose concentration below 2.5 mmol/L (45 mg/dl) should produce no increase in acid secretion.

TREATMENT OF HYPERSECRETION

Drugs, such as ranitidine (Zantac) and cimetidine (Tagamet) compete with histamine for the H_2 receptors, so directly reducing acid secretion. The initial clinical response is usually good but relapse may occur when treatment is stopped.

Post-gastrectomy Syndromes

There may be some degree of malabsorption after gastrectomy (p.**252**). Rapid passage of the contents of the small gastric remnant into the duodenum may be associated with:

- the '*early dumping syndrome*'. Soon after a meal the patient may experience abdominal discomfort and feel faint and nauseated. These symptoms may be caused by the rapid passage of hypertonic fluid into the duodenum. Before this abnormally large load can be absorbed, water passes along the osmotic gradient from the extracellular space into the lumen. The reduced plasma volume causes faintness and the large volume of fluid causes abdominal discomfort.

- the '*late dumping syndrome*' (or post-gastrectomy hypoglycaemia). If a meal containing a high glucose concentration passes quickly into the duodenum glucose absorption is very rapid stimulating a surge in insulin secretion. The resultant 'overswing' of plasma glucose concentration may cause hypoglycaemic symptoms, typically occurring about *two hours after a meal*. This is a form of reactive hypoglycaemia (p.**213**).

Both these disabilities can be minimized if meals low in carbohydrate are taken little and often.

PANCREATIC FUNCTION

Pancreatic secretions can be divided into endocrine and exocrine components. The endocrine function which controls the plasma glucose concentration is discussed in Chapter 10.

The exocrine secretions are made up of two components, the alkaline pancreatic fluid and the digestive enzymes. The alkaline fluid is primarily responsible for neutralizing gastric acid secretions, thus providing an optimal environment for duodenal digestive enzyme activity. These enzymes include the *proteases*, trypsin and chymotrypsin, and *amylase* and *lipase*. Some of the proteases are secreted as precursors and are converted to the active form within the intestinal lumen.

Gut peptides, released from the duodenum in response to a rise in the hydrogen ion concentration or to the presence of food, control pancreatic secretion. They include:

- *secretin* which stimulates the release of a high volume of alkaline fluid;

- *cholecystokinin* which stimulates the release of a fluid rich in enzymes.

TESTS OF EXOCRINE PANCREATIC FUNCTION

Plasma enzyme measurements are of limited value in assessing exocrine function. Such measurements include:

- *plasma trypsin concentrations*, which may be used to screen for cystic fibrosis during the first six weeks of life when full pancreatic function should be established. Blockage of pancreatic ductules by sticky mucus secretion causes high plasma trypsin concentrations. After about six weeks plasma concentrations may fall as pancreatic insufficiency develops; normal levels do not exclude the diagnosis;

- *plasma amylase activity*. This enzyme consists of two forms, of salivary gland and pancreatic origin respectively. Because the salivary isoenzyme is the principal form in plasma, total enzyme activity is not significantly lowered when the pancreatic secretory cell mass is reduced by chronic pancreatic disease. However, in acute pancreatitis total plasma amylase activity is usually significantly increased due to release from damaged cells.

Duodenal enzymes. Measurement of pancreatic enzymes and the bicarbonate concentration in duodenal aspirates before and after stimulation with cholecystokinin and secretin is not very suitable for routine use because of the difficulty in positioning the duodenal tube and in quantitative sampling of the secretions.

'*Tubeless tests*' have been developed that avoid the need for intubation and that overcome the difficulties of sample collection.

- *The PABA test.* A synthetic peptide, labelled with *p*-aminobenzoic acid (PABA), is taken orally. After PABA has been split from the peptide by chymotrypsin, it is absorbed and excreted in the urine. Urinary excretion of PABA is significantly reduced in chronic pancreatitis. Abnormal results may occur if there is renal glomerular dysfunc-

tion, liver disease, or malabsorption even in the presence of normal pancreatic function. The effect of these conditions is assessed by repeating the test with unconjugated PABA, which eliminates the need for digestion before absorption. This test is rarely necessary and is only performed in special centres.

- *The pancreolauryl test.* A similar, but technically simpler, test uses fluorescein dilaurate. Fluorescein is released and absorbed and the amount excreted in a timed urine sample is measured.

Disorders of the Pancreas rarely Associated with Malabsorption

Absence of pancreatic secretions may, by impairing digestion, cause malabsorption. However, there are three relatively common pancreatic diseases that are only rarely associated with malabsorption

- **Acute pancreatitis**, due to necrosis of pancreatic cells, is associated with the release of enzymes into the retroperitoneal space and blood stream. The presence of pancreatic juice in the peritoneal cavity causes *severe abdominal pain and shock.* A vicious cycle is set up as more pancreatic cells are digested by the released enzymes. Acute pancreatitis is most commonly idiopathic but may follow obstruction of the pancreatic duct, or regurgitation of bile along this duct. Other predisposing factors include *excess alcohol ingestion and biliary tract disease.* Trauma to the pancreas, by damaging the cells, may initiate the vicious cycle. Hypercalcaemia and hypertriglyceridaemia may also precipitate acute pancreatitis.

Some causes of a raised plasma amylase are shown in Table 12.1 and discussed more fully in Chapter 15. Typically plasma amylase

Table 12.1 Some causes of a raised plasma total amylase activity

---

Marked increase
  acute pancreatitis
  perforated peptic ulcer
  diabetic ketoacidosis

Moderate increase
  acute abdominal disorders
    perforated peptic ulcer
    acute cholecystitis
    intestinal obstruction
    abdominal trauma
    ruptured ectopic pregnancy
  salivary gland disorders
    mumps
    salivary calculi
    Sjögren's syndrome
  morphine administration–spasm of sphincter
  severe glomerular dysfunction–retention of amylase
  myocardial infarction
  diabetic ketoacidosis
  macroamylasaemia (p.**305**)

activity increases about five-fold in acute pancreatitis but plasma enzyme activities of up to, and even above, this value may be reached in a number of other disorders, in particular after gastric perforation into the lesser sac. Occasionally the plasma enzyme activity in acute pancreatitis may not be very high and usually falls rapidly as the enzyme is excreted in the urine. Consequently a *high plasma amylase activity is only a rough guide to the presence of acute pancreatitis and normal or only slightly raised values do not exclude the diagnosis.*

- **Chronic pancreatic failure** is not always associated with steatorrhoea. It rarely follows a severe attack of acute pancreatitis but is more likely after repeated acute or subacute attacks. Pancreatic calcification may sometimes be seen on radiographic examination of the abdomen.
- **Carcinoma of the pancreas** is very difficult to diagnose by laboratory tests unless the lesion is in the head of the organ and causes obstructive jaundice; extensive gland destruction may cause late-onset diabetes mellitus.

Malabsorption Syndromes

Malabsorption is usually, but not always, associated with impaired fat absorption (steatorrhoea). *No biochemical test is sensitive enough for the early detection, or precise enough for the differential diagnosis, of steatorrhoea;* endoscopy and ultrasound have reduced the need for laboratory tests. However, biochemical tests are important in detecting and monitoring treatment of the metabolic effects of prolonged and severe malabsorption and include:

- *faecal fat estimation.* Steatorrhoea is defined as a daily faecal fat excretion consistently more than 18 mmol (5 g) of fat, measured as fatty acids. This is usually associated with a faecal stool weight greater than 60 g. Whatever the aetiology, unequivocal steatorrhoea can only be demonstrated when the disease is extensive and has usually already been elucidated by radiological or histopathological means. Gross steatorrhoea causes foul smelling, bulky, pale, greasy stools which are difficult to flush away in the toilet. There may be diarrhoea;
- *triolein breath test.* Absorbed fat is ultimately metabolized to CO_2 and water.

If ^{14}C-labelled triglyceride (triolein) is given by mouth the ratio of $^{14}CO_2$ to unlabelled CO_2 can be measured in expired air. A low ratio usually indicates impaired fat absorption. Various assumptions have to be made when interpreting results; the assay uses expensive isotopes and requires special expertise. Although the results correlate with faecal fat measurements, the limitations discussed have prevented its widespread adoption.

Generalized Malabsorption Associated with Steatorrhoea

Generalized malabsorption may result from either intestinal or pancreatic disease.

- In *intestinal* malabsorption *fat digestion is normal*, but absorption of the products of digestion is impaired.

- In *pancreatic* steatorrhoea the *absorptive capacity is normal* but fat cannot be digested because there is deficiency of digestive enzymes.

REDUCTION OF ABSORPTIVE AREAS OR GENERALIZED IMPAIRMENT OF TRANSPORT MECHANISMS

Villous atrophy. Malabsorption may be caused by a reduction of the absorptive area because of flattened intestinal villi, demonstrated by microscopic examination of a mucosal biopsy specimen. Causes include:

- **coeliac disease (gluten-sensitive enteropathy)** is caused by sensitivity to the protein α-gliadin, present in gluten in wheat and rye. The condition is characterized by *villous atrophy*, mainly in the proximal small intestine, which is usually reversible following gluten withdrawal from the diet. Clinical symptoms usually become evident at about one year of age with failure to thrive and diarrhoea, but may present at any age. Antibodies to α-gliadin may be detected in plasma and their measurement used to monitor compliance with a gluten free diet. Long term prognosis is good although patients diagnosed during adult life have a increased susceptibility of developing lymphomas;
- **tropical sprue** in which villous atrophy does not respond to a gluten-free diet. There may be a bacterial cause because the condition sometimes responds to broad-spectrum antibiotics. Folate should also be given;
- **'idiopathic steatorrhoea'**. This term should be reserved for those cases of steatorrhoea associated with flattened villi, which respond neither to a gluten-free diet nor to broad-spectrum antibiotics.

Extensive surgical resection of the small intestine may so reduce the absorptive area as to cause malabsorption.

Extensive infiltration or inflammation of the small intestinal wall, for example caused by Crohn's or Whipple's disease, or to small intestinal lymphoma, may impair absorption; malabsorption may be aggravated by alteration of the bacterial flora due to reduced intestinal motility.

INCREASED RATE OF TRANSIT THROUGH THE SMALL INTESTINE

Food passes through the intestine more rapidly than usual:

- *after gastrectomy*, when normal mixing of food with fluid, acid and pepsin does not occur in the stomach, resulting in impaired enzyme activity within the small intestine. An increased rate of transit through the duodenum may contribute to the malabsorption. However post-gastrectomy malabsorption is rarely severe, although iron deficiency is a relatively common complication;
- *in the carcinoid syndrome* (p.**396**), which is associated with excessive production of 5-hydroxytryptamine (5-HT; serotonin) by tumours of argentaffin cells usually arising in the small intestine, or by their metastases, usually in the liver. *This is a rare disorder*. It may occasionally present with malabsorption which is probably the result of increased intestinal motility due to the concomitant release of a gut peptide, Substance P.

IMPAIRED DIGESTIVE ENZYME ACTIVITY

Failure of digestive enzyme secretion. Pancreatic dysfunction may cause malabsorption by reducing secretion of digestive enzymes.

- **Chronic pancreatitis** may present insidiously or may remain undetected. It is commonest in alcoholics. Glucose intolerance may develop due to reduced islet cell mass. If pancreatic disease causes obstructive jaundice, as in carcinoma of the head of the pancreas, there may be mild steatorrhoea due to impairment of lipase activity because of bile salt deficiency (p.**245**). Pancreatic lipase activity can be reduced by up to 75 per cent before chemical steatorrhoea occurs.

- **Cystic fibrosis (CF)** is an autosomal, recessively inherited, disorder of chloride transport affecting exocrine glandular secretions (p.**249**). It may present in the newborn with intestinal symptoms, such as meconium ileus, (failure to pass the first faeces containing bile, intestinal debris and mucus), or in early childhood with recurrent respiratory infections; it may however not be diagnosed until the patient is an adult. Thick, viscous pancreatic and bronchial secretions may cause malabsorption and chronic lung disease respectively. Cirrhosis of the liver may develop. The diagnosis is made clinically and by measuring the pilocarpine-induced sweat electrolyte concentrations; the chloride and sodium concentrations are about twice normal. The detection of albumin in meconium or a raised plasma trypsin concentration during the first six weeks of life may be used to screen for the disorder.

Over 200 different mutations have been identified, the commonest having a prevalence of about 70 per cent. Prenatal diagnosis is available in some countries using chorionic villus sampling at eight to 10 weeks, but is only offered if the gene defect has already been established within the family, usually following the identification of an affected child. There is no correlation between the gene mutation and the clinical course of the disorder.

Inactivation of pancreatic enzymes by acid. The increased intestinal hydrogen ion

activity in the Zollinger-Ellison syndrome (p.**257**) may inactivate pancreatic lipase and cause precipitation of bile salts within the gut lumen, so resulting in malabsorption.

PROTOZOAL INFESTATION (GIARDIASIS).

Giardia lamblia, contracted following the ingestion of contaminated water, may cause acute diarrhoea or malabsorption following more chronic infestation. Diagnosis may be made by histological examination of the intestinal mucosa in which the organism may be demonstrated. Villous atrophy may be seen.

Differential Diagnosis of Generalized Intestinal and Pancreatic Malabsorption (Table 12.2)

The diagnosis of malabsorption is usually made by clinical, haematological, histological and radiological means, and supplemented by biochemical tests. Malabsorption of fat occurs both in generalized intestinal and in pancreatic disease.

Anaemia is rarer in pancreatic than in intestinal malabsorption since iron, vitamin B_{12} and folate do not depend on pancreatic enzymes for absorption. The blood and bone-marrow films typically show a mixed iron deficiency and megaloblastic picture

Table 12.2 Differential diagnosis and investigation of causes of steatorrhoea

	Upper small intestinal disease	**Pancreatic disease**	**'Contaminated bowel' syndrome**
Anaemia	Dimorphic picture (mixed megaloblastic and iron deficiency common)	Rare	Megaloblastic common
Intestinal biopsy	Flattened villi or other cause	Normal	Normal
Xylose absorption	Reduced	Normal	Usually normal

(p.**275**). Anaemia may be aggravated by protein deficiency.

Differences in carbohydrate metabolism. Polysaccharide absorption is impaired in both conditions but hypoglycaemia is rare. In pancreatic malabsorption, in which neither disaccharidase activity nor active monosaccharide absorption is affected, both monosaccharides and disaccharides can be absorbed. Hyperglycaemia suggests that pancreatic disease is the cause of malabsorption, but *it is by no means diagnostic of it.*

Xylose absorption test. Xylose is a pentose that, like glucose, can be absorbed without digestion, but the metabolism of which is not controlled by hormones; therefore unlike glucose it is not affected by insulin secretion. An oral dose of xylose is absorbed by normally functioning upper small intestinal cells. Metabolism of the absorbed pentose is very slow and, because it is freely filtered by the glomeruli, most of it appears in the urine. In the xylose absorption test either the amount excreted in the urine during a fixed period, or, in children, the plasma concentration at a defined time after the dose, is measured.

- Intestinal disease impairs xylose absorption and therefore reduces excretion.
- Pancreatic disease does not affect either.

Unfortunately, there are several sources of imprecision in the test (p.**260**).

- Xylose is absorbed mostly from the upper small intestine and absorption may therefore be normal despite significant ileal dysfunction, for example in Crohn's disease.
- The urine test depends on accurate collections over a short time interval and therefore even more significant errors may occur than in 24-hour collections (p.**427**).
- Mildly impaired renal function decreases glomerular filtration of xylose and may give falsely low results in the urine tests, or a falsely high plasma concentration. This is a common cause of misleading results in the elderly. *The xylose absorption test should not be performed if glomerular function is even only marginally impaired.*

- Both plasma concentrations and urine excretion depend partly on the volume of distribution of the absorbed xylose. In oedematous or very obese patients results may be falsely low.

Failure of Absorption of Specific Substances

Altered intestinal bacterial flora may cause malabsorption of vitamin B_{12} and fat. Such conditions include:

- *contaminated bowel ('blind loop') syndrome*, which is caused by bacterial proliferation due to impaired intestinal motility and stagnation of intestinal contents. It occurs when the 'blind loops' are the result of surgery or in the presence of small intestinal diverticula. Some bacteria may cause malabsorption by catalysing the deconjugation of bile salts (p.**246**). Since more vitamin B_{12} and folate may be used by the bacteria *megaloblastic anaemia* is common;
- *treatment with broad-spectrum antibiotics* may, by altering the small intestinal bacterial flora, cause a similar syndrome.

Abnormal bacterial growth may sometimes be diagnosed by:

- *culture of organisms* from a specimen collected into a special anaerobic microbiological medium after intubation of the upper small intestine. The test is only useful if intubation is performed by an expert;
- *the ^{14}C-glycocholate breath test.* ^{14}C-glycocholate is taken orally. The intestinal bacteria split the cholate from the labelled glycine; the latter is absorbed and metabolized; $^{14}CO_2$ is measured in the expired air. False positive results may occur in patients with disorders of the terminal ileum.

Biliary obstruction causes malabsorption of fat and of fat-soluble substances by preventing the secretion of bile salts into the intestinal lumen; steatorrhoea results. The diagnosis is usually clinically obvious due to the presence of jaundice. Retention of bile salts, such as may occur in primary biliary cirrhosis, may cause intense skin irritation.

Local diseases or surgery of the small intestine may cause selective malabsorption of substances absorbed predominantly at those sites. Diseases involving the terminal ileum, such as Crohn's disease or tuberculosis, may impair absorption of bile salts and vitamin B_{12}. Vitamin B_{12} absorption may also be impaired because of intrinsic factor deficiency caused either by damage to gastric parietal cells in pernicious anaemia, or to total gastrectomy or extensive malignant infiltration of the stomach. Malabsorption of vitamin B_{12} may be demonstrated using the Schilling test (p.**261**).

Disaccharidase deficiency may occur in generalized disorders of the intestinal wall because the enzymes are localized on the brush border of the enterocyte. This deficiency is relatively unimportant compared with that due to general malabsorption. Tests for these syndromes are therefore useful only in the absence of steatorrhoea, when selective rather than generalized malabsorption of carbohydrate may be present.

The symptoms of disaccharidase deficiency are due to the effects of unabsorbed, osmotically active sugars in the intestinal lumen. They include *faintness, abdominal discomfort* and *severe diarrhoea* after ingestion of the offending disaccharide (compare with the 'dumping syndrome'; p.**249**). Diarrhoea may be severe enough to cause volume depletion in infants. Stools are typically acid because bacteria metabolize sugars to acids. Unabsorbed sugars may be detectable in the faeces and some disaccharides, which may be absorbed intact, may be detectable in the urine.

Lactase deficiency may be caused by several disorders.

- *Acquired lactase deficiency* is commoner than the congenital form and is probably the commonest type of disaccharidase deficiency. It may not present until child-

hood, or even adult life, possibly in genetically predisposed individuals. It may also present in association with other intestinal disorders, such as coeliac disease and inflammatory bowel disease.

- *Lactase deficiency associated with prematurity* may resemble the congenital form. However, the sensitivity to milk usually disappears when lactase is synthesized within a few days of birth.
- *Congenital lactase deficiency* is very rare. Infants present with severe diarrhoea or colicky abdominal pain, soon after the introduction of milk feeds. The syndrome is treated by removing milk and milk products from the diet.

Sucrase and isomaltase deficiency usually coexist.

- *Congenital sucrase-isomaltase deficiency* is more common than congenital lactase deficiency.
- *Acquired sucrase-isomaltase deficiency and maltase deficiency* of any kind are very rare.

The diagnosis of disaccharidase deficiency may be confirmed by:

- estimating the relevant enzymes in intestinal biopsy tissue. This is the most reliable test and no others may be needed;
- measuring the plasma glucose concentration, as in the glucose tolerance test, after giving an oral load of the particular disaccharide. If the disaccharide cannot be hydrolysed the constituent monosaccharides cannot be absorbed and the concentrations of plasma glucose rise very little. The result should be compared with that of a glucose tolerance test (p.**218**). If this is also flat the abnormal response to disaccharides is not diagnostic. If the patient experiences typical symptoms, or if disaccharides are excreted in the urine when the offending sugar is given, the comparison need not be made.

Radiological examination may help to make the diagnosis of disaccharidase deficiency. Barium is administered first without, and then with, the disaccharide. The osmotic effect of the unabsorbed sugar causes flocculation of the barium.

Protein-losing enteropathy. In many cases of malabsorption protein is lost through the gut due to failure to digest and absorb that entering it in intestinal secretions and by cell desquamation. *Isolated protein-losing entero-pathy is a very rare syndrome* in which absorption is normal, but the intestinal wall is abnormally permeable to large molecules, a condition similar to that of the glomeruli in the nephrotic syndrome. It occurs in a variety of conditions in which there is ulceration of the bowel or abnormal lymphatic drainage. The clinical picture, like that of the nephrotic syndrome (p.**331**), is due to hypoalbuminaemia.

If there is no evidence of generalized malabsorption and the disorder is suspected, the diagnosis can be made after the intravenous administration of a radiolabelled protein such as albumin or transferrin by measuring its recovery in a timed stool collection. Alternatively, the concentration of α_1-antitrypsin, a protein resistant to proteolytic degradation, can be measured in a known weight of faeces; false positive results may be caused by gastrointestinal bleeding. Typically the serum protein electrophoretic pattern is similar to that found in the nephrotic syndrome (p.**332**); the relatively high molecular weight components of the α_2-fraction are retained and all other fractions are reduced.

Metabolic Consequences of Malabsorption

The following findings may occur after very prolonged disease but are not necessary for the diagnosis of malabsorption.

Fat-soluble vitamin deficiency (p.**268**) may be a consequence of impaired fat absorption due to steatorrhoea.

- *Vitamin D deficiency* causes impaired calcium absorption and sometimes leads to rickets or osteomalacia. The low plasma free-ionized calcium concentration stimulates parathyroid hormone secretion causing secondary hyperparathyroidism (p.**181**).
- *Vitamin K* is needed for hepatic synthesis of prothrombin and other clotting factors. A bleeding tendency, associated with a prolonged prothrombin time, may develop. This prothrombin deficiency, unlike that due to liver disease, can be reversed by parenteral administration of vitamin K.
- *Vitamin A deficiency* is rarely evident clinically, although malabsorption of an oral dose of vitamin A can sometimes be demonstrated.

Amino acid and peptide malabsorption occur in intestinal disease, due to impaired intestinal transport mechanisms; in pancreatic disease the digestion of protein is severely impaired. In either case prolonged disease may cause:

- generalized muscle and tissue wasting and osteoporosis (p.**184**);
- reduced concentration of all plasma proteins. The low plasma albumin concentration may cause *oedema* and reduced antibody formation (immunoglobulins) may predispose to *infection*.

Anaemia is rarer in pancreatic than in intestinal malabsorption; iron, vitamin B_{12} and folate do not depend on pancreatic enzymes for absorption. The blood and bone-marrow films typically show a mixed iron deficiency and megaloblastic picture. Anaemia may be aggravated by protein deficiency.

The presenting clinical features in *severe and long-standing generalized malabsorption*, whether intestinal or pancreatic, may include:

- bulky, fatty stools, with or without diarrhoea;
- generalized wasting and malnutrition (protein deficiency);
- osteoporosis and osteomalacia (protein and calcium deficiency);
- oedema (hypoalbuminaemia due to protein deficiency);
- tetany (hypocalcaemia due to vitamin D and calcium deficiency);

- recurrent infections (immunoglobulin deficiency).

Tumours of the Enteropancreatic System Secreting Gut Hormones

These tumours are very rare. They are usually found in the pancreatic islets and cause well-recognized clinical and pathological syndromes. Because of their rarity no attempt has been made to describe them all.

Gastrinomas, usually in the pancreatic islets, secrete large quantities of gastrin despite high gastric hydrogen ion levels and may cause the *Zollinger-Ellison syndrome*. About 60 per cent of gastrinomas are malignant. Of the remaining 40 per cent only about a third (13 per cent of the total) are single, resectable adenomas, the rest being multiple. The very high rate of gastric acid secretion causes ulceration in the stomach and proximal small intestine with severe diarrhoea; inhibition of pancreatic lipase activity by the low pH may cause steatorrhoea. This syndrome may be associated with benign, and usually non-functioning, adenomas elsewhere, for example, in the anterior pituitary, parathyroid, and thyroid glands and in the adrenal cortex (multiple endocrine neoplasia, p.**397**).

- Fasting plasma gastrin concentrations are up to 30 times the upper reference limit in the *Zollinger-Ellison syndrome*.
- High plasma gastrin concentrations may also be caused by *hypochlorhydria* and this condition must be excluded before making a diagnosis, based on the results of a plasma gastrin concentration alone.

Glucagonomas usually arise from the α-cells of the pancreatic islets. The presenting clinical feature is a *bullous rash*, known as *necrolytic migratory erythema*, often accompanied by psychiatric disturbances, thromboembolism, glossitis, weight loss, impaired glucose tolerance, anaemia and a raised erythrocyte sedimentation rate. High plasma glucagon concentrations could explain the impaired glucose tolerance, but the cause of the other features, all of which are cured by resection of the tumour, is not clear. Diagnosis can be made by finding a very high plasma glucagon concentration.

VIPomas are *extremely rare tumours*, usually of the pancreatic islet cells, secreting large amounts of vasoactive intestinal peptide (VIP), a hormone that increases intestinal motility. They cause a syndrome in which there is *very profuse, watery diarrhoea*, the Verner-Morrison or WDHA (Watery Diarrhoea, Hypokalaemia and Achlorhydria) syndrome.

Summary

Normal Intestinal Absorption

1. Normal intestinal absorption depends on adequate digestion of food and therefore on normal pancreatic function, and on a normal area of functioning cells.
2. Normal digestion and absorption of fat depends on the presence of bile salts as well as of lipase.
3. Absorption of cholesterol, phospholipids and fat-soluble vitamins depends on normal triglyceride absorption.

Gastric Function

1. Hypersecretion of acid is associated with duodenal ulceration and the Zollinger-Ellison syndrome.
2. Hyposecretion of acid is associated with pernicious anaemia and extensive gastric infiltration.
3. The vagal stimulation of gastric secretion can be tested by inducing hypoglycaemia with insulin.

Pancreatic Function

1. Acute pancreatitis is associated with a short-lived rise in plasma amylase activity. This enzyme may also be raised in many acute abdominal disorders and in renal glomerular failure. The assay of total amylase activity is useless for detecting chronic pancreatic disease.

Malabsorption Syndromes

1. In intestinal malabsorption there is malabsorption of small molecules, usually due to a reduced absorptive area.
2. In pancreatic malabsorption there is malabsorption of fats, proteins and polysaccharides, but small molecules are usually absorbed normally.

3. An abnormal small intestinal bacterial flora may cause steatorrhoea because of deconjugation of bile salts, and megaloblastic anaemia because of bacterial competition for vitamin B_{12} and folate.
4. There may be steatorrhoea in biliary obstruction, because of lack of bile salts in the intestinal lumen.
5. Selective malabsorption of vitamin B_{12} occurs in pernicious anaemia due to deficiency of intrinsic factor.
6. Selective disaccharidase deficiency causes malabsorption of disaccharides. These deficiencies are more commonly acquired than congenital in origin.

Peptide-secreting Tumours of the Enteropancreatic System

1. All these tumours are very rare.
2. Gastrinomas cause the Zollinger-Ellison syndrome. Gastric hyperacidity causes peptic ulceration, diarrhoea and sometimes steatorrhoea.
3. Glucagonomas are associated with necrolytic migratory erythema and nonspecific symptoms and signs.
4. VIPomas (tumours secreting vasoactive intestinal peptide) may cause the Verner-Morrison syndrome – very severe watery diarrhoea which often causes hypokalaemia (WDHA).

*I*NVESTIGATION OF SUSPECTED MALABSORPTION

This proposed scheme for the investigation of suspected malabsorption discusses only laboratory tests. These tests are relatively insensitive and often unsatisfactory and have largely been replaced by other non-chemical tests.

Malabsorption may be suspected if the patient presents with:

- a history of chronic diarrhoea of unknown origin;
- a history of weight loss;
- clinical, radiological, haematological and/or biochemical findings suggestive of malnutrition with no obvious cause.

1. Has the patient a history which may suggest alteration in the intestinal bacterial flora?

   - Has he been on long-term broad-spectrum antibiotics?
   - Has he had gastrointestinal surgery, which may have resulted in 'blind loops'?
   - Has he travelled in the tropics or possibly drunk contaminated water? If so, consider the possibility of tropical sprue.

2. What is the appearance of the stool?

   - Bulky, pale, greasy stools suggest steatorrhoea.
   - Constipation with hard dry stools makes the diagnosis of malabsorption highly improbable.
   - Watery stools, especially if blood-stained, suggest colonic disease such as ulcerative colitis. The possibility of purgative abuse must always be considered.

3. Plasma electrolyte abnormalities, especially severe hypokalaemia, and signs of extracellular volume depletion without obvious evidence of malnutrition, favour colonic disease as a cause of diarrhoea rather than a small intestinal malabsorption syndrome.

4. Anaemia is more likely to be due to intestinal than to pancreatic disease:

   - a hypochromic, microcytic picture may be the result of blood loss at any level of the gastrointestinal tract;
   - a normochromic, normocytic picture is a nonspecific finding in any chronic disease;
   - *a dimorphic (mixed iron deficiency and macrocytic) picture is very suggestive of intestinal malabsorption*;
   - low red cell folate and/or plasma vitamin B_{12} concentrations suggest intestinal malabsorption.

5. If any or all of the above investigations suggest steatorrhoea a cause should be sought. The most definitive tests are:

   - endoscopy, with histological examination of an intestinal biopsy specimen. Flattened villi suggest:
     gluten-sensitive enteropathy;
     idiopathic steatorrhoea;
     tropical sprue.
   - *Giardia lamblia* may be detected microscopically.
   - radiological examination, which may detect infiltration of the mucosa.

6. If doubt remains faecal fat estimation *may* help. However, because of the difficulty of obtaining an accurately timed faecal collection, only very high results are of unequivocal significance; in such cases steatorrhoea will probably be obvious visually. For this reason many hospital laboratories no longer perform this test.

7. If steatorrhoea is obvious on clinical grounds and after visual inspection of the stool, and if the intestinal histological picture is normal, the most likely possibilities are:

- localized intestinal disease, such as Crohn's disease;
- contaminated small bowel (blind loop) syndrome;
- pancreatic disease. This is a rare cause of malabsorption unless there has been a history of recurrent attacks of acute pancreatitis.

Tests such as abdominal ultrasound or CT scanning may help, especially if pancreatic carcinoma is suspected.

8. The xylose absorption test is rarely helpful. If it is unequivocally normal an upper intestinal lesion is unlikely. Such a result does not, however, exclude ileal or pancreatic disease, contaminated bowel syndrome, or even some cases of gluten-sensitive enteropathy.
9. A pancreolauryl test may help confirm the presence of pancreatic insufficiency (p.**250**).
10. If malabsorption is proven, and if there is laboratory evidence of malnutrition, blood haemoglobin and plasma calcium, phosphate and albumin concentrations and alkaline phosphatase activity should be monitored to assess the efficacy of treatment.

FAECAL FAT ESTIMATION

Faecal fat excretion should represent the difference between the fat absorbed and that entering the gastrointestinal tract from the diet and from the body (p.**244**). Absorption of fat, and more importantly the addition of fat to the intestinal contents, occurs throughout the small intestine. A single 24-hour collection of faeces gives very inaccurate results for two reasons.

- the transit time from the duodenum to the rectum is variable;
- rectal emptying is variable and may not be complete.

Consecutive 24-hour collections give faecal fat results that may vary by several hundred per cent. The longer the period of collection the more accurate the calculated daily mean result; it is desirable to collect stools for a minimum of three days but preferably five. The precision may be increased by collecting between 'markers', usually dyes or radiopaque pellets taken orally. The dye can be detected by visual inspection and the pellets by radiological visualization of the stools.

Procedure: This protocol is for a five-day collection using carmine markers.

Day 0. The first 'marker' (usually four capsules of carmine) is given. *As soon as this marker appears in the stool the collection is started*. This marker will gradually disappear in subsequent stools.

Day 5 after the first marker. The second marker is given. *As soon as this marker appears in the stool the collection is stopped*.

Fat is estimated in all the specimens passed between the appearance of the two markers, including only one of the marked stools.

It is very important that all stool samples be collected. The patient must use only bedpans during the test period, and all samples must be appropriate labelled with the date, time and number of the specimen in the series.

Before starting the test make sure that the patient is not to be discharged, operated on (except in an emergency) and does not receive enemas or aperients; any patient needing aperients is most unlikely to have steatorrhoea at that time. Neither a barium enema nor a barium meal should be performed for a few days before or during the collection because barium interferes with the estimation.

Interpretation: A mean daily fat excretion of clearly more than 18 mmol (5 g) indicates steatorrhoea. The result is not affected by diet within very wide limits, because in the normal subject almost all the fat is of endogenous origin. However, if the patient is on a very low fat diet mild steatorrhoea may not be detected.

XYLOSE ABSORPTION TEST

The result of the xylose absorption test is invalidated if there is poor renal function and oedema in which the total body water is increased and the xylose concentration therefore diluted.

The test is imprecise because of the problems of urine collection (p.**427**).

A dose of 5 g of xylose is preferable to one of 25 g because a high xylose concentration within the intestinal lumen may, like a large dose of glucose (p.**255**), have an osmotic effect that causes symptoms and affects the results.

Procedure: The patient fasts overnight.

08.00 hours. The bladder is emptied and the specimen discarded. *5 g of xylose dissolved in 200 ml of water is given orally.* All specimens passed between 08.00 hours and 10.00 hours are put into a bottle labelled Number 1.

10.00 hours. The bladder is emptied and the specimen *put into Bottle 1*, which is now complete. All specimens passed between 10.00 hours and 13.00 hours are put into a bottle labelled Number 2.

13.00 hours. The bladder is emptied and the specimen *put into Bottle 2*, which is now complete. Both bottles are sent to the laboratory for analysis.

Interpretation: In the normal subject more than 23 per cent of the dose (1.5 g) should be excreted during the five hours. About fifty per cent or more of the total excretion should occur during the first two hours. In mild intestinal malabsorption the total five-hour excretion may be normal, but delayed absorption is reflected in a two- to five-hour ratio of less than 40 per cent. In pancreatic malabsorption the result should be normal (p.**254**).

The considerable limitations of this test are discussed on p.**254**.

THE SCHILLING TEST

Procedure: A small dose of radiolabelled vitamin B_{12} is given orally and its excretion measured in urine. A flushing dose of non-radiolabelled vitamin is given parenterally at the same time as, or just after, the labelled dose to ensure quantitative urinary excretion. Haematological tests, such as examination of blood and bone marrow films, should have been completed before the vitamin B_{12} is given.

Interpretation: If malabsorption of the vitamin is due to pernicious anaemia, administration of the labelled vitamin with intrinsic factor restores normal absorption; if it is due to intestinal disease malabsorption persists.

LABORATORY TESTS TO IDENTIFY SOME METABOLIC COMPLICATIONS

The laboratory investigations on plasma to identify some of the metabolic complications of generalized malabsorption include:

- anaemia:
    haematological investigations;
    folate and vitamin B_{12}.
- rickets/osteomalacia (vitamin D deficiency):
    calcium with albumin, phosphate with urea;
    alkaline phosphatase activity.
- prolonged bleeding time (vitamin K deficiency):
    prothrombin time.
- infection:
    immunoglobulins.

Principles of Intravenous Feeding

The principles of carbohydrate and lipid metabolism and gastrointestinal digestion and absorption, discussed in Chapters 10, 11 and 12, all have important applications in the management of nutrition, and of intravenous (parenteral) nutrition in particular. The principles, including those of fluid and electrolyte homeostasis, must be fully understood in order to manage patients receiving parenteral nutrition.

The metabolism of carbohydrate, fat and, to a lesser extent, the carbon chains of some amino acids, supplies the energy needs of the body by coupling the breakdown of their energy-rich bonds with ATP synthesis. Some of the constituent elements, carbon, hydrogen and oxygen, leave the body as carbon dioxide and water.

Daily energy loss as heat is about 120 kJ (30 kcal) per kg body weight in a normal adult. In addition there is a daily protein turnover of about 3 g per kg body weight (about 0.5 g of nitrogen), of which about 0.15 g of nitrogen per kg body weight is excreted (1 g of nitrogen is derived from about 6.25 g of protein). These losses are usually balanced by dietary intake of equivalent amounts of energy, as carbohydrate, fat, and protein. Excess energy is stored as glycogen and triglyceride. If expenditure exceeds intake these energy stores are drawn upon. In a well-nourished adult, enough energy is stored as hepatic glycogen to last at least a day and therefore postoperative patients without complications do not need intravenous feeding. Once this store has been depleted energy is derived from triglyceride, and later from body tissue components such as the proteins of cells including those of muscle. This may cause severe ketosis from the metabolism of fats and ketogenic amino acids and increase nitrogen turnover and loss. *The daily energy and nitrogen requirements are not constant.* They are significantly increased in ill, catabolic patients, in whom stress-induced hormonal responses impair insulin activity, resulting in impaired glucose tolerance and increased protein breakdown (*catabolic phase*). Under such circumstances there is failure to use dietary energy and nitrogen efficiently until the factors causing negative balance have been corrected.

Method of Administration of Parenteral Nutrition

If possible all patients should be fed by mouth (enterally); it is simpler than parenteral feeding and causes fewer complications. However, if enteral feeding is contraindicated, for example after major abdominal surgery, or if there is persistent vomiting, parenteral feeding may be essential. It can be given through a peripheral vein or through a central venous catheter into a large vessel. The amount of energy that can be given into a peripheral vein is limited because glucose and amino acid solutions are hyperosmolar and cause irritation to small vessel walls, sometimes causing thrombophlebitis. Hyperosmolar solutions infused through a central venous catheter minimizes the risk of thrombophlebitis. The choice depends partly on the length of time for which parenteral feeding is required, but more importantly on the expertise available for the insertion of the central venous catheter.

The principles of carbohydrate, lipid and protein metabolism, and those of fluid and electrolytes, must be fully understood in order to manage patients receiving parenteral nutrition.

Principles of Prescribing Parenteral Nutrition

If prolonged fasting is anticipated intravenous feeding should be used from the beginning and be given preferably through a central venous catheter inserted into a large vessel. Intravenous feeding should not, if possible, be stopped suddenly; the patient should gradually be weaned on to enteral feeding. The regime depends on the clinical condition of the patient and the volume that can safely be infused.

The energy source can be either glucose- or fat-containing fluids (for example 'Intralipid' soybean emulsion, KabiVitrum Ltd). The composition of some of these solutions is shown in Table 2.8 (p.**54**). At least 50 per cent of the energy requirements should be given as:

- *glucose.* Severe illness may cause insulin resistance and administration of large amounts of glucose may be inadvisable unless exogenous insulin is given. Glucose infusion should not be stopped suddenly;

insulin must be stopped first or hypoglycaemia may occur. Glucose should preferably be infused throughout the 24 hours.
- *fat.* The fat particles in Intralipid are similar in size to, and are metabolized in the same way as, chylomicrons (p.**227**). Providing that some carbohydrate is given at a constant rate, there is no risk of significant ketoacidosis. A grossly lipaemic plasma may interfere with some laboratory analyses, particularly that of plasma sodium (p.**38**). This problem can be avoided if non-lipid-containing solutions are infused for a few hours before sampling. If lipaemia then persists it suggests that the rate of administration is faster than the rate at which the fat can be metabolized, and the infusion should be slowed.

Giving energy as glucose and fat minimizes the use of amino acids for gluconeogenesis and reduces urinary nitrogen loss.

Nitrogen supplementation, supplied in solutions containing essential amino acids, is needed to replace the daily nitrogen loss and to promote tissue healing. The assessment of nitrogen requirements is difficult. A normal

Table 12.3 Examples of daily intravenous feeding solutions for adult patients with normal renal function and in fluid and electrolyte balance, requiring either basal or increased nitrogen intake. Additional water, fat-soluble vitamins and trace elements should be given, if necessary.

	Volume (ml)	Energy (kJ)	Nitrogen (g)	Na^+ (mmol)	K^+ (mmol)	Ca^{2+} (mmol)	PO_4^{2-} (mmol)	Mg^{2+} (mmol)	Zn^{2+} (μmol)
Basal requirements supplying 800 kJ/g N									
Synthamin 9 (Travenol)	1000		9.1	73	60		30	5.0	
Glucose 20%	1500	5000							
Intralipid 10% (KabiVitrum)	500	2300					7		
Addamel	10					5		1.5	20
	3010	7300	9.1	73	60	5	37	6.5	20
Increased requirements supplying 775 kJ/g N									
Synthamin 14 (Travenol)	1000		14.0	73	60		30	5.0	
Glucose 20%	1000	3350							
Glucose 50%	500	4200							
Intralipid 10% (KabiVitrum)	500	2300					7		
Addamel	10					5		1.5	20
	3010	9850	14.0	73	60	5	37	6.5	20

adult patient needs about 9 g of nitrogen a day, but this increases as the catabolic rate increases, for example in stress and infection, to up to 20 g of nitrogen a day. During the catabolic phase amino-acid infusion is unnecessary, as the body cannot use administered nitrogen efficiently, and much of it is excreted in the urine as urea or free amino acids. About 840 kJ (200 kcal) of energy per gram of nitrogen are needed by a normal adult to synthesize protein from amino acids. This proportion decreases slightly as the catabolic rate and nitrogen requirements increase.

The estimation of the 24-hour urinary nitrogen output can, if glomerular function is normal, be used as a rough guide to replacement. However, once tissue repair predominates, use of amino acid increases (*anabolic phase*) and urinary nitrogen loss may fall suddenly; this indicates an increased, not a decreased, need for nitrogen. Conversely during the catabolic phase increasing nitrogen intake may result in an increased urinary loss because it cannot be used (p.**265**).

Vitamin, mineral and trace element supplementation must be given during very long-term parenteral feeding in addition to the nitrogen and energy requirements. Tissue destruction leads to loss of intracellular constituents, such as phosphate and some trace elements, such as zinc and copper. It may be necessary to add phosphate to the infusion. Urinary trace metal loss is high during the catabolic phase, but falls as anabolism becomes predominant. If parenteral feeding has been very prolonged deficiencies may become apparent and weight gain may be impaired if supplements are not given.

The composition of fluids used as part of an intravenous feeding regime are shown in Tables 2.7, 2.8, and 2.9 (p.**54**, p.**54**, and p.**55**), and examples of feeding regimes for patients with normal renal function and who are in electrolyte balance are given in Table 12.3. Daily parenteral nutrition solutions are frequently prepared in 3 litre bags that contain the appropriate daily nitrogen, energy, vitamin and trace element require-

Table 12.4 Some clinical and metabolic complications of long-term parenteral nutrition

Complications of central line
   malposition
   infection
Hyper/hypoglycaemia
Acid-base and electrolyte disturbances
Hypophosphataemia
Cholestatic type of liver disease
Essential vitamin and mineral deficiencies (long-term only)
Misinterpretation of laboratory results associated with lipid infusion
   pseudohyponatraemia

ments in addition to those of sodium and potassium.

Monitoring of Long-term Intravenous Feeding

Some clinical and metabolic complications associated with long-term parenteral feeding are shown in Table 12.4. One of the most important complications is infection of the central line and careful nursing attention is therefore essential. The biochemical investigations that may be used to prevent the onset of these complications, are discussed below.

Initially results of daily plasma sodium, potassium, TCO_2 and urea concentrations help in the assessment of water and electrolyte needs and renal function. Plasma glucose concentrations must be monitored carefully as patients may develop stress related glucose intolerance with *hyperglycaemia*, consequent cell dehydration and polyuria or rapid *hypoglycaemia* if glucose infusion is stopped with continued insulin infusion. Plasma calcium, phosphate, magnesium and albumin concentrations should be measured weekly to detect possible metabolic complications. Blood haemoglobin, MCV and MCHC and the prothrombin time should also be monitored at least weekly. Plasma concentrations of trace elements, in particular zinc and copper, should be measured every two weeks.

Daily estimation of the 24-hour output of urinary nitrogen may help to assess nitrogen use and the amount that should be replaced. If urea excretion increases quantitatively when nitrogen intake is increased it indicates that the nitrogen cannot be used, and supplements should *not* be increased. If nitrogen loss falls while supplements are being given it indicates that anabolism is increasing, and supplements *should be* increased until urinary excretion increases. Once the patient has been established on long-term feeding the frequency of monitoring can be reduced.

A *cholestatic type of liver disorder* may develop in some patients receiving intravenous feeding. The plasma alkaline phosphatase activity increases, with a later rise in the plasma transaminase activities. Unless significant symptoms occur, this is not an indication to stop parenteral feeding because liver dysfunction usually resolves when the parenteral feeding is stopped.

Vitamins

13

Because they were thought to be amines when first discovered, the term 'vitamines', was coined for substances found to be, like protein, fat and carbohydrates essential for life, but, unlike them, needed in only minute amounts.

Vitamins are now known to be organic compounds, not necessarily amines, essential for normal growth and development; they must be taken in the diet because the body either cannot synthesize them at all, or in sufficient amounts for its needs; vitamin D, for example, can be synthesized in the skin from 7-dehydrocholesterol by the action of ultraviolet light, but, for various reasons, the amount of sunlight reaching the skin may be insufficient to provide the required amount.

A normal mixed diet provides adequate amounts of vitamins and supplementation is then unnecessary. Deficiencies are rarely seen in affluent populations except in:

- those with an inadequate dietary intake, because they:
    are, especially if elderly or disabled, unable to afford a suitable diet or to prepare food properly;
    have anorexia nervosa;
    are food faddists.
- those in whom, despite an adequate intake, absorption is impaired;
- those on long-term unsupplemented artificial diets or parenteral nutrition;
- chronic alcoholism.

Some vitamins (notably A and D) are toxic if taken in excess. Because of the increase in self-administration encouraged by misleading media publicity, unscrupulous advertising and ready availability in 'Health Food' shops, vitamin overdosage has become commoner than previously.

The biochemical functions of many vitamins are known but it is not easy to relate these to the clinical features found in some deficiency states.

Testing for deficiency should be carried out as soon as the diagnosis is suspected; results of laboratory tests usually rapidly revert to normal once the patient has started eating a normal diet, for example after admission to hospital, and it may then be impossible to confirm the original diagnosis.

CLASSIFICATION OF VITAMINS

Vitamins are classified into two groups on the basis of their solubilities, one group being fat-soluble and the other water-soluble.

The distinction is of clinical importance, because steatorrhoea may be associated with deficiency of fat-soluble, with relatively little clinical evidence of lack of most of the water-soluble vitamins except B_{12} and folate.

FAT-SOLUBLE VITAMINS

The fat-soluble vitamins are:

- A (retinol);
- D (calciferol);
- K (2-methyl-1,4-naphthoquinone);
- E (α-tocopherol).

Each of these has more than one active chemical form, but variations in structure are very slight and in the following discussion each vitamin is considered as a single substance.

Vitamin A (retinol)

SOURCES OF VITAMIN A

Precursors of vitamin A (the carotenes) are found in the yellow and green parts of plants and are especially abundant in carrots. The active vitamin is formed by hydrolysis of β-carotene in the intestinal mucosa; each molecule can produce two molecules of vitamin A, which are absorbed as retinol esters and stored in the liver. The yield of the vitamin is much less than the theoretical maximum, especially in children. Retinol is transported to tissues bound to the α-globulin, retinol-binding protein

Vitamin A is stored in animal tissues, particularly in the liver, which is an important source of the preformed vitamin; it is also present in milk products and eggs.

FUNCTIONS OF VITAMIN A

Rhodopsin (visual purple), the retinal pigment that is *necessary for vision in dim light* (scotopic vision) consists of a protein (opsin) combined with vitamin A. In bright light rhodopsin is destroyed. It is partly regenerated in the dark, but, because the regeneration is not quantitatively complete, vitamin A is needed to maintain retinal levels.

Vitamin A is also essential for normal:

- *mucopolysaccharide synthesis*;
- *mucus secretion.*

CLINICAL EFFECTS OF VITAMIN A DEFICIENCY

The clinical effects of vitamin A deficiency are:

- due to rhodopsin deficiency:
  'night blindness'. Deficiency is associated with poor vision in dim light, especially if the eyes have recently been exposed to bright light. It is uncommon for the patient to complain of this.
- due to deficient mucus secretions:
  drying and squamous metaplasia of ectodermal tissue;

follicular hyperkeratosis. Skin secretion is diminished and there may be hyperkeratosis of hair follicles; dry, horny papules, varying in size from a pinhead to a quarter-inch in diameter, are found mainly on the extensor surfaces of the thighs and forearms. Squamous metaplasia of the bronchial epithelium has also been reported and may be associated with a tendency to chest infection; *xerosis conjunctivae and xerophthalmia.* The conjunctiva and cornea become dry and wrinkled, with squamous metaplasia of the epithelium and keratinization of the tissue, resulting from deficiency of mucus secretion. *Bitot's spots,* seen in more advanced cases, are elevated white patches, composed of keratin debris, found in the conjunctivae. Prolonged deficiency leads to *keratomalacia* with ulceration and infection and consequent scarring of the cornea, causing blindness. Keratomalacia is an important cause of blindness in the world as a whole, but is rarely seen in affluent countries.

- *anaemia*, which responds to vitamin A, but not to iron therapy.

CAUSES OF VITAMIN A DEFICIENCY

Hepatic stores of vitamin A are so large that clinical signs only develop after many months, or even years, of dietary deficiency. Such prolonged deficiency is very rare in affluent communities. In steatorrhoea clinical evidence of vitamin A is rare although plasma concentrations may be low. By contrast, deficiency is relatively common in less affluent countries, especially in children, and is a common cause of blindness.

DIAGNOSIS AND TREATMENT OF VITAMIN A DEFICIENCY

There is a poor correlation between the eye changes and the biochemical findings. The diagnosis should be made on clinical criteria; very low plasma vitamin A concentrations usually confirm deficiency. In conditions such as non-cirrhotic liver disease, in which plasma concentrations of retinol-binding protein are low, those of vitamin A may be decreased despite normal liver stores. In cirrhosis of the liver the stores may be very low.

High doses of vitamin A, in fish liver oil, should be given to treat xerophthalmia and advanced skin lesions. Night blindness and early retinal and corneal changes respond very rapidly to treatment; corneal scarring is irreversible.

HYPERVITAMINOSIS A

Vitamin A in large doses is toxic. Acute intoxication has been reported in Arctic regions as a result of eating polar bear liver, which has a very high vitamin A content, but more commonly overdosage is due to excessive use of vitamin preparations, often without medical advice.

- In acute poisoning symptoms include nausea and vomiting, abdominal pain, drowsiness and headache.
- Chronic hypervitaminosis A causes fatigue, insomnia, bone pain, loss of hair and desquamation and discoloration of the skin.

Vitamin D (Calciferol)

The metabolism and functions of vitamin D, and the effects and treatment of its deficiency, are discussed in Chapter 9.

Overdosage may cause hypercalcaemia and its accompanying dangers (p.**177**). In chronic overdosage stores of cholecalciferol are large and therefore hypercalcaemia may persist, or even progress, for several weeks after stopping ingestion.

Vitamin K

Vitamin K, like many of the B vitamins, can be synthesized by bacteria in the ileum, from which it can be absorbed; dietary deficiency does not occur. However, deficiency may occur:

- in patients with steatorrhoea; the vitamin, whether taken in the diet or produced by intestinal bacteria, cannot be absorbed normally;
- after administration of some broad-spectrum antibiotics which may alter the intestinal bacterial flora and so reduce the synthesis of vitamin K, especially in children.

Vitamin K is needed for synthesis of prothrombin and coagulation factors VII, IX and X in the liver, and deficiency is accompanied by a bleeding tendency with a prolonged prothrombin time. If these findings are due to deficiency of the vitamin they can be corrected by parenteral administration (p.**256**).

In the newborn plasma vitamin K concentrations are lower than in adults because:

- very little can be transported across the placenta;
- the neonatal gut is only gradually colonized by bacteria capable of synthesizing vitamin K;
- protein synthesis has not yet reached full adult capacity, particularly in premature infants.

Deficiency may be severe enough to cause *haemorrhagic disease of the newborn*, a condition which may present within two to three days of birth.

Vitamin E (α-tocopherol)

Newborn infants are deficient in vitamin E, a potent antioxidant, and this may be associated with haemolytic anaemia, particularly in those born prematurely. There is some evidence that vitamin E deficiency, due to prolonged and severe fat malabsorption, may cause neurological symptoms in adults.

WATER-SOLUBLE VITAMINS

The water-soluble vitamins are:

- the B complex:
  - thiamine (B$_1$);
  - riboflavine (B$_2$);
  - nicotinamide (niacin);
  - pyridoxine (B$_6$);
  - folate (pteroylglutamate);
  - the vitamin B$_{12}$ complex (cobalamins);
  - biotin and pantothenate (probably of no clinical significance in man).
- ascorbate (vitamin C).

Thiamine, folate, vitamin B$_{12}$ and ascorbate are actively absorbed from the intestinal tract and the rest diffuse passively through the intestinal mucosal wall.

The B Complex

A group of food factors were originally classified together as the B group, with the exception of vitamin B$_{12}$ and folate, which were discovered later. Most of these act as enzyme cofactors, but it is not easy to relate the clinical findings to the underlying biochemical lesion.

Many are synthesized by colonic bacteria. Opinions vary as to the importance of this source in man but, because absorption of water-soluble vitamins from the large intestine is poor, probably most of those synthesized within the colon are unavailable to the body.

Clinical deficiency is rare in affluent communities. When deficiency does occur it is usually multiple, involving most of the B group, and is associated with protein malnutrition; for this reason it may be difficult to decide which signs and symptoms are specific for an individual vitamin and which are part of a general malnutrition syndrome.

Thiamine (B$_1$)

SOURCES OF THIAMINE AND CAUSES OF DEFICIENCY

Thiamine cannot be synthesized by animals, including man. It is found in most dietary components; wheat germ, oatmeal and yeast are particularly rich in the vitamin. Adequate amounts are present in a normal diet and deficiency is commonest in alcoholics and in patients with anorexia nervosa.

FUNCTIONS OF THIAMINE

Thiamine is a component of thiamine pyrophosphate, which is an essential cofactor for decarboxylation of 2-oxoacids; one such reaction is the conversion of pyruvate to acetyl CoA. In thiamine deficiency pyruvate cannot be metabolized and accumulates in the blood. Thiamine pyrophosphate is also an essential cofactor for transketolase in the pentose-phosphate pathway.

CLINICAL EFFECTS OF THIAMINE DEFICIENCY

Deficiency of thiamine causes *beriberi*, in which anorexia and emaciation, neurological lesions (motor and sensory polyneuropathy; Wernicke's encephalopathy) and cardiac arrhythmias may occur; this form is called 'dry' beriberi. In 'wet' beriberi there is peripheral oedema, sometimes associated with cardiac failure. Some of these findings may be due to protein rather than to thiamine deficiency.

Beriberi may be aggravated by a high carbohydrate diet, possibly because this leads to an increased rate of glycolysis and therefore of pyruvate production.

LABORATORY DIAGNOSIS OF THIAMINE DEFICIENCY

Probably the most reliable test for thiamine deficiency is estimation of erythrocyte transketolase activity, with and without added thiamine pyrophosphate. A reduced activity, if due to thiamine deficiency, becomes normal after addition of the cofactor. This test is rarely indicated and should not be requested once a normal diet, or vitamin supplementation, has been started because plasma concentrations are rapidly corrected.

Riboflavine (B₂)

SOURCES OF RIBOFLAVINE

Riboflavine is found in large amounts in yeasts and germinating plants such as peas and beans, and in smaller amounts in fish, poultry and meat, especially offal.

FUNCTIONS OF RIBOFLAVINE

Riboflavine activity is present in many naturally occurring flavoproteins, most incorporating riboflavine in the form of flavine mononucleotide (FMN) and flavine adenine dinucleotide (FAD). FMN and FAD are reversible *electron carriers* in biological oxidation systems which are, in turn, oxidized by cytochromes (Fig. 13.1).

CLINICAL EFFECTS OF RIBOFLAVINE DEFICIENCY

Riboflavine deficiency (*ariboflavinosis*) causes a rough, scaly skin, especially on the face, cheilosis (red, swollen, cracked lips), angular stomatitis and similar lesions at the mucocutaneous junctions of the anus and vagina, and a swollen, tender, red tongue which is described as magenta coloured. Congestion of conjunctival blood vessels may be visible if the eye is examined with a slit lamp.

LABORATORY DIAGNOSIS OF RIBOFLAVINE DEFICIENCY

Riboflavine acts as a cofactor for *glutathione reductase*. The finding of a low erythrocyte activity of this enzyme, which increases by about 30 per cent after the addition of FAD, suggests riboflavine deficiency.

Nicotinamide (Niacin)

SOURCES OF NICOTINAMIDE

Nicotinamide can be formed in the body from nicotinic acid. Both substances are plentiful in animal and plant foods although much of that in plants is bound in an unabsorbable form. *Some nicotinic acid can also be synthesized in man from tryptophan.* Probably both dietary and endogenous sources are necessary to provide enough nicotinamide for normal metabolism.

FUNCTIONS OF NICOTINAMIDE

Nicotinamide is the active constituent of nicotinamide adenine dinucleotide (NAD⁺), and its phosphate (NADP⁺), which are important cofactors in *oxidation-reduction reactions*. Reduced NAD⁺ and NADP⁺ are, in turn, reoxidized by flavoproteins, and the functions of riboflavine and nicotinamide are closely linked (Fig. 13.1). NAD⁺ and NADP⁺ and their reduced forms are essential for glycolysis and oxidative phosphorylation, and for many synthetic processes.

CLINICAL EFFECTS OF NICOTINAMIDE DEFICIENCY

It may be difficult to distinguish between the clinical features due to coexistent deficiencies, such as of pyridoxine, and those specifically due to nicotinamide. However, nicotinamide deficiency is probably the most important factor precipitating the clinical syndrome of *pellagra*. The symptoms are

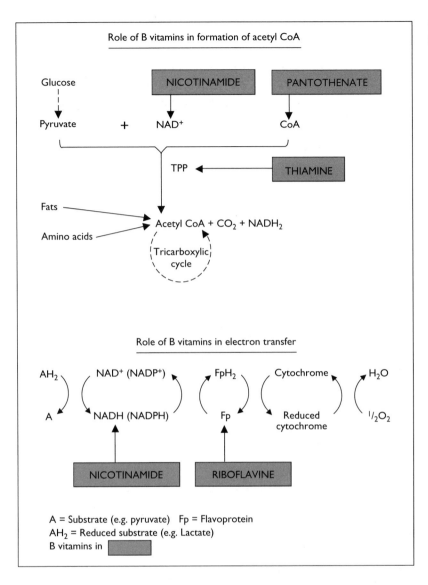

Fig. 13.1 Some biochemical interrelations of the B vitamins.

often remembered by the mnemonic 'three Ds' – dermatitis, diarrhoea and dementia.

- *Dermatitis* is a sunburn-like erythema, especially severe in areas exposed to the sun, which may progress to pigmentation and to thickening of the skin; 'pellagra' literally means 'rough skin'.
- *Diarrhoea* is due to widespread inflammation of the mucosal membranes of the gastrointestinal tract; anorexia may aggravate weight loss.
- *Dementia*, with delusions, may be preceded by irritability and depression.

Other features include achlorhydria, stomatitis and vaginitis.

CAUSES OF NICOTINAMIDE DEFICIENCY

Dietary deficiency of nicotinamide, like that of the other B vitamins, is rare in affluent communities.

Hartnup disease is due to a rare inborn error of metabolism involving the renal, intestinal and other cellular transport mechanisms for the monoamino-monocarboxylic amino acids, including tryptophan (p.**360**). Subjects with the disorder may present with a pellagra-like rash that can be cured by giving between 40 and 200 mg of nicotinamide daily. If the endogenous supply of tryptophan is reduced, then dietary nicotinic acid is probably insufficient to supply the body's needs over long periods of time; under these circumstances only a slight reduction of intake may precipitate pellagra. A similar clinical picture has been reported as a rare complication of the *carcinoid syndrome*, when tryptophan is diverted to the synthesis of large amounts of 5-hydroxy-tryptamine (p.**396**).

Nicotinic acid (but not nicotinamide) may reduce hepatic secretion of VLDL and therefore plasma concentrations of VLDL and LDL (p.**237**).

LABORATORY DIAGNOSIS OF NICOTINAMIDE DEFICIENCY

If a normal diet has not been started the diagnosis can sometimes be made by measuring nicotinic acid concentrations in body fluids.

Pyridoxine (B₆)

SOURCES OF PYRIDOXINE AND CAUSES OF DEFICIENCY

Pyridoxine (pyridoxol), its aldehyde (pyridoxal) and amine (pyridoxamine) are widely distributed in food; dietary deficiency is very rare. The antituberculous drug *isoniazid* (isonicotinic hydrazide) and possibly L-dopa have been reported to produce the picture of pyridoxine deficiency, probably by competing with it in metabolic pathways.

FUNCTIONS OF PYRIDOXINE

Pyridoxal phosphate, formed in the liver from pyridoxine, pyridoxal and pyridoxamine, is a cofactor mainly for the *transaminases*, and for *decarboxylation of amino acids*.

CLINICAL EFFECTS

Deficiency may cause roughening of the skin, peripheral neuropathy and a sore tongue. A rare hypochromic, microcytic anaemia, with increased iron stores (sideroblastic anaemia) responds to large doses of pyridoxine even when there is no evidence of vitamin deficiency ('pyridoxine-responsive' anaemia).

LABORATORY DIAGNOSIS OF PYRIDOXINE DEFICIENCY

Pyridoxal phosphate is needed for conversion of tryptophan to nicotinic acid. In pyridoxine deficiency this pathway is impaired. *Xanthurenic acid* is the excretion product of 3-hydroxykynurenic acid, the metabolite before the 'block'; in pyridoxine deficiency it is found in abnormally high amounts in the urine after an oral *tryptophan load*.

The urinary metabolite of pyridoxal phosphate, 4-pyridoxic acid, may also be measured.

The increase in the activity of *erythrocyte aspartate transaminase* after addition of pyridoxal phosphate may be measured. The more severe the pyridoxine deficiency the greater the increase in enzyme activity after addition of the vitamin.

Biotin and Pantothenate

Lack of these two vitamins probably does not produce a clinical deficiency syndrome.

- *Biotin* is produced by intestinal bacteria; it is also present in eggs, but large amounts of raw egg white in experimental diets have caused loss of hair and dermatitis thought to be due to biotin deficiency. Probably the protein *avidin*, present in egg white, combines with biotin and prevents its absorption. Biotin is a cofactor in carboxylation reactions.

- *Pantothenate* is a component of coenzyme A (CoA), which is essential for fat and carbohydrate metabolism (Fig. 13.1). The vitamin is very widely distributed in foodstuffs.

Note that, as a general rule, deficiency of the group of B vitamins already discussed results in lesions of the skin, mucous membranes and the nervous system.

Folate and B₁₂

Folate is included in the B group. Both folate and B₁₂ are essential for the normal maturation of erythrocytes; deficiency of either causes megaloblastic anaemia. Their effects are so closely interrelated that they are usually considered together. A fuller discussion of the haematological diagnosis and treatment of megaloblastic anaemia will be found in haematology textbooks.

Folate is present in green vegetables and some meats. It is easily destroyed during cooking and *dietary deficiency* may occasionally occur. It is absorbed throughout the small intestine and, in contrast to most of the other B vitamins (except B₁₂), clinical deficiency is relatively common in *intestinal malabsorption syndromes*, especially in the 'contaminated bowel' syndrome (p.**254**). In these conditions, and during pregnancy and lactation, low red-cell folate concentrations may be associated with megaloblastic anaemia.

The active form of the vitamin is tetrahydrofolate, which is essential for the transfer of one-carbon units: it is particularly important in purine and pyrimidine, and therefore DNA and RNA, synthesis. Methotrexate, a cytotoxic analogue of folate, competes with it for metabolism and therefore inhibits DNA synthesis.

The vitamin B₁₂ group includes several cobalamins, found in animal products but *not* in green vegetables. Dietary deficiency is rare. The cobalamins are transported in plasma by a specific carrier protein, transcobalamin II. Deoxyadenosyl- and methylcobalamin have,

like folate, coenzyme activity in nucleic acid synthesis. Hydroxocobalamin is the form most commonly used in treatment, and both it and cyanocobalamin are converted to cofactor forms in the body. All forms are absorbed mainly in the terminal ileum, combined with *intrinsic factor* derived from the gastric parietal cells. In pernicious anaemia antibodies to gastric parietal cells or to intrinsic factor cause malabsorption of vitamin B₁₂. The relation between intestinal dysfunction and vitamin B₁₂ deficiency is discussed in Chapter 12.

Deficiency of vitamin B₁₂, like that of folate, causes megaloblastic anaemia. However, unlike that of folate it can cause *subacute combined degeneration of the spinal cord*. Although the megaloblastic anaemia of vitamin B₁₂ deficiency can be reversed by folate, this treatment should never be given in pernicious anaemia because it does not improve, and may even aggravate, the neurological lesions, causing permanent disability.

The known biological functions and the clinical syndromes associated with deficiencies of the B vitamins are summarized in Table 13.1. As a general rule deficiencies of this group cause lesions of skin, mucous membranes and the nervous system.

Ascorbate (Vitamin C)

SOURCES OF ASCORBATE

Ascorbate is found in fruit, particularly citrus fruits, and vegetables. A quantitatively significant dietary source is ascorbate added to other foods as a preservative. It cannot by synthesized by man, other primates, or the guinea pig.

FUNCTIONS OF ASCORBATE

Ascorbate can be reversibly oxidized in biological systems to dehydroascorbate and, although its functions in man are not certain, it probably acts as a hydrogen carrier. It

Table 13.1 The biochemical functions and clinical deficiency syndromes associated with the B vitamins

Name	Synonym	Biochemical function	Clinical deficiency syndrome
Thiamine	Aneurin Vitamin B_1	Cocarboxylase (as thiamine pyrophosphate)	Beriberi (neuropathy) Wernicke's encephalopathy
Riboflavine	Vitamin B_2	In flavoproteins (electron carriers as FAD and FMN)	Ariboflavinosis (affecting skin and eyes)
Nicotinamide	PP factor Niacin	In NAD^+ and $NADP^+$ (electron carriers)	Pellagra (dermatitis, diarrhoea, dementia)
Pyridoxine	Adermin Vitamin B_6	Cofactor in decarboxylation and deamination (as phosphate)	? Pyridoxine responsive anaemia ? Dermatitis
Biotin Pantothenate		Carboxylation cofactor In Coenzyme A	} Probably unimportant clinically
Folate	Pteroyl glutamate	Metabolism of purines and pyrimidines	Megaloblastic anaemia
Cobalamins	Vitamin B_{12} group	Cofactor in synthesis of nucleic acid	Megaloblastic anaemia Subacute combined degeneration of the spinal cord

seems to be necessary for normal collagen formation.

CAUSES OF ASCORBATE DEFICIENCY

Deficiency of ascorbate causes *scurvy* which was commonly seen on long sea voyages in the 16th, 17th and 18th centuries during which period fresh fruit and vegetables were unavailable.

Dehydroascorbate is easily and irreversibly oxidized and loses its biological activity in the presence of oxygen; this reaction is catalysed by heat.

Deficiency occurs most commonly in the elderly, especially those who do not eat fresh fruit and vegetables and who tend to cook in frying pans; the combination of heat and the large area of food in contact with air irreversibly oxidizes the vitamin. Ascorbate deficiency can occur in iron overload (p.**418**).

CLINICAL EFFECTS OF ASCORBATE DEFICIENCY

Many of the signs and symptoms of scurvy are related to deficient collagen formation. These include:

- *fragility of vascular walls* causing a bleeding tendency, often with a positive Hess test, petechiae and ecchymoses, swollen, tender, spongy, bleeding gums and, occasionally, haematuria, epistaxis and retinal haemorrhages. In infants subperiosteal bleeding and haemarthroses are extremely painful and may lead to permanent joint deformities;
- *poor wound healing*;
- *deficiency of bone matrix causing osteoporosis* and poor healing of fractures. In children bone formation is impaired at the epidiaphyseal junctions, which look 'frayed' radiologically;
- *anaemia*, possibly due to impaired erythropoiesis. This may sometimes be cured by ascorbate alone. Bleeding aggravates the anaemia.

This florid form of scurvy *is rarely seen nowadays* and the patient most commonly presents complaining that bruising occurs after only minor trauma.

All the signs and symptoms are dramatically and rapidly cured by the administration of ascorbate.

DIAGNOSIS OF ASCORBATE DEFICIENCY

The laboratory confirmation of the clinical diagnosis of ascorbate deficiency can only be made *before* therapy has started. Once ascorbate has been given it is difficult to prove that deficiency was previously present.

Although leucocyte ascorbate assay was said to be more reliable in confirming the diagnosis than that of plasma, levels probably alter in parallel; plasma assay is technically more satisfactory but chemical estimations are rarely indicated.

Summary

1. Vitamins have important biochemical functions, most of which are now well understood. Unfortunately the relationship of these to clinical syndromes is not always obvious.
2. The fat-soluble vitamins, especially vitamin D, may be deficient in steatorrhoea. Both vitamin A and vitamin D are stored in the body and deficiency takes some time to develop.
3. Vitamin A is necessary for the formation of rhodopsin (visual purple) and for normal mucopolysaccharide synthesis. Deficiency is associated with poor vision in dim light and with drying and metaplasia of epithelial surfaces, especially those of the conjunctiva and cornea
4. Vitamin D, as 1,25-dihydroxyvitamin D, is necessary for normal calcium metabolism; deficiency causes rickets in children and osteomalacia in adults.
5. Both vitamin A and vitamin D are toxic in excess.
6. Vitamin K is necessary for prothrombin formation and deficiency is associated with a bleeding tendency.
7. Thiamine deficiency causes beriberi.
8. Riboflavine deficiency causes ariboflavinosis.
9. Nicotinamide can be synthesized from tryptophan in the body; dietary deficiency causes a pellagra-like syndrome, which may also be found in Hartnup disease, when tryptophan absorption is deficient, and in the carcinoid syndrome, when tryptophan is used in excess for 5-hydroxytryptamine synthesis.
10. Pyridoxine-responsive anaemia may occur.
11. Folate and vitamin B_{12} deficiencies produce megaloblastic anaemia and deficiency of vitamin B_{12} can also cause subacute combined degeneration of the spinal cord. Compared with the other B vitamins, deficiencies of these are relatively common in malabsorption syndromes, and vitamin B_{12} and folate deficiency can be features of the 'contaminated bowel' syndrome. Pernicious anaemia is due to intrinsic factor deficiency with consequent malabsorption of vitamin B_{12}.
12. Ascorbate deficiency causes scurvy.

The liver and Gall stones

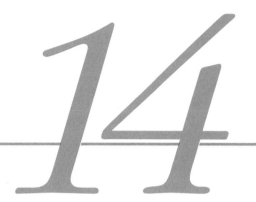

14

The Liver

Outline of the Functions of the Liver

The liver has important synthetic and metabolic functions. It also detoxifies and, like the kidneys, excretes end products of metabolism.

The main blood supply to the liver is from the *portal vein*, which is formed from the superior mesenteric and splenic veins and so drains the intestinal tract. Oxygen is supplied by the hepatic artery. The organ is made up of hexagonal lobules of cells (Fig 14.1). Rows of hepatocytes radiate from the central hepatic vein and are separated by sinusoidal spaces, along the walls of which are interspersed hepatic macrophages, the Kupffer cells. These cells are part of the reticuloendothelial system and are phagocytic and so have an important detoxifying function. At the corners of each lobule are the portal tracts that contain branches of the hepatic artery, the portal vein and bile ducts. Blood flows from the portal tracts towards the central hepatic vein. Therefore:

- hypoxia and toxins that are metabolized in the liver cause damage to the centrilobular area first;
- toxins that do not depend on hepatic metabolism primarily affect the periphery of the lobule.

Almost all nutrients from the gastrointestinal tract except fat micelles pass through the sinusoidal spaces before entering the systemic circulation. Distortion of this architectural arrangement, as in cirrhosis (fibrosis) of the liver, may allow blood to pass directly from the portal to the central and then into the hepatic vein, so bypassing the hepatocytes and therefore significantly reducing the detoxifying capacity.

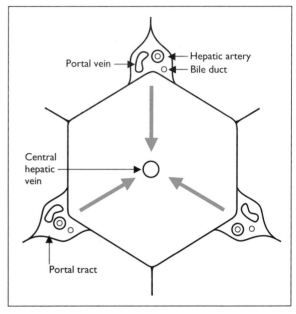

Fig. 14.1 Diagrammatic representation of a cross-section of a hepatic lobule showing the relation between the central hepatic vein and the portal tracts. Blood flows towards the central vein as indicated by the arrows.

GENERAL METABOLIC FUNCTIONS

When the glucose concentration is high in the portal vein, it is converted to glycogen and the carbon skeletons of fatty acids which are transported to adipose tissue as very low density lipoprotein (VLDL) (Fig. 10.2; p.**199**).

During fasting the systemic plasma glucose concentration is maintained by the breakdown of glycogen (glycogenolysis) or by the synthesis of glucose from substrates such as glycerol, lactate and amino acids (gluconeogenesis). Fatty acids reaching the liver from fat stores may be metabolized in the tricarboxylic acid cycle, converted to ketones or incorporated into triglycerides (Fig. 10.3, p.**201**).

SYNTHETIC FUNCTIONS

Hepatocytes synthesize:

- plasma proteins, except immunoglobulins and complement;
- most coagulation factors, including fibrinogen and factors II (prothrombin), V, VII, IX, X, XI, XII and XIII. Of these prothrombin (II) and factors VII, IX and X cannot be synthesized without vitamin K;
- the lipoproteins, VLDL and HDL (Chapter 11);
- primary bile acids.

The liver has a very large functional reserve. Deficiencies in synthetic function can only be detected if liver disease is extensive; such abnormalities are more often due to non-hepatic factors. For example, before a fall in plasma albumin concentration is attributed to advanced liver disease extrahepatic causes must be excluded, such as the loss of protein through the kidney, gut or skin, or across capillary membranes into the interstitial space as in even mild inflammation or infection.

Prothrombin levels, assessed by measuring the prothrombin time, may be reduced because of impaired hepatic synthesis, whether due to failure to absorb vitamin K or to hepatocellular damage. If hepatocellular function is adequate, parenteral administration of vitamin K will reverse the abnormality (p.**256**).

EXCRETION AND DETOXIFICATION

The excretion of *bilirubin* is considered in more detail below. Other substances that are inactivated and excreted by the liver include:

- *amino acids*, which are deaminated in the liver. Amino groups, and the ammonia produced by intestinal bacterial action and absorbed into the portal vein, are converted to urea;
- *cholesterol*, which is excreted in the bile either unchanged or after conversion to bile acids (p.**293**);
- *steroid hormones*, which are metabolized and inactivated by conjugation with glucuronate and sulphate and excreted in the urine in these water-soluble forms;

- *many drugs*, which are metabolized and inactivated by enzymes of the endoplasmic reticulum system; some are excreted in the bile;
- *toxins*. The reticuloendothelial Kupffer cells in the hepatic sinusoids are well placed to extract toxic substances which have been absorbed from the gastrointestinal tract.

Efficient excretion of the end-products of metabolism and of bilirubin depends on:

- normally functioning liver cells;
- normal blood flow through the liver;
- patent biliary ducts.

Efficient detoxification depends on the Kupffer cell function.

Because of the very large hepatic reserve tests for impairment of metabolic, including synthetic and secretory, function are relatively insensitive indicators of liver disease.

Bilirubin Metabolism and Jaundice

Jaundice only becomes clinically apparent when the plasma bilirubin concentration reaches about 35 μmol/L (2 mg/dl), twice the upper reference limit. It occurs when bilirubin production exceeds the hepatic capacity to excrete it. This may be because:

- an increased rate of bilirubin production exceeds normal excretory capacity of the liver (*prehepatic jaundice*);
- the normal load of bilirubin cannot be conjugated and/or excreted by damaged liver cells (*hepatic jaundice*);
- the biliary flow is obstructed, so that conjugated bilirubin cannot be excreted into the intestine and is regurgitated into the systemic circulation (*posthepatic jaundice*).

FORMATION AND EXCRETION OF BILIRUBIN

At the end of their lifespan red blood cells are broken down by the reticuloendothelial system, mainly in the spleen. The released haemoglobin is split into globin, which enters the general protein pool and haem, which is converted to bilirubin after removal of iron, which is reused (p.**376**).

About 80 per cent of bilirubin is derived from haem within the reticulo-endothelial system. Other sources include the breakdown of immature red cells in the bone marrow and of compounds chemically related to haemoglobin, such as myoglobin and the cytochromes.

Bilirubin is transported to the liver bound to albumin and accounts for most of that found in normal plasma. In this form it is called *unconjugated bilirubin* which is lipid-soluble and therefore, if not protein bound, can cross cell membranes including those forming the 'blood-brain barrier'; it is potentially toxic. However, at physiological concentrations it is all protein bound.

In the adult about 300 µmol (180 mg) of bilirubin reaches the liver where it is transferred from plasma albumin, through the permeable vascular sinusoidal membrane. The hepatocytes can handle a much greater load than this. It is bound to *ligandin* (Y protein). From there it is actively transported to the smooth endoplasmic reticulum where it is conjugated with glucuronate by a process catalysed by uridyl diphosphate (UDP) glucuronyl transferase. Bilirubin monoglucuronide passes to the canalicular surfaces of the hepatocytes where, after addition of a second glucuronate molecule, it is secreted by active processes into the bile canaliculi. This process is largely dependent on active secretion of bile acids from hepatocytes. These energy-dependent steps are the ones most likely to be impaired by liver damage (hypoxia and septicaemia) and by increased pressure in the biliary tract. Other anions, including drugs, may compete for binding to ligandin and so impair bilirubin conjugation and therefore excretion.

The metabolism and excretion of bilirubin are summarized in Fig. 14.2.

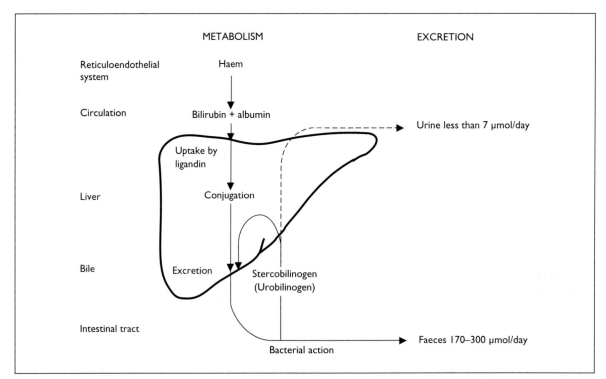

Fig. 14.2 Metabolism and excretion of bilirubin.

RETENTION OF BILIRUBIN IN PLASMA: JAUNDICE

Unconjugated hyperbilirubinaemia occurs if there is:

- a marked increase in the bilirubin load as a result of haemolysis, or of the breakdown of large amounts of blood after haemorrhage into the gastrointestinal tract or, for example, under the skin due to extensive bruising;
- impaired binding of bilirubin to ligandin or impaired conjugation with glucuronate in the liver.

In some pathological conditions plasma unconjugated bilirubin levels may increase so much that they exceed the protein-binding capacity. The lipid-soluble, unbound bilirubin damages brain cells (*kernicterus*). This is most likely to occur in newborn, particularly premature, infants in whom the hepatic conjugating mechanisms are immature (p.**342**). In addition, the proportion of unbound, unconjugated bilirubin, and therefore the risk of cerebral damage, increases if:

- plasma albumin concentrations are low;
- unconjugated bilirubin is displaced from binding sites by:
    - high levels of free fatty acids;
    - drugs such as salicylates or sulphonamides.

Unconjugated bilirubin is normally all protein-bound, is not water soluble and therefore cannot be excreted in the urine. *Patients with unconjugated hyperbilirubinaemia do not have bilirubinuria* ('acholuric jaundice').

Conjugated bilirubinaemia is one of the earliest manifestations of impaired hepatic excretion. In most cases of jaundice in adults both conjugated and unconjugated fractions of bilirubin are increased in plasma but conjugated bilirubin predominates. Conjugated bilirubin is water-soluble, is less strongly protein-bound than the unconjugated form, and therefore can be excreted in the urine. *Bilirubinuria is always pathological.* Dark urine may be an early sign of some forms of hepatobiliary disease.

UROBILIN

Conjugated bilirubin enters the gut lumen in bile where it is broken down by bacteria in the distal ileum and the colon into a group of products, known as stercobilinogen (faecal urobilinogen). Some is absorbed into the portal circulation, most of which is re-excreted in bile (*enterohepatic circulation*). A small fraction enters the systemic circulation and is excreted in the urine as *urobilinogen*, which can be oxidized to a coloured pigment, *urobilin.*

Urobilinogen, in contrast to bilirubin, is often detectable in the urine of normal people by testing with commercial strips, particularly if the urine, and therefore the urobilinogen, is concentrated. Urinary urobilinogen is increased when:

- *haemolysis* is very severe. Large amounts of bilirubin enter the intestinal lumen and are converted to stercobilinogen. An increased amount of urobilinogen is formed and absorbed. If the hepatic capacity to resecrete it is exceeded, it is passed in the urine;
- *liver damage* impairs re-excretion of normal amounts of urobilinogen into the bile.

Urinary urobilinogen excretion is so variable in normal subjects that only very high urinary levels, found during acute haemolytic episodes, may occasionally be of diagnostic significance.

The colourless unabsorbed stercobilinogen is oxidized to stercobilin, a pigment which contributes to the brown colour of faeces. Pale stools may, therefore, suggest biliary obstruction.

Urobilin and stercobilin are coloured ('bile pigments').

Biochemical Tests for Liver Disease

The changes in plasma bilirubin concentration in various types of liver disorders have already been outlined.

CELL DAMAGE

Several tests are often misleadingly called 'liver function tests'. However, plasma enzyme activities indicate liver cell membrane damage rather than function. Because these enzymes are also present in other tissues, changes in plasma activities may reflect damage to those tissues rather than to the liver (Chapter 15; Plasma enzymes in diagnosis).

Transaminases (alanine (ALT; GPT) and aspartate (AST; GOT) transaminases). A rise in plasma transaminase activities is a sensitive indicator of damage to cytoplasmic and/or mitochondrial membranes. Plasma enzyme activities rise when the membranes of only very few cells are damaged. Liver cells contain more AST than ALT, but ALT is confined to the cytoplasm in which its concentration is higher than that of AST.

- *In inflammatory or infective conditions*, such as viral hepatitis, the cytoplasmic membrane sustains the main damage; leakage of cytoplasmic contents causes a relatively greater increase in plasma ALT than AST activities.
- *In infiltrative disorders* in which there is damage to both mitochondrial and cytoplasmic membranes, there is a proportionally greater increase in plasma AST activity than ALT.

The relative plasma activities of ALT and AST may help to indicate the type of cell damage.

SYNTHETIC FUNCTION

The measurement of the prothrombin time and plasma albumin concentration may be used to assess function in certain conditions. The hepatic synthetic and secretory capacities are large; only severe and usually prolonged liver disease demonstrably impairs prothrombin and albumin synthesis.

- *Albumin.* Hypoalbuminaemia is such a common finding in many severe illnesses that it is a less specific indicator of impaired synthetic capacity than a prolonged prothrombin time.

- *The prothrombin time* may be prolonged due to *cholestasis*; fat-soluble vitamin K cannot be absorbed normally if fat absorption is impaired due to intestinal bile salt deficiency (p.**256**). The abnormality is then corrected by parenteral administration of the vitamin. A prolonged prothrombin time may also result from severe impairment of synthetic ability if the liver cell mass is greatly reduced; in such cases it is *not* corrected by parenteral administration of vitamin K.

EXCRETORY FUNCTION

A high plasma conjugated bilirubin concentration indicates impaired hepatic excretory function; this may be accompanied by a high plasma alkaline phosphatase activity.

OTHER TESTS FOR LIVER DISEASE

Alkaline phosphatase (ALP) is derived from a number of different tissues including the liver, the osteoblasts in bone and the placenta (p.**306**). Plasma activities rise in cholestatic liver disease because ALP synthesis is increased and the enzyme within the biliary tract is regurgitated into plasma.

Gamma-glutamyltransferase (GGT) is an enzyme derived from the endoplasmic reticulum of the cells of the hepatobiliary tract. As this reticulum proliferates, for example in response to prolonged intake of alcohol and of drugs such as phenobarbitone and phenytoin, synthesis of the enzyme is induced and plasma GGT activity increases. *Therefore raised plasma activities do not necessarily indicate hepatocellular damage.*

Biochemical investigations can be used to investigate hepatic disorders, the mechanisms underlying which can be divided into three main groups; these often coexist, but one usually predominates in any particular condition.

- *Liver-cell damage* is characterized by release of enzymes (aspartate (AST; GOT) and alanine (ALT; GPT) transaminases) from damaged hepatocytes. *Plasma ALT and AST activities are increased.*

- *Cholestasis* is characterized by retention of conjugated bilirubin and of alkaline phosphatase (ALP), and by increased ALP synthesis at the sinusoidal surface. *Plasma conjugated bilirubin levels and alkaline phosphatase activities are increased.*

- Reduced mass of functioning cells, if considerable, is characterized by a reduction in prothrombin and albumin synthesis. *The prothrombin time is prolonged and plasma albumin concentration is reduced.*

Diseases of the Liver

Cholestasis

Cholestasis may be either:

- *intrahepatic*, in which bile secretion from the hepatocytes into the canaliculi is impaired, due to:
  viral hepatitis;
  drugs such as chlorpromazine or toxins such as alcohol;
  inflammation of the biliary tract (cholangitis);
  autoimmune disease (primary biliary cirrhosis);
  cystic fibrosis.
- *extrahepatic*, due to obstruction to the flow of preformed bile through the biliary tract by:
  biliary stones;
  inflammation of the biliary tract;
  pressure on the tract from outside by malignant tissue, usually of the head of the pancreas;
  biliary atresia (rare).

It is essential to distinguish between intra- and extrahepatic causes of cholestasis as surgery is often indicated for the latter but is usually contraindicated for intrahepatic lesions. The biochemical findings are similar. Unless the cause is clinically obvious, evidence of dilated ducts due to extrahepatic obstruction should be sought using ultrasound, CT scanning or cholangiography.

- *Bilirubin* concentrations in plasma may be normal if only part of the biliary system is involved by intrahepatic lesions such as cholangitis, early primary biliary cirrhosis or primary or secondary tumours (p.**286**). Bilirubin can be secreted by the unaffected areas.
- *Alkaline phosphatase* activity is the most sensitive test for cholestasis. Increased synthesis of ALP in the affected ducts increases the activity of this enzyme in plasma. If this is the only abnormal finding, and if the cause is not obvious on other grounds, it must be shown to be of hepatic origin before it is assumed to indicate liver disease (p.**306**).

Patients with prolonged, and more widespread cholestasis may present with severe jaundice and itching due to deposition of retained bile salts in the skin; the plasma bilirubin concentration may be as high as 850 μmol/L (50 mg/dl). More rarely there is bleeding due to malabsorption of vitamin K, with consequent prothrombin deficiency. Cholesterol retention may cause hypercholesterolaemia. Dark urine and pale stools suggest biliary retention of conjugated bilirubin, although steatorrhoea may contribute to the latter finding.

The jaundice caused by extrahepatic obstruction due to malignant tissue is typically painless and progressive, but there may be a history of vague persistent back pain and weight loss. By contrast, intraluminal obstruction by a gall stone may cause severe pain which, like the jaundice, is often intermittent. Gall stones may not always cause such symptoms. If a large stone lodges in the lower end of the common bile duct the picture may be indistinguishable from that of malignant obstruction.

Although most of the findings are directly attributable to cholestasis, back pressure may damage hepatocytes and plasma transaminase activities may increase slightly.

Primary biliary cirrhosis is a rare disorder of unknown aetiology which occurs most commonly in middle-aged women. Destruction and proliferation of the bile ducts produce a predominantly cholestatic picture, with itching and a plasma ALP activity which may be very high. However, because there is a variable degree of hepatocellular destruction, in the early stages the clinical symptoms and histological findings may resemble those of chronic active hepatitis (p.**288**). Jaundice develops late in most patients. Mitochondrial antibodies are detectable in the serum of over 90 per cent of cases; the serum IgM concentration is usually raised.

Prolonged parenteral nutrition may be associated with a progressive increase in plasma ALP activity and a subsequent rise in the plasma transaminases. The cause is not known and the biochemical changes usually return to normal when the parenteral feeding is discontinued. This finding is rarely an indication to stop this treatment.

Acute Hepatitis

The biochemical findings in acute hepatitis are predominantly those of cell membrane damage with an increase in plasma ALT activity greater than that of AST. There may be a superimposed cholestatic picture and, in very severe cases, impaired prothrombin synthesis.

Viral hepatitis may be associated with many viral infections, such as *infectious mononucleosis, rubella and cytomegalovirus*. However, the term is most commonly used to describe three principal types of viral infection in which the clinical features of the acute illness are very similar, although with a different incubation period.

- *Hepatitis A ('infectious hepatitis')*, transmitted by the faecal-oral route as a foodborne infection, is relatively common in schools and other institutions and has an incubation period of between 15 and 45 days. Relapses may occur but it rarely progresses to chronic hepatitis.
- *Hepatitis B ('serum hepatitis')* is transmitted by blood products and other body fluids; it occurs more sporadically than hepatitis A. It has a longer incubation period of between 40 and 180 days. Some patients may be anicteric, some may develop fulminant hepatitis or chronic active hepatitis (p.**288**) and later cirrhosis. They may become asymptomatic carriers of the disease.
- *Hepatitis C (non-A, non-B hepatitis)*, which is usually the result of transfusion of blood or blood products, has an incubation period of between 15 and 50 days. About half the patients develop chronic hepatitis sometimes progressing to cirrhosis.

In all types there may be a three or four day history of anorexia, nausea and tenderness or discomfort over the liver before the onset of jaundice. Some patients remain anicteric. Plasma transaminase activities are very high from the onset of symptoms; they peak about four days later, when jaundice becomes detectable but may remain elevated for several months. Once jaundice appears some of the initial symptoms improve.

In the early stages there is often a *cholestatic element*, with *pale stools*, due to reduced intestinal bilirubin, and *dark urine* due to a *rise in plasma conjugated bilirubin concentration*; unconjugated bilirubin concentrations also increase due to impaired hepatocellular conjugation. Unless cholestasis is severe, in which case the biochemical picture may resemble that described on p.**285**, *plasma bilirubin concentrations rarely exceed 350 μmol/L (about 20 mg/dl) and the plasma ALP activity is only moderately raised or even normal.* If hepatocellular damage is severe and extensive the *prothrombin time may be increased,* and, in cases with cholestasis, malabsorption of vitamin K may be a contributory factor.

Serological findings. Testing for viral antigens, or for antibodies synthesized in response to the virus, can be used to diagnose viral hepatitis.

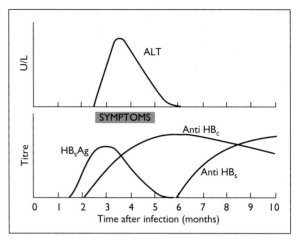

Fig. 14.3 Serological and biochemical changes following infection with hepatitis B virus.

- *Hepatitis A* viral (HAV) antibodies of the IgG class are detectable in the serum of patients at the onset of symptoms. The presence of an IgM anti-HAV antibody is suggestive of previous infection. Most cases of hepatitis A recover completely.
- *Hepatitis B* (HBV) infection, during the prodromal illness, can be diagnosed by the presence in the serum of a viral surface antigen (HB$_s$Ag) and an HB$_e$ antigen, an internal component of the virus. These antigens are short-lived. During the next few weeks an antibody response occurs with the appearance of serum antibodies to the viral core, anti-HB$_c$, to HB$_e$ and finally to the surface antibody, anti-HB$_s$ which may be used to document previous infection (Fig. 14.3).

  The presence of the HB$_e$ antigen correlates with infectivity and its disappearance is a good prognostic sign. HB$_s$Ag may persist, especially in patients with an impaired immune response, and indicates chronicity, associated with raised plasma transaminase activities.
- *Hepatitis C* (HCV; non-A, non-B hepatitis) infection is diagnosed by exclusion. Anti-HCV antibodies may be detected in serum about 12 weeks after exposure to the virus in about half the patients.

Acute alcoholic hepatitis occurs in heavy drinkers, often after a period of increased alcohol intake. Although the clinical features may mimic acute viral hepatitis, the plasma transaminase activities and bilirubin concentration are not usually as markedly

elevated. The finding of a raised plasma γ-glutamyltransferase (GGT) activity, associated with macrocytosis, hyperuricaemia and hypertriglyceridaemia, is suggestive of chronic alcohol ingestion. *None of these findings is diagnostic of alcoholism*; moreover, an alcoholic has an equal chance of developing viral hepatitis as the rest of the population. Alcoholic hepatitis may progress to cirrhosis.

Some drugs and other toxins are hepatotoxic, sometimes directly and sometimes due to a hypersensitivity reaction; in the latter case the damage is not dose-related. The clinical picture may resemble that of acute viral hepatitis. *A drug history is an essential part of the assessment of a patient presenting with liver disease.* Table 14.1 lists some of these drugs.

Chronic Hepatitis

The finding of persistent, usually only slightly, raised plasma transaminase activities, sometimes with chronic or recurrent symptoms suggesting liver disease, may be caused by several disorders. It may be the only abnormal biochemical finding.

Table 14.1 Some drug effects on the liver

	Hepatic necrosis	Hepatitis-like reaction	Chronic hepatitis	Cholestasis
α-methyldopa	+	+	+	+
Carbamazepine				+
Chlorambucil		+		+
Chlordiazepoxide		+		
Chlorpromazine				+
Chlorpropamide				+
Chlortetracycline	+			
Cytotoxic drugs	+*			
Erythromycin				+
Ferrous sulphate	+*			
Halothane	+	+		+
Indomethacin				+
Isoniazid		+	+	
Monoamine oxidase inhibitors (MAO)		+		
Methotrexate			+	
Nitrofurantoin		+	+	+
Oxyphenisatin		+	+	
Para-amino salicylic acid		+		+
Paracetamol (acetaminophen)	+*		+	
Phenothiazines				+
Phenylbutazone		+		+
Phenytoin		+		
Salicylate (aspirin)	+*			
17 α-alkylated steroids (oral contraceptives)				+
Tolbutamide				+
Valproate	+			+

*Indicates that the damage is dose-dependent and predictable.

Chronic persistent hepatitis is a term used to describe the finding of slightly raised plasma transaminase activities without clinical signs or symptoms and without a significant change in their activities over many years. They rarely exceed three times the upper reference limits. Jaundice is unusual. The biochemical findings may be discovered by chance. The condition is probably benign.

Chronic active hepatitis is caused by active hepatocellular destruction with episodes of relapses and remissions. It may progress to cirrhosis. It occurs at any age but is most common in young women. It may:

- be associated with, or a consequence of viral infections, such as HBV or HCV or may be drug-induced;
- be part of an autoimmune process that sometimes involves more than one organ;
- have no obvious cause.

The earliest findings that differentiate it from chronic persistent hepatitis are an increasing plasma IgG concentration, perhaps detected by a rising plasma γ-globulin concentration, and the presence of *smooth muscle and antinuclear antibodies*. As the disease progresses more cells are destroyed and the *plasma AST activity may rise to or exceed that of ALT*; slight jaundice may develop. If there is significant hepatocellular destruction the plasma albumin concentration falls.

Cirrhosis

Cirrhosis is the end result of many inflammatory and metabolic diseases involving the liver, including prolonged toxic damage most usually due to alcohol. In 'cryptogenic cirrhosis' the cause is unknown.

The fibrous scar tissue distorts the hepatic architecture and regenerating nodules of hepatocytes disrupt the blood supply, sometimes increasing the pressure in the portal vein, causing portal hypertension. Blood may be shunted from the portal into the hepatic vein, bypassing the liver.

- In the early stages there may be no abnormal biochemical findings.
- During phases of active cellular destruction the plasma AST, and sometimes ALT, activities rise slightly.
- In advanced cases, the biochemical findings are mostly associated with a reduced functioning cell mass (p.**284**). The vascular shunting allows antigenic substances, which have been absorbed from the intestine, to bypass the normal hepatic sinusoidal filtering process, and to stimulate increased synthesis of IgG and IgA, producing the typical serum protein electrophoretic pattern of β-γ-fusion (p.**317**).

Portal hypertension and impaired lymphatic drainage lead to the accumulation of fluid in the peritoneal cavity (*ascites*). This may be aggravated by hypoalbuminaemia, which may also cause peripheral oedema. In advanced cirrhosis the findings of hepatocellular failure develop.

Primary hepatocellular carcinoma may develop in a cirrhotic liver.

Hepatocellular Failure

Liver damage severe enough to cause obvious clinical signs of impaired hepatocellular function may be caused by severe hepatitis, advanced cirrhosis, or follow an overdose of a liver toxin such as paracetamol (acetaminophen). The biochemical findings may include any or all of those of acute hepatitis. Jaundice is progressive. In the final stage the number of hepatocytes, and so the *total* amount of transaminases released, may

be so reduced that plasma activities fall despite continuing damage to the remaining cells. This finding should not be interpreted as a sign of recovery. Other features may include:

- *hypovolaemia and hypotension* which are due to loss of circulating fluid in ascites and in the oedema fluid formed because of hypoalbuminaemia (p.**35**), and which may be aggravated by vomiting. The resultant low renal blood flow may have two consequences:
  secondary hyperaldosteronism, causing *electrolyte disturbances*, *especially hypokalaemia*, and sometimes dilutional hyponatraemia (p.**48**);
  renal circulatory insufficiency (p.**13**), causing oliguria, a high plasma creatinine concentration and uraemia despite reduced urea synthesis.
- *impaired hepatic deamination of amino acids*, causing accumulation of amino acids in plasma with overflow aminoaciduria and sometimes *hyperammonaemia*. If the reduced formation of urea from amino acids is not balanced by renal retention due to the decrease in GFR, the plasma urea concentration may be low;
- *impairment of hepatic gluconeogenesis* may occasionally cause *hypoglycaemia*.

Hepatic Invasion or Infiltration

Invasion of the liver by secondary carcinoma, or infiltration by lymphoma or granulomas such as sarcoidosis, may be associated with abnormal biochemical tests; sometimes the only abnormal finding is a raised plasma AST activity; the ALT may also be raised to a lesser extent. The picture may reflect cholestasis, with or without jaundice. Metabolic function is rarely demonstrably impaired. If a primary hepatocellular carcinoma develops, either in a cirrhotic liver or *de novo*, the plasma transaminase and ALP activities usually rise rapidly, and plasma α-fetoprotein concentrations are often very high; this latter finding is *not* diagnostic of primary hepatic malignancy (p.**400**).

Metabolic Liver Disease

A group of rare metabolic disorders, most of which are inherited, is associated with liver disease, especially cirrhosis.

α₁-antitrypsin deficiency (p.**326**) is associated with neonatal hepatitis which progresses to cirrhosis in childhood. Often there is basal emphysema.

Diagnosis. This can be confirmed by demonstrating a low plasma α_1-antitrypsin concentration and by identifying the phenotype.

Galactosaemia an autosomal recessive disorder, due most commonly to a deficiency of *hexose-1-phosphate uridylyltransferase* (galactose-1-phosphate uridyltransferase), may cause cirrhosis of the liver if untreated. Liver transplantation may be indicated, if hepatocellular carcinoma, a complication of cirrhosis, develops.

Galactose is necessary for the formation of cerebrosides, of some glycoproteins and, during lactation, of milk. Excess is rapidly converted into glucose. The symptoms of galactosaemia only become apparent if the infant is taking milk; the plasma galactose concentrations then rise. The main features include:

* vomiting and diarrhoea, with failure to thrive;
* prolonged prothrombin time;
* hepatosplenomegaly with jaundice and cirrhosis;
* cataract formation;
* mental retardation;
* renal tubular damage due to deposition of galactose-1-phosphate in the tubular cells (Fanconi syndrome).

Galactose is a reducing substance. The urine may give a positive reaction with Clinitest tablets. This feature may be absent if the subject is not receiving milk and therefore galactose. Tubular damage may cause a generalized aminoaciduria.

Diagnosis. This is made by identifying the reducing substance as galactose by thin-layer chromatography and by demonstrating a deficiency of the enzyme in erythrocytes.

Treatment. Galactose in milk and milk-products should be eliminated from the diet. Sufficient galactose for the body's needs can be synthesized endogenously as UDP-galactose. This will reverse the acute symptoms but not some of the chronic long-term neurological complications.

Wilson's disease (p.**361**) is a rare recessively inherited disorder caused by reduced biliary excretion of copper and by impaired hepatic incorporation of copper into caeruloplasmin. The symptoms are due to excessive accumulation of copper in the liver, brain and kidneys and present with evidence of acute liver failure, chronic hepatitis or cirrhosis in children or in young adults.

Diagnosis. This may be made by finding low plasma copper and caeruloplasmin concentrations and an increased urinary copper excretion. Histological examination with the demonstration of an increased copper content of a liver biopsy specimen is essential to confirm the diagnosis.

Reye's syndrome. This rare disorder presents as acute hepatitis, associated with marked encephalopathy, severe metabolic acidosis and hypoglycaemia in children between the ages of three to about 12 years. There is acute fatty infiltration of the liver. The plasma transaminase activities are high, but plasma bilirubin levels are only slightly raised. The aetiology is uncertain, but the condition may be precipitated by viral infections, such as influenza A or B, drugs such as salicylates and sodium valproate and certain toxins; in some countries it has been recommended that children are not given aspirin.

A number of inherited metabolic disorders, particularly those involving fatty acid oxidation, may present with a Reye-like syndrome in children under about three years.

Haemochromatosis (p.**382**). Idiopathic haemochromatosis is a genetically determined disorder in which slightly increased intestinal absorption of iron over many years produces large iron deposits of parenchymal distribution. It presents, usually in middle age, as cirrhosis with *diabetes mellitus, hypogonadism* and *increase in skin pigmentation*. Because of the darkening of the skin, due to an increased in melanin rather than to iron deposition, the condition has been referred to as 'bronzed diabetes', although the colour is grey rather than bronze. Cardiac manifestations may be prominent, particularly in younger patients, many of whom die of cardiac failure. In about 10 to 20 per cent of cases hepatocellular carcinoma develops.

Idiopathic haemochromatosis has an autosomal recessive mode of inheritance. The gene for this disorder is closely associated with the HLA gene locus, a fact of importance in family studies. Those members of a family with an HLA haplotype identical with that of the patient are likely to develop the disease.

Factors such as alcohol abuse may hasten the accumulation of iron and the development of liver damage.

Diabetes mellitus and hypogonadism may occur in both idiopathic haemochromatosis and alcoholic cirrhosis so that it may be difficult to distinguish between them. The incidence of these complications is higher in idiopathic haemochromatosis but this does not help in the diagnosis of the individual case. Examination of liver biopsy specimens may further confuse the issue. The liver in cases of alcoholic cirrhosis not infrequently contains increased stainable iron. Not only do some alcoholic drinks, notably wines, contain significant amounts of iron, but there is evidence that in cirrhosis there may be increased iron absorption due possibly to the effect of alcohol. However, the majority of patients with cirrhosis do not have increased iron stores as shown by chemical testing, and the liver biopsy specimen shows that the iron is mainly present in the portal tracts. The clinical, histological and biochemical changes of cirrhosis are usually more obvious than those of iron accumula-tion; this contrasts with the picture in haemochromatosis with an apparently equivalent load.

Diagnosis. This may be made by measuring plasma iron concentration and total iron-binding capacity (TIBC), as an indicator of transferrin concentration, with almost total saturation.

Family studies. Relatives of patients with proven idiopathic haemochromatosis must be investigated. Plasma iron concentration and percentage saturation of TIBC are the most sensitive indicators of the disease.

Treatment of End Stage Liver Disease

Liver transplantation may be the only possible treatment for end stage liver disease. Complications include graft failure, hepatic artery thrombosis, infection and acute and chronic rejection. Both acute rejection, which occurs in up to 80 per cent of recipients, and chronic rejection, occurring in about 10 per cent of cases, are associated with a rise in plasma bilirubin concentration and alkaline phosphatase activity; chronic rejection is usually irreversible.

Haemolytic Jaundice

Haemolytic jaundice has been discussed on p.**283**. In adults, unconjugated hyperbilirubinaemia is usually mild because of the large reserve hepatic secretory capacity. The plasma bilirubin concentration is usually less than 70 µmol/L (4 mg/dl). Erythrocytes contain a high concentration of AST and lactate dehydrogenase (LD_1 and LD_2) (p.**303**). After or during severe haemolysis a rise in plasma activities of these enzymes should not be misinterpreted as evidence of myocardial damage or of liver disease.

Jaundice in the Newborn

Red-cell destruction, together with immature hepatic handling of bilirubin, may cause a high plasma level of unconjugated bilirubin in the newborn; so-called 'physiological jaundice' is common (p.**343**). As a result of haemolytic disease, the plasma concentration of unconjugated bilirubin may be as high as 500 µmol/L (30 mg/dl) and exceed the plasma protein-binding capacity; free-unconjugated bilirubin may be deposited in the brain, causing *kernicterus*. Neonatal jaundice and its treatment are discussed more fully on p.**342**.

The course and severity of jaundice may be aggravated by drugs.

- Those, such as sulphonamides and salicylates, which by *displacing bilirubin from plasma albumin*, increase the risk of deposition in the brain. Salicylates should not, in any case, be prescribed for children because of the association with Reye's syndrome.
- Novobiocin *inhibits glucuronyl transferase*, thus exacerbating unconjugated hyperbilirubinaemia.
- Any drug causing *haemolysis* aggravates hyperbilirubinaemia.

The Inherited Hyperbilirubinaemias

There is a group of inherited disorders in which either unconjugated or conjugated hyperbilirubinaemia is the only detectable abnormality.

UNCONJUGATED HYPERBILIRUBINAEMIA

Gilbert's syndrome is a relatively common, familial condition which may be present at any age, but usually after the second decade. Plasma unconjugated bilirubin concentrations are usually between 20 and 40 µmol/L (1.2 and 2.5 mg/dl) and rarely exceed 80 µmol/L

(5 mg/dl). They fluctuate and may rise during intercurrent illness or fasting. The condition is harmless but must be differentiated from haemolysis and hepatitis. It often becomes evident when plasma bilirubin concentrations fail to return to normal after an attack of hepatitis, or during any mild illness which, because of the jaundice, may be misdiagnosed as hepatitis. Although some patients do have shortened red-cell survival, the reason for the hyperbilirubinaemia is not clear and may be due to several factors involved in the hepatic uptake and conjugation of bilirubin.

The other inherited hyperbilirubinaemias are rare.

Crigler–Najjar syndrome, due to deficiency of hepatic glucuronyl transferase, is more serious. It usually presents at birth. The plasma unconjugated bilirubin concentration may increase to concentrations that exceed the binding capacity of albumin and so cause kernicterus. The defect may be:

- *complete* (Type I) and inherited as an autosomal recessive condition;
- *partial* (Type II) and inherited as an autosomal dominant condition. In Type II the plasma bilirubin concentration may be reduced by drugs that induce enzyme synthesis, such as phenobarbitone.

CONJUGATED HYPERBILIRUBINAEMIA

Dubin–Johnson syndrome is harmless and is due to defective excretion of conjugated bilirubin, but not of bile acids, and is characterized by slightly raised plasma conjugated bilirubin levels that tend to fluctuate. Because the bilirubin is conjugated it may be detectable in the urine. Plasma alkaline phosphatase activities are normal. There may be hepatomegaly and the liver is dark brown in appearance due to the presence of a pigment with the staining properties of lipofuscin. The diagnosis may be confirmed by the characteristic staining of a specimen obtained by liver biopsy.

Rotor syndrome is similar in most respects to the Dubin-Johnson syndrome but liver cells are not pigmented.

Bile and Gall Stones

Bile Acids and Bile Salts

Four bile acids are produced in man. Two of these, *cholic acid* and *chenodeoxycholic acid* are synthesized in the liver from cholesterol and are called *primary bile acids*. They are secreted in bile as sodium salts, conjugated with the amino acids glycine or taurine (*primary bile salts*). These are converted by bacteria, within the intestinal lumen, to the *secondary* bile salts, *deoxycholate* and *litho-cholate* respectively (Fig. 14.4).

Secondary bile salts are partly absorbed from the terminal ileum and colon and are re-excreted by the liver (enterohepatic circulation of bile salts). Therefore, bile contains a mixture of primary and secondary bile salts.

Deficiency of bile salts in the intestinal lumen leads to impaired micelle formation and malabsorption of fat (p.**245**). Such deficiency may be caused by cholestatic liver disease (failure of bile salts to reach the intestinal lumen) or by ileal resection or disease (failure of reabsorption causing a reduced bile-salt pool).

FORMATION OF BILE

Between one and two litres of bile are produced by the liver daily. This hepatic bile contains bilirubin, bile salts, phospholipids and cholesterol, as well as electrolytes in concentrations similar to those in plasma. Small amounts of protein are also present.

In the gallbladder there is active reabsorption of sodium, chloride and bicarbonate, together with an isosmotic amount of water. Consequently, gallbladder bile is ten times more concentrated than hepatic bile; sodium is the major cation and bile salts the major anions. The concentrations of other nonabsorbable molecules, such as conjugated bilirubin, cholesterol and phospholipids, also increase.

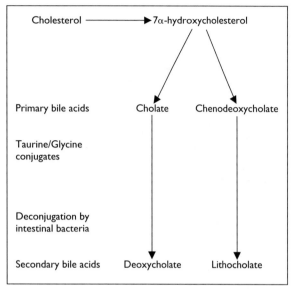

Fig. 14.4 Synthesis of bile acids in the liver and their conversion to secondary bile salts in the intestine.

Gall Stones

Although most gallstones contain all biliary constituents, they consist predominantly of one. Only about 10 per cent contain enough calcium to be radiopaque and in this way differ from renal calculi.

Pigment stones are found in such *chronic haemolytic states* as hereditary spherocytosis. Increased breakdown of haemoglobin increases bilirubin formation and therefore biliary secretion. The stones consist mostly of bile pigments, with variable amounts of calcium. They are small, hard and dark green or black, and are usually multiple. Rarely they contain enough calcium to be radiopaque.

Cholesterol stones. Cholesterol is most likely to precipitate if bile is supersaturated with it; further precipitation on a nucleus of crystals causes progressive enlargement. Not all patients with a high biliary cholesterol concentration suffer from bile stones. Changes in the relative concentrations of different bile salts may favour precipitation. The stones may be single or multiple. They are described as mulberry-like and are either white or yellowish; the cut surface appears crystalline.

There is no association between hyper-cholesterolaemia and the formation of cholesterol gall stones. However, there is an increased incidence in patients taking some lipid lowering drugs, such as the fibric acid derivative clofibrate (p.**237**).

Mixed stones. Most gall stones contain a mixture of bile constituents, usually with a cholesterol nucleus as a starting point. They are multiple, faceted, dark brown stones with a hard shell and a softer centre. They may contain enough calcium to be radiopaque.

Cholesterol and mixed stones are said to be commonest in multiparous women but may be found in either sex or at any age.

CONSEQUENCES OF GALL STONES

Gall stones may remain silent for an indefinite length of time and be discovered only at laparotomy for an unrelated condition. They may, however, lead to several clinical consequences.

- *Biliary colic.*
- *Acute cholecystitis.* Obstruction of the cystic duct by a gallstone causes chemical irritation of the gall bladder mucosa by trapped bile and secondary bacterial infection.
- *Chronic cholecystitis* may also be associated with gallstones.
- *Obstruction of the common bile duct* occurs if a stone lodges in the bile duct. The patient may present with biliary colic, obstructive jaundice which is usually intermittent, or acute pancreatitis if the pancreatic duct is also occluded.
- Extremely rarely gallstones may be associated with *carcinoma of the gall bladder.*

TREATMENT OF GALL STONES

The commonest treatment for symptomatic gall stones is cholecystectomy. Additional approaches include:

- dissolving the gall stone. The bile acid *urodeoxycholic acid* reduces the relative saturation of bile with cholesterol and so facilitates dissolving cholesterol stones, particularly small uncalcified ones;
- shock-wave lithotripsy in which the stone is shattered into tiny fragments and can then pass through the cystic duct.

Summary

Liver Disease

1. The liver has a central role in many metabolic processes.
2. Bilirubin, derived from haemoglobin, is conjugated in the liver and excreted in the

bile. Conversion to stercobilinogen (faecal urobilinogen) takes place in the intestinal lumen. Some reabsorbed urobilinogen is excreted in the urine.
3. Bilirubin metabolism may be assessed by measuring plasma concentrations of bilirubin and by visual inspection of the stool and urine.

4. Jaundice is due to a raised plasma bilirubin concentration either of the unconjugated fraction only, or, in adults, most commonly of both fractions.

5. The results of initial biochemical tests may be characteristic of one or more of three underlying pathological processes:

   • liver cell damage (high transaminases);
   • cholestasis (high alkaline phosphatase);
   • reduced functioning tissue mass (low plasma albumin concentration or prolonged prothrombin time).

   Jaundice may or may not be present with any of these processes.

6. Unconjugated, without conjugated, hyperbilirubinaemia is usually due to haemolysis. In the newborn it may, if severe, exceed the plasma protein-binding capacity, and free unconjugated bilirubin may enter brain cells and cause kernicterus.

7. A group of inherited conditions are characterized by hyperbilirubinaemia. Most are relatively harmless, but the Crigler-Najjar syndrome may cause kernicterus.

Bile and Gall Stones

1. Bile secreted by the liver is concentrated in the gall bladder before passing into the intestinal lumen.

2. Pigment stones may occur in chronic haemolytic states.

3. Cholesterol stones are the commonest and may occur when cholesterol crystals precipitate from supersaturated bile. The initiating factors are unknown.

HANDLING OF SAMPLES FROM PATIENTS WITH POSSIBLE HEPATITIS OR ACQUIRED IMMUNE DEFICIENCY SYNDROMES (AIDS)

All samples received by laboratory staff should be considered infectious.

Anyone handling a specimen known to be infected (whether medical, nursing, portering or laboratory staff), is at risk. *It is the responsibility of the clinician sending the blood to identify it clearly as potentially dangerous.* This is particularly important for samples from patients:

- with viral hepatitis;
- undiagnosed jaundice;
- positive test for HB$_s$Ag;
- known or suspected HIV (AIDS);
- at risk because they are in a dialysis unit.

The sample must be sent to the laboratory in leak-proof tubes in a sealed plastic bag and be clearly labelled as a biohazard. Strict adherence to the local safety policy is mandatory. In many countries national guidelines have been produced for the handling of infectious specimens. It is strongly recommended that investigations should not be carried out if these guidelines are contravened.

INVESTIGATION OF SUSPECTED LIVER DISEASE

The commonly available laboratory tests for the diagnosis of liver disease are measurement of plasma levels of:

- bilirubin – excretory function;
- transaminases (ALT and/or AST) – hepatocellular damage;
- alkaline phosphatase (ALP) – cholestasis;
- albumin and/or prothrombin time – synthetic function.

The initial selection of investigations depends on the age of the patient, the history and clinical features. Different diseases may, however, present in a similar way and a single disorder may present in more than one way. In this section we will consider the differential diagnosis of clinical problems.

JAUNDICE AS A PRESENTING FEATURE

Whereas a patient with chronic liver disease may present with jaundice, the differential diagnosis of jaundice with bilirubinuria (due to conjugated bilirubin) in a previously well patient is usually between acute hepatocellular damage and cholestasis.

1. When taking the history pay special attention to:

   - recent exposure to hepatitis or infectious mononucleosis;
   - recent administration of blood or blood-products;
   - oral drug and alcohol intake;
   - intravenous drug abuse;
   - associated symptoms such as abdominal pain, pruritus, weight loss or anorexia and nausea;
   - recent changes in the colour of the urine or stools.

2. On examination look for:

   - hepatomegaly;
   - signs of liver decompensation such as liver flap, 'liver palms' etc.;

- a marked increase in urinary urobilino-gen without bilirubinuria, in the presence of jaundice. This suggests haemolysis as a cause. Inspect the colour of the urine and stools. Dark yellow or brown urine and pale stools suggest biliary obstruction. Fresh urine containing only urobilinogen is initially of normal colour.

The examination of a *fresh* urine sample may be included as part of the physical examination of the patient. This test may confirm the presence of bilirubin, and so of conjugated hyperbilirubinaemia. Reagent strips are available for testing for bilirubin and urobilinogen.

- **Ictostix** includes stabilized, diazotized 2,4-dichloraniline, which reacts with biliru-bin to form azobilirubin. These reagents are incorporated in multiple test sticks. The test will detect about 3 μmol/L (0.2 mg/dl) of *bilirubin*. Drugs, such as large doses of chlorpromazine, may give false positive results.
- **Urobilistix** includes paradimethylamino-benzaldehyde, also incorporated in multi-ple test sticks, which reacts with *urobilinogen*. Urobilistix does not react with porphobilinogen. This test will detect urobilinogen in urine from some normal subjects. *False positive* results may occur after taking drugs such as *p*-aminosalicylic acid and some sulphonamides.

All reagent strips must be stored, and the tests performed strictly according to the manufacturer's instructions.

3. Whatever the results of the urine and stool inspection and testing, request plasma transaminase and alkaline phosphatase assays:

- *in hepatitis*, there is a predominant increase in the plasma transaminases; the plasma ALT activity is higher than the AST. If hepatitis or infectious mononucleosis is suggested by the history, request serological tests (p.**287**);

- *in cholestasis*, there is predominant elevation of the plasma ALP activity. Bile duct dilation should be sought using ultrasound or radiological tests:
  if the bile ducts are dilated there is obstruction that may require surgery; if the plasma ALP activity is high but dilated ducts are not demonstrated there is probably intrahepatic cholestasis. Request serological tests for hepatitis, smooth muscle, mitochondrial and nuclear antibodies and immunoglobulin levels.

If the diagnosis is still in doubt, and if the prothrombin time is normal (a prolonged prothrombin time increases the chance of bleeding), a liver biopsy may be indicated.

4. If acute alcoholic hepatitis is suspected contributory evidence may be the finding of a disproportionately high plasma gamma-glutamyltransferase activity compared with those of transaminases, and of macrocytosis, hypertriglyceridaemia and hyperuricaemia.

None of these findings is diagnostic.

SUSPECTED CHRONIC LIVER DISEASE, WITH OR WITHOUT JAUNDICE

1. Relevant points in the clinical evaluation are:

- a previous history of hepatitis;
- alcohol intake;
- the presence, or history, of other autoimmune disorders;
- pruritus or features of malabsorption.

2. Request plasma transaminases and alkaline phosphatase assays.

- A plasma ALT activity higher than that of the AST may be due to reversible alcoholic hepatitis, to chronic persistent hepatitis, or to early chronic active hepatitis;
- A plasma AST activity higher than that of ALT may be due to cirrhosis or severe chronic active hepatitis;
- A high plasma ALP activity suggests cholestasis.

3. A high blood alcohol concentration, despite denial of drinking by the patient suggests, but *does not prove*, an alcoholic aetiology.
4. Detectable plasma mitochondrial or smooth-muscle antibodies suggest a non-alcoholic cause.
5. Serum protein electrophoresis and immunoglobulin assay may help in the diagnosis of:

- cirrhosis, high serum IgG and IgA concentrations causing β-γ fusion on the electrophoretic strip;
- chronic active hepatitis, a high serum IgG concentration and normal IgA;
- primary biliary cirrhosis, a high serum IgM concentration.

HEPATIC INVASION AND INFILTRATION

1. Significant infiltration of the liver by tumour cells, or by granulomas such as sarcoidosis, may occur without detectable biochemical abnormality, or there may be any of the changes described on p.**289**. In this situation measurement of the plasma AST activity, usually the most sensitive test, may be high despite a normal plasma ALT activity.
2. If primary hepatocellular carcinoma is suspected, the plasma ALP activity and α-fetoprotein level may also be high.
3. Radionuclide scans or other imaging procedures, or a liver biopsy, may be indicated.

UNCONJUGATED HYPERBILIRUBINAEMIA

Predominantly unconjugated hyperbilirubinaemia with plasma conjugated bilirubin levels less than about 10 per cent of the total, and with little or no bilirubinuria, may be due to:

- an increased bilirubin load. If there is no obvious cause, such as extensive bruising, haematological tests for haemolysis are indicated;
- inherited defects of bilirubin uptake or conjugation (p.**292**). Other tests for liver disease are usually normal, and the diagnosis is made by the exclusion of evidence for haemolysis.

A greatly increased bilirubin load may result in an increased urinary urobilinogen excretion (p.**283**).

Plasma Enzymes in Diagnosis

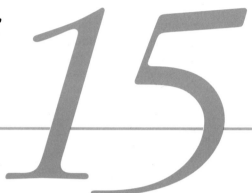

15

An enzyme is a protein that catalyses one or more specific biochemical reactions. It is easier to measure enzyme *activity* in body fluids, by monitoring changes in either substrate or product concentrations, than to measure enzyme protein concentration directly. Very low concentrations result in a large increase in rate of substrate utilization and product formation *in vitro*. However measurement of the protein concentration is more specific and less prone to analytical variation but is significantly more expensive.

Most enzymes are present in cells at much higher concentrations than in plasma. Some occur predominantly in cells of certain tissues, where they may be located in different cellular compartments such as the cytoplasm or the mitochondria. 'Normal' plasma enzyme levels reflect the balance between the rate of synthesis and release into plasma during cell turnover, and the rate of clearance from the circulation.

The enzyme activity in plasma may be:

- *increased* due to proliferation of cells, an increase in the rate of cell turnover or damage or in enzyme synthesis (induction), or to reduced clearance from plasma;
- *lower than normal*, very occasionally due to reduced synthesis, congenital deficiency or the presence of inherited variants of relatively low biological activity; examples of the latter are the cholinesterase variants (p.**311**).

Changes in plasma enzyme activities may sometimes help to detect and localize tissue cell damage or proliferation, or to monitor treatment and progress of disease.

Assessment of Cell Damage and Proliferation

Plasma enzyme levels depend on:

- the rate of release from damaged cells which, in turn, depends on the rate at which damage is occurring;
- the extent of cell damage.

In the absence of cell damage the rate of release depends on:

- the rate of cell proliferation;
- the degree of induction of enzyme synthesis.

These factors are balanced by:

- the rate of enzyme clearance from the circulation.

Acute cell damage, for example in viral hepatitis, may cause very high plasma enzyme activities that fall as the condition resolves. By contrast, the liver may be much more extensively involved in advanced cirrhosis but the *rate* of cell damage is often low and consequently plasma enzyme activities may be only slightly raised or be within the reference range. In very severe liver disease plasma enzyme activities may even fall terminally, when the number of hepatocytes is grossly reduced.

It is not known how most enzymes are removed from, or their action inhibited in, the circulation. Relatively small peptides, such as α-amylase, can be cleared by the kidneys; most enzymes are large proteins and are probably catabolized by plasma proteases before being taken up by the reticuloendothelial system. In health each enzyme has a fairly constant and characteristic biological half-life; a knowledge of this half-life may be of help in assessing the time since the onset of an acute illness. After a myocardial infarction, for example, plasma levels of creatine kinase and aspartate transaminase fall to normal before those of lactate dehydrogenase, which has a longer half-life. The half-life may be lengthened if there is circulatory impairment.

Renal glomerular impairment may delay the rate of fall of those plasma enzymes cleared through the kidneys. For example plasma amylase activity may be high due to renal glomerular impairment, rather than to pancreatic damage.

Localization of Damage

Most of the enzymes commonly measured to assess tissue damage are present in nearly all cells, although their relative concentrations in certain tissues may differ. Measurement of the plasma activity of an enzyme known to be in high concentration within cells of a particular tissue may indicate an abnormality of those cells, but the results will rarely enable a specific diagnosis to be made. For example, if there is circulatory failure after a cardiac arrest very high plasma levels of enzymes originating from many tissues may occur because of hypoxic damage to cells and reduced rates of clearance; the raised plasma levels of 'cardiac' enzymes do not necessarily mean that a myocardial infarct caused the arrest.

The diagnostic precision of plasma enzyme analysis may be improved by:

- *estimation of more than one enzyme.* Many enzymes are widely distributed, but their relative concentrations may vary in different tissues. For instance, although both alanine and aspartate transaminases are abundant in the liver, the concentration of aspartate transaminase is much greater than that of alanine transaminase in heart muscle;
- *isoenzyme determination.* Some enzymes exist in more than one form; these isoenzymes may be separated by their different physical or chemical properties. If they originate in different tissues such identification will give more information than the measurement of plasma total enzyme activity; for example, creatine kinase may be derived from skeletal or cardiac muscle, but one of its isoenzymes is found predominantly in the myocardium;
- *serial enzyme estimations.* The rate of change of plasma enzyme activity is related to a balance between the rate of entry and the rate of removal from the circulation. A persistently raised plasma enzyme activity is suggestive of a chronic

disorder or occasionally of impaired clearance.

The distribution of enzymes within cells may differ. Alanine transaminase and lactate dehydrogenase are predominantly located in cytoplasm and glutamate dehydrogenase in mitochondria, whereas aspartate transaminase occurs in both these cellular compartments. Different disease processes in the same tissue may affect the cell in different ways, causing alteration in the relative plasma enzyme activities (p.**284**).

Non-specific Causes of Raised Plasma Enzyme Activities

Before attributing a change in plasma enzyme activity to a specific disease process it is important to exclude the presence of factitious or nonspecific causes.

Slight rises in plasma aspartate transaminase activities are common, non-specific findings in many illnesses. Moderate exercise, or a large intramuscular injection, may lead to a rise in plasma creatine kinase activity; isoenzyme determination may identify skeletal muscle as the tissue of origin (p.**304**).

Some drugs, such as the anticonvulsants phenytoin and phenobarbitone, may induce synthesis of the microsomal enzyme, gamma-glutamyltransferase, and so increase its plasma activity in the absence of disease.

Plasma enzyme activities may be raised if the rate of clearance from the circulation is reduced. In the absence of hepatic or renal disease this may occur if, for example, the plasma enzyme forms:

- macromolecules (aggregates), such as in macroamylasaemia (p.**305**);
- complexes with immunoglobulins, as occasionally occur with lactate dehydrogenase, alkaline phosphatase or creatine kinase.

Factors Affecting Results of Plasma Enzyme Assays

Analytical factors affecting results. The total concentration of all plasma enzyme proteins is less than 1 g/L. Results of enzyme assays are not usually expressed as concentrations, but as activities. Changes in concentration may give rise to proportional changes in catalytic activity, but the results of such measurements depend on many analytical factors. These include the concentrations of the substrate and product, the pH and temperature at which the reaction is carried out, the type of buffer, and the presence of activators or inhibitors. *Because the definition of 'international units' does not take these factors into account, results from different laboratories, apparently expressed in the same units, may not be directly comparable.* Therefore, plasma enzyme activities must be interpreted in relation to the reference ranges from the issuing laboratory.

Physiological factors affecting enzyme activities, include for example:

- *age*:
    plasma aspartate transaminase activity is moderately higher during the neonatal period than in adults;
    plasma alkaline phosphatase activity of bony origin is higher in children than in adults and peaks during the pubertal bone growth spurt before falling to adult levels.
- *sex*:
    plasma γ-glutamyltransferase activity is higher in men than in women (p.**308**).
- *physiological conditions*:
    plasma alkaline phosphatase activity rises during the last trimester of pregnancy because of the presence of the placental isoenzyme;
    several enzymes, such as the transaminases and creatine kinase, rise moderately in plasma during and immediately after labour or strenous exercise.

Plasma enzyme activities must be interpreted in relation to the sex- and age-matched reference ranges of the issuing laboratory.

ABNORMAL PLASMA ENZYME ACTIVITIES

In the following section individual enzymes of clinical importance will be considered. Applications of their assays in defined clinical situations will be discussed later in the chapter.

tor, pyridoxal phosphate for optimal activity. They are widely distributed in the body.

Transaminases

The transaminases are enzymes involved in the transfer of an amino group from a 2-amino- to a 2-oxoacid; they need the cofac-

Aspartate Transaminase (AST)

AST (glutamate oxaloacetate transaminase, GOT) is present in high concentrations in cells of cardiac and skeletal muscle, liver, kidney and erythrocytes. Damage to any of these tissues may increase plasma AST levels.

CAUSES OF RAISED PLASMA AST ACTIVITIES

- *Artefactual*:
    due to *in vitro* release from erythrocytes if there is haemolysis or if separation of plasma from cells is delayed.
- *Physiological*:
    during the neonatal period (about 1.5 times the upper adult reference limit).
- *Marked increase* (10 to 100 times the upper adult reference limit):
    circulatory failure with 'shock' and hypoxia (p.**301**);
    myocardial infarction (p.**308**);
    acute viral or toxic hepatitis (p.**286**).
- *Moderate increase*:
    cirrhosis (may be normal, but may rise to twice the upper adult reference limit);
    infectious mononucleosis (due to liver involvement);
    cholestatic jaundice (up to 10 times the upper adult reference limit);
    malignant infiltration of the liver (may be normal, but may rise to twice the upper reference limit);
    skeletal muscle disease (p.**310**);
    after trauma or surgery (especially after cardiac surgery);
    severe haemolytic episodes (of erythrocyte origin).

Alanine Transaminase (ALT)

ALT (glutamate pyruvate transaminase, GPT) is present in high concentrations in liver and, to a lesser extent, in skeletal muscle, kidney and heart.

CAUSES OF RAISED PLASMA ALT ACTIVITIES

- *Marked increase* (10 to 100 times the upper limit of the adult reference range):

circulatory failure with 'shock' and hypoxia;
acute viral or toxic hepatitis.
- *Moderate increase:*
    cirrhosis (may be normal or up to twice the upper adult reference limit);
    infectious mononucleosis (due to liver involvement);
    liver congestion secondary to congestive cardiac failure;
    cholestatic jaundice (up to 10 times the upper reference limit in adults);
    surgery or extensive trauma and skeletal muscle disease (much less affected than AST).

Lactate Dehydrogenase (LD)

LD catalyses the reversible interconversion of lactate and pyruvate. The enzyme is widely distributed in the body, with high concentrations in cells of cardiac and skeletal muscle, liver, kidney, brain and erythrocytes; measurement of plasma total LD activity is therefore a non-specific marker of cell damage.

CAUSES OF RAISED PLASMA TOTAL LD ACTIVITY

- *Artefactual*:
    due to *in vitro* haemolysis or delayed separation of plasma from whole blood.
- *Marked increase* (more than 5 times the upper reference limit in adults):
    circulatory failure with 'shock' and hypoxia;
    myocardial infarction (p.**308**);
    some haematological disorders. In blood diseases such as megaloblastic anaemia, acute leukaemias and lymphomas, very high levels (up to 20 times the upper reference limit in adults) may be found. Smaller increases occur in other disorders of erythropoiesis such as thalassaemia, myelofibrosis and haemolytic anaemias;

renal infarction, or occasionally during rejection of a renal transplant.
- *Moderate increase*:
  viral hepatitis;
  malignancy of any tissue;
  skeletal muscle disease;
  pulmonary embolism;
  infectious mononucleosis.

ISOENZYMES OF LD

Five isoenzymes can be detected by electrophoresis and are referred to as LD_1 to LD_5. LD_1, the fraction which migrates fastest towards the anode, predominates in cells of cardiac muscle, erythrocytes and kidneys. The slowest moving isoenzyme, LD_5, is the most abundant form in the liver and in skeletal muscle. Whereas in many conditions there is an increase in all fractions, the finding of certain patterns is of diagnostic value.

- Predominant elevation of LD_1 and LD_2 (LD_1 greater than LD_2) occurs after myocardial infarction, in megaloblastic anaemia and after renal infarction.
- Predominant elevation of LD_2 and LD_3 occurs in acute leukaemia; LD_3 is the main isoenzyme elevated due to malignancy of many tissues.
- Elevation of LD_5 occurs after damage to the liver or skeletal muscle.

It is rarely necessary to quantify LD isoenzyme activity. A rise in LD_1 is most significant in the diagnosis of myocardial infarction. However as LD_1 and, to a lesser extent LD_2 and LD_3, can use 2-hydroxybutyrate as well as lactate as substrate some laboratories assay hydroxybutyrate dehydrogenase (HBD) as an index of LD_1 activity (p.**309**). Immunological methods for the specific measurement of LD_1 are available but are relatively expensive.

Creatine Kinase (CK)

CK is most abundant in cells of cardiac and skeletal muscle and in brain, but also occurs in other tissues such as smooth muscle.

CAUSES OF RAISED PLASMA CK ACTIVITIES

- *Artefactual*:
  due to *in vitro* haemolysis, using most methods;
- *Physiological*:
  neonatal period (slightly raised above the adult reference range);
  during and for a few days after parturition;
- *Marked increase*:
  'shock' and circulatory failure;
  myocardial infarction (p.**308**);
  muscular dystrophies (p.**310**) and rhabdomyolysis (breakdown of skeletal muscle);
- *Moderate increase*:
  muscle injury;
  after surgery (for about a week);
  physical exertion. There may be a significant rise in plasma activity after only moderate exercise, muscle cramp or following an epileptic fit;
  after an intramuscular injection;
  hypothyroidism (thyroxine may influence the catabolism of the enzyme);
  alcoholism (possibly partly due to alcoholic myositis);
  some cases of cerebrovascular accident and head injury;
  some patients predispose to malignant hyperpyrexia (p.**363**).

Plasma CK activity is raised in all types of muscular dystrophy, but not usually in neurogenic muscle diseases such as poliomyelitis, myasthenia gravis, multiple sclerosis or Parkinson's disease.

ISOENZYMES OF CK

CK consists of two protein subunits, M and B, which combine to form three isoenzymes, BB (CK-1), MB (CK-2) and MM (CK-3). CK–MM is the predominant isoenzyme in skeletal and cardiac muscle and is detectable in the plasma of normal subjects.

CK–MB accounts for about 35 per cent of the total CK activity in cardiac muscle and less than five per cent in skeletal muscle; its plasma activity is always high after myocardial infarction. The use and limitations of CK–MB estimation are considered on p.**309**. It may be detectable in the plasma of patients with a variety of other disorders in whom the total CK activity is raised, but this accounts for less than six per cent of the total.

CK–BB is present in high concentrations in the brain and in the smooth muscle of the gastrointestinal and genital tracts. Raised plasma activities may occur during parturition. Although they have also been reported after brain damage and in association with malignant tumours of the bronchus, prostate and breast, measurement is not of proven value for diagnosing these conditions. In malignant disease plasma total CK activity is usually normal.

α-*amylase*

Amylase breaks down starch and glycogen to maltose. It is present at a high concentration in pancreatic juice and in saliva and may be extracted from such other tissues as the gonads, Fallopian tubes, skeletal muscle and adipose tissue. In normal subjects most plasma amylase is derived from the pancreas and salivary glands. Being of relatively low molecular weight, it is excreted in the urine.

Estimation of plasma amylase activity is mainly requested to help in the diagnosis of acute pancreatitis, in which the plasma activity may be very high. However, it may also be raised in association with other intra- and extra-abdominal conditions that cause similar acute abdominal pain; a high result is not a specific diagnostic marker for acute pancreatitis.

CAUSES OF RAISED PLASMA AMYLASE ACTIVITY

- *Marked increase* (five to 10 times the upper reference limit):
    acute pancreatitis;
    severe glomerular impairment;

    severe diabetic ketoacidosis;
    perforated peptic ulcer especially if there is perforation into the lesser sac.
- *Moderate increase* (up to five times the upper reference limit):
    other acute abdominal disorders:
        perforated peptic ulcer;
        acute cholecystitis;
        intestinal obstruction;
        abdominal trauma;
        ruptured ectopic pregnancy.
    salivary gland disorders:
        mumps;
        salivary calculi;
        Sjögren's syndrome;
        after injection of contrast medium into salivary ducts for sialography.
    morphine administration (spasm of the sphincter of Oddi);
    severe glomerular dysfunction (may be markedly raised);
    myocardial infarction (occasionally);
    acute alcoholic intoxication;
    diabetic ketoacidosis (may be markedly raised);
    macroamylasaemia.

Macroamylasaemia. In some patients a high plasma amylase activity is due to a low renal excretion of the enzyme, despite normal glomerular function. The condition is symptomless; it is thought that either the enzyme is bound to a high molecular weight plasma component such as protein, or that the amylase molecules form large polymers that cannot pass through the glomerular membrane. This harmless condition may be confused with other causes of hyperamylasaemia.

Pancreatic pseudocyst. If the plasma amylase activity fails to fall after an attack of acute pancreatitis there may be leakage of pancreatic fluid into the lesser sac (a pancreatic pseudocyst). Urinary amylase levels are high, differentiating it from macroamylasaemia. This is one of the few indications for estimating urinary amylase activity, which is inappropriately low relative to the plasma activity if there is glomerular impairment or macroamylasaemia.

ISOENZYMES OF AMYLASE

Plasma amylase is derived from the pancreas and salivary glands. It is rarely necessary to identify the isoenzyme components in plasma, but they can be distinguished by electrophoresis, or by using an inhibitor derived from wheat germ. Possible indications for isoenzyme determination include:

- the coexistence of mumps or renal failure, which complicate the interpretation of high activities due to acute pancreatitis;
- the possibility of chronic pancreatic disease, in which low activities may be found.

Some laboratories now measure the plasma 'pancreatic' amylase activity using a method that incorporates wheat germ rather than starch. The different substrates affect the results and *it is important to interpret the result against the reference range from the same laboratory.*

Alkaline Phosphatase (ALP)

The alkaline phosphatases are a group of enzymes that hydrolyse organic phosphates at high pH. They are present in most tissues but are in particularly high concentration in the osteoblasts of bone and the cells of the hepatobiliary tract, intestinal wall, renal tubules and placenta. The exact metabolic function of ALP is unknown but it is probably important for calcification of bone.

In adults plasma ALP is derived mainly from bone and liver in approximately equal proportions; the proportion due to the bone fraction is increased when there is increased osteoblastic activity that may be physiological.

CAUSES OF RAISED PLASMA ALP ACTIVITY

- *Physiological*:
  during the last trimester of pregnancy the plasma total ALP activity rises due to the contribution of the placental isoenzyme;
  in preterm infants plasma total ALP activity is up to five times the upper reference limit in adults, and consists predominantly of the bone isoenzyme;
  in children the total activity is about 2.5 times, and increases to up to five times, this upper limit during the pubertal bone growth spurt. There is a gradual increase in the proportion of liver ALP with age;
  in the elderly the plasma bone isoenzyme activity may increase slightly.
- *Bone disease*:
  rickets and osteomalacia (p.**181**);
  Paget's disease of bone (may be very high);
  secondary malignant deposits in bone;
  osteogenic sarcoma, only if very extensive;
  primary hyperparathyroidism with extensive bone disease (usually normal but may be slightly elevated) (p.**179**);
  secondary hyperparathyroidism (p.**181**).
- *Liver disease*:
  intra- or extrahepatic cholestasis (p.**285**);
  space-occupying lesions, tumours, granulomas, and other causes of hepatic infiltration.
- *Malignancy*:
  bone or liver involvement or direct tumour production.

A placental-like, so-called 'Regan', isoenzyme may occasionally be identified in plasma in patients with malignant disease, especially carcinoma of the bronchus.

Transient very high levels of ALP have been recorded in children under three years, but the clinical significance of this finding is unknown.

Plasma total ALP activity is not usually increased in myelomatosis despite the X-ray appearance of multiple 'punched-out' osteolytic lesions. The lesions are in the marrow cavity, not the bone substance, and osteoblastic activity is not stimulated. However, ALP activity may be raised if there is liver involvement, or, more rarely, if there is healing of very extensive pathological fractures.

POSSIBLE CAUSES OF LOW PLASMA ALP ACTIVITY

- *Arrested bone growth*:
  achondroplasia;
  cretinism;
  severe ascorbate deficiency.
- *Hypophosphatasia*, an autosomal recessive disorder, associated with rickets or osteomalacia.

ISOENZYMES OF ALKALINE PHOSPHATASE

Bone disease with increased osteoblastic activity, or liver disease with involvement of the biliary tracts, are the commonest causes of an increased total alkaline phosphatase activity.

Rarely the cause is not apparent and further tests may be helpful. The isoenzymes originating from cells of bone, liver, intestine and placenta may be separated by electrophoresis, but interpretation may be difficult if the total activity is only marginally raised. The placental and 'Regan' isoenzymes are more stable at 65°C than the bone, liver and intestinal isoenzymes, and heat inactivation may help to differentiate the heat-stable from the heat-labile fraction.

The placental isoenzyme does not cross the placenta and is therefore not detectable in the plasma of the newborn.

Acid Phosphatase (ACP)

Acid phosphatase is found in cells of the prostate, liver, erythrocytes, platelets and bone. The main indications for estimation are to help diagnose prostatic carcinoma and to monitor its treatment. The estimation is gradually being replaced by the measurement of *plasma prostate specific antigen* (PSA), a protein derived from the prostate. This test is more specific and sensitive for diagnosis and monitoring treatment. However, it may be raised in similar circumstances to those affecting prostatic ACP and is more expensive to estimate.

Normally acid phosphatase drains from the prostate, through the prostatic ducts, into the urethra and very little can be detected in plasma. In extensive prostatic carcinoma, particularly if it has spread extensively or has metastasized, plasma acid phosphatase activity rises, probably because of the increased number of prostatic acid phosphatase-containing cells. If the tumour is small, or is too undifferentiated to synthesize the enzyme, plasma activities may be normal. For this reason the assay is more useful for monitoring the treatment of a known case of disseminated prostatic carcinoma than for making the diagnosis.

SAMPLING FOR ACID PHOSPHATASE ASSAY

Opinions differ about whether rectal examination increases the serum activity by pressure on prostatic cells. The effect is certainly rare if the examination is performed by an experienced clinician. However, we have found that the serum ACP activity can rise to two or three times the upper reference limit in some cases, and that it only falls to its basal level after several days (p.**424**). It is obvious that prostatectomy will release large amounts of the enzyme into the plasma and the assay should not be requested for at least a week after the operation. Heparin inhibits ACP activity, and therefore clotted rather than heparinized blood must be used. The enzyme is unstable and specimens for assay should be sent to the laboratory without delay. Haemolysed specimens must not be assayed, partly because the enzyme is released from blood cells *in vitro*.

ISOENZYMES OF ACID PHOSPHATASE

Release of acid phosphatase from blood cells *in vitro* may occur even in unhaemolysed samples and many methods have been devised in an attempt to measure only the prostatic fraction, without complete success. One method makes use of the fact that L-tartrate inhibits prostatic acid phosphatase; the assay is performed with and without the addition of L-tartrate; the difference in activity between the results, the *tartrate-labile* fraction, is mainly *prostatic* acid phosphatase. Other methods measure the prostatic enzyme protein concentration directly by immunoassay.

Causes of raised serum acid phosphatase activity

- *Tartrate-labile*:
  artefactually following rectal examination, acute retention of urine or passage of a catheter, due to pressure on prostatic cells; disseminated carcinoma of the prostate.
- *Total*:
  artefactually in a haemolysed specimen, or following rectal examination;
  acute retention of urine or passage of a catheter;
  disseminated carcinoma of the prostate;
  Paget's disease of bone;
  some cases of metastatic bone disease, especially with osteosclerotic lesions;
  Gaucher's disease (probably from Gaucher cells);
  occasionally in thrombocythaemia.

The assay is not of diagnostic value in the last four conditions.

Gamma-glutamyl-transferase (GGT)

Gamma-glutamyltransferase occurs mainly in the cells of liver, kidneys, pancreas and prostate. Plasma GGT activity is higher in men than in women.

Causes of raised plasma GGT activity

- *Induction of enzyme synthesis*, without cell damage, by drugs or alcohol. Many drugs, most commonly the anticonvulsants, phenobarbitone and phenytoin, and alcohol induce proliferation of the endoplasmic reticulum.
- *Cholestatic liver disease*, when changes in GGT activity usually parallel those of alkaline phosphatase. In the cholestatic jaundice of pregnancy plasma GGT activities do not increase.
- *Hepatocellular damage*, such as that due to infectious hepatitis; measurement of plasma transaminase activities is a more sensitive indicator of such conditions.

Slightly or moderately raised activities (up to about three times the upper reference limit) are particularly difficult to interpret. Very high plasma GGT activities, out of proportion to those of the transaminases, may be due to:

- alcoholic hepatitis;
- induction by anticonvulsant drugs or by chronic alcohol intake;
- cholestatic liver disease.

A patient should never be labelled an alcoholic because of a high plasma GGT activity alone.

*P*LASMA ENZYME PATTERNS IN DISEASE

Myocardial Infarction

The diagnosis of a myocardial infarction is usually made on the clinical presentation, electrocardiographic findings and confirmed by the characteristic changes in plasma enzyme activities. The plasma enzyme estimations of greatest value are CK, LD (or HBD) and AST. The choice of estimation depends on the time which has elapsed since the suspected infarction. An approximate guide to the sequence of changes is given in Table 15.1.

All plasma enzyme activities (including that of CK–MB) may be normal until at least

Table 15.1 The time sequence of changes in plasma enzymes after myocardial infarction

Enzyme	Starts to rise (hours)	Time after infarction of peak elevation (hours)	Duration of rise (days)
CK (total)	4–6	24–48	3–5
AST	6–8	24–48	4–6
LD (HBD)	12–24	48–72	7–12

four hours after the onset of chest pain due to a myocardial infarction; *blood should not be taken for enzyme assay until this time has elapsed.* If the initial plasma CK activity is normal, a second sample should be taken about four to six hours later. A rise in the plasma CK activity supports the diagnosis of an infarction. The simultaneous measurement of plasma CK–MB activity, which is shown to exceed six per cent of the total CK activity, may occasionally help in the early diagnosis; a raised plasma CK–MB activity or concentration alone is not diagnostic of an infarction. *Once the diagnosis has been confirmed further blood sampling is rarely required.*

The indications for thrombolytic treatment, which must be given early after an infarction, are usually based on the clinical presentation and ECG changes; they very rarely depend on the measurement of plasma cardiac enzymes.

Most of the CK released after a myocardial infarction is the MM isoenzyme, which is found in both skeletal and myocardial muscle and has a longer half-life than the MB fraction. After about 24 hours the finding of a high MM and undetectable MB does not exclude myocardial damage as a cause of high total CK activities; by this time the plasma HBD activity is usually raised. In most cases of suspected myocardial infarction measurement of plasma total CK and LD_1 (HBD) activities, together with the clinical and ECG findings, are adequate to make a diagnosis. Plasma total CK activity alone can be very misleading.

A raised plasma total CK activity, due entirely to the MM isoenzyme, may follow recent intramuscular injection, exercise or surgery; this is more likely if associated with a normal plasma LD_1 (HBD) or AST activity.

Plasma enzyme activities are raised in about 95 per cent of cases of myocardial infarction and are sometimes very high. The degree of rise is a very rough indicator of the size of the infarct, but is of limited prognostic value. The prognosis often depends more on the site than on the size of the infarct. A second rise of plasma enzyme activities after their return to normal may indicate extension of the damage.

Plasma enzyme activities do not usually rise significantly after an episode of angina pectoris without infarction.

The sequence of changes in plasma AST activity after myocardial infarction are similar to those of CK (Table 15.1), although it rises significantly less with respect to the upper reference limit. Even a small myocardial infarct does cause some hepatic congestion due to right-sided heart dysfunction, and this may contribute to the rise of plasma AST activity. This is rarely a diagnostic problem because the increase in plasma AST activity following an infarction is usually much greater. If there is primary hepatic dysfunction, congestive cardiac failure without infarction or pulmonary embolism (which, by impairing pulmonary blood flow, usually causes some hepatic congestion), plasma AST rises whereas LD_1 (HBD), but not total LD, activity usually remains normal.

At the time of writing the measurement of plasma concentrations of cardiac troponin T, a peptide derived from cardiac muscle, is being evaluated as an early and specific marker of acute myocardial infarction.

Liver Disease

Plasma enzyme changes in liver disease are discussed in Chapter 14.

Muscle Disease

In the muscular dystrophies plasma levels of the muscle enzymes, CK and the transaminases, are increased, probably because of leakage from the diseased cells. Results of plasma CK estimation are the more specific. Points to consider in interpretation are:

- activities are *highest* (up to 10 times the upper reference limit or more) in the *early stages of the disease*. Later, when much of the muscle has wasted, they are lower and may even be normal;
- activities are *higher following muscular activity which has been taken immediately after rest* (because of release of CK built up in muscle during rest) than after prolonged activity;
- activities are *higher in the newborn than in adults*.

Similar, but less marked, changes are found in many patients with myositis.

The clinical diagnosis of the Duchenne type of muscular dystrophy can be confirmed by measuring the plasma CK activity, examining a muscle biopsy specimen and by DNA analysis in the majority of cases.

Carriers of the disorder can often be detected by DNA analysis and by finding raised plasma CK activities. The rise is only moderate, and non-specific causes of raised enzyme activities must be excluded (p.**304**). The specimen should be collected:

- at a time when normal plasma activities would be expected to be highest, that is *late in the day after ordinary physical activity* (levels may be normal in known carriers in the morning);

- *not during pregnancy* (levels may be falsely low in early pregnancy);
- at a time when release from normal skeletal muscle is not abnormally high, that is:
  not for 48 hours after severe or prolonged exercise;
  not for 48 hours after an intramuscular injection.

The assay must be performed on a fresh or appropriately stored specimen, preferably on three separate occasions, to minimize errors of interpretation due to random variations in plasma levels. The laboratory should be informed *before* the blood is taken.

Although plasma enzyme activities are usually *normal* in *neurogenic muscular atrophy*, the number of false positives makes such tests unreliable in differentiating these conditions from primary muscle disease.

Enzymes in Malignancy

Plasma total enzyme activities may be raised, or an abnormal isoenzyme detected, in several neoplastic disorders.

- Serum prostatic (tartrate-labile) acid phosphatase activity rises in some cases of malignancy of the prostate gland.
- Any malignancy may be associated with a non-specific increase in plasma LD_1 (HBD) and, occasionally, transaminase activity.
- Plasma transaminase and alkaline phosphatase estimations may be of value to monitor treatment of malignant disease. Raised levels may indicate secondary deposits in liver or, of alkaline phosphatase, in bone. Liver deposits may also cause an increase in plasma LD or GGT.
- Tumours occasionally produce a number of enzymes, such as the 'Regan' ALP isoenzyme, LD (HBD) or CK–BB, assays of which may be used as an aid to diagnosis or for monitoring treatment.

Haematological Disorders

Very high activities of LD (HBD) may be found in megaloblastic anaemias and leukaemias and in other conditions in which bone marrow activity is abnormal. Typically there is much less change in the plasma AST than in the LD (HBD) activities.

Severe *in vivo* haemolysis produces changes in both AST and LD (HBD) activities which mimic those of myocardial infarction.

Plasma Cholinesterase and Suxamethonium Sensitivity

There are normally two isoenzymes of cholinesterase:

- cholinesterase ('pseudocholinesterase'), found in plasma and synthesized mainly in the liver;
- acetylcholinesterase, found predominantly in erythrocytes and nervous tissue.

Causes of decreased plasma cholinesterase activity

- Hepatic parenchymal disease (reduced synthesis).
- Ingestion, or absorption through the skin, of such anticholinesterases as organophosphates.
- Inherited abnormal cholinesterase variants, with low biological activity.

Causes of increased plasma cholinesterase activity

- Recovery from liver damage (actively growing hepatocytes).
- Nephrotic syndrome.

SUXAMETHONIUM SENSITIVITY

The muscle relaxant suxamethonium (succinyl choline; 'scoline') is usually broken down by plasma cholinesterase, and this limits the duration of its action. Giving suxamethonium to patients with a low cholinesterase activity, usually due to an enzyme variant, is often followed by a prolonged period of apnoea ('scoline apnoea'); such patients may need ventilatory support after operation.

The abnormal cholinesterase variants may be classified by measuring the percentage inhibition of the enzyme activity by dibucaine (dibucaine number) or by fluoride (fluoride number).

- A normal dibucaine number despite a low plasma activity suggests that synthesis has been impaired, but does not completely exclude a genetic abnormality.
- A low dibucaine number with a very low activity is usually due to the presence of an abnormal gene.
- Intermediate dibucaine numbers result from other genetic abnormalities, whether homozygous or heterozygous, and the variants may have normal or low activities.

Identification of patients susceptible to suxamethonium, and of their affected relatives, is important. All blood relatives should be traced and investigated to identify their genotype, and so to predict the chance of later anaesthetic risk. All affected individuals should carry a warning card, or should wear some other form of warning (for example, a 'Medic Alert' bracelet).

Summary

1. Enzyme concentrations are high in cells. Natural decay of these cells releases enzymes into the plasma. Plasma activities are usually low but measurable.

2. Plasma enzyme assays are most useful in the detection of raised levels due to cell damage.

3. Assays of selected enzymes may help to identify the damaged tissues, and isoenzyme studies may increase the specificity. In general, a knowledge of the patterns of enzyme changes, together with the clinical and other findings, are needed if a useful interpretation is to be made.

4. Non-specific causes of raised enzyme activities include peripheral circulatory insufficiency, trauma, malignancy and surgery.

5. Artefactual increases may occur in haemolysed samples.

6. Enzyme estimations may be of value in the diagnosis and monitoring of:

- myocardial infarction (CK, LD and its isoenzymes such as HBD, and sometimes AST);
- liver disease (transaminases, ALP and sometimes GGT);
- bone disease (ALP);
- prostatic carcinoma (tartrate-labile ACP);
- acute pancreatitis (α-amylase);
- muscle disorders (CK).

Proteins in Plasma and Urine

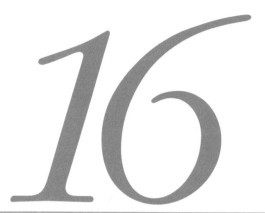

Plasma Proteins

Plasma contains a mixture of proteins differing in origin and function.

METABOLISM OF PROTEINS

The amount of protein in the vascular compartment depends on the balance between the rate of synthesis and the rate of catabolism or loss and the relative distribution between the intra- and extravascular compartments; the *concentration* depends on the relative amounts of protein and water in the vascular compartment. Abnormal concentrations do not necessarily reflect abnormalities in protein metabolism.

- *Synthesis.* Hepatocytes synthesize many plasma proteins; those of the complement system are synthesized both in these cells and by macrophages. Immunoglobulins are mainly derived from the B cells of the immune system.
- *Catabolism and loss.* Most plasma proteins are taken up by pinocytosis into *capillary endothelial cells or mononuclear phagocytes* where they are *catabolized*. Small proteins are *lost passively* through the *renal glomeruli* and *intestinal wall*. Some are reabsorbed, either directly by renal tubular cells or after digestion in the intestinal lumen; some are catabolized by renal tubular cells.

FUNCTIONS OF PLASMA PROTEINS

The following is an outline of the main functions of the plasma proteins. However, the function of many has not yet been identified. Peptide hormones and blood clotting factors contribute quantitatively relatively small, but physiologically important, amounts of plasma protein. Only a few circulating enzymes are functional; most originate from cell breakdown.

- *Inflammatory response and control of infection.* The immunoglobulins and the complement proteins form part of the immune system and the latter, together with a group of proteins known as 'acute-phase reactants', are involved in the inflammatory response.
- *Transport.* Albumin and specific binding proteins transport many hormones, vitamins, lipids, bilirubin, calcium, trace metals and drugs. Combination with protein allows poorly water-soluble substances to be transported in plasma. The protein-bound fraction of many of these is physiologically inactive, unlike the unbound fraction.
- *Control of extracellular fluid distribution.* Distribution of water between the intra- and extravascular compartments is influenced by the colloid osmotic effect of plasma proteins, especially that of albumin (p.**35**).

Methods of Assessing Plasma Proteins

The concentrations of plasma proteins may be expressed either as concentrations (for example g/L) or as activities of those proteins that have defined functions, as for example, clotting times for prothrombin. The distinction is important when abnormal forms of protein are present at normal concentration but with impaired function as, for example, C_1 inhibitor (p.**326**).

Total Proteins

Total protein estimation is of limited clinical value. Acute changes in concentration, like those of all proteins, reflect the ratio of protein to fluid in the vascular compartment. As in the case of sodium (p.**38**), acute changes are more likely to be due to loss from, or gain by, the vascular compartment of protein-free fluid than of protein. Only marked changes of major constituents, such as albumin and immunoglobulins, are likely to alter total protein concentrations significantly.

Plasma total protein concentrations may be misleading for other reasons. They may be normal in the presence of quite marked changes in the constituent proteins. For example:

- a fall in plasma albumin concentration may roughly be balanced by a rise in immunoglobulin concentrations. This is quite common;
- most individual proteins except albumin contribute little to the total protein concentration; quite a large percentage change in the concentration of one may not cause a detectable change in the total protein concentration.

Raised plasma total protein concentrations may be due to:

- loss of protein-free fluid, or excessive stasis during venepuncture (p.**424**);
- a major increase in one or more of the immunoglobulins.

Low plasma total protein concentrations may be due to:

- dilution, for example if blood is taken near the site of an intravenous infusion;
- hypoalbuminaemia (p.**318**);
- profound immunoglobulin deficiency.

Qualitative Methods

ELECTROPHORESIS

Electrophoresis, which separates proteins according to their different electrical charges, is usually performed by applying a small amount of serum to a strip of cellulose acetate or agarose and passing a current across it for a standard time. In this way five main groups of proteins, albumin and the α_1-, α_2-, β-, and γ-globulins, may be distinguished after staining and may be visually compared with those in a normal control serum. Each of the globulin fractions contains several proteins (Fig. 16.1). Changes in electrophoretic patterns are most obvious when:

- the concentrations of protein, such as albumin, which is usually in high concentration, are abnormal;
- there are parallel changes in several proteins in the same fraction;
- a band not present in normal serum is visible.

The following description applies to the normal appearance, in adults, of the principal bands seen after electrophoresis on cellulose acetate:

- **albumin**, usually a single protein, makes up the most obvious band;
- α_1-**globulins** consist almost entirely of α_1-*antitrypsin*;
- α_2-**globulins** consist mainly of α_2-*macroglobulin* and *haptoglobin*;
- β-**globulins** often separate into two; β_1 consists mainly of *transferrin* with a contribution from LDL and β_2 consists of the C_3 *component of complement*;
- γ-**globulins** are *immunoglobulins*. Some immunoglobulins are also found in the α_2 and β regions.

If *plasma* rather than serum is used, *fibrinogen* appears as a distinct band in the β–γ region. This may make interpretation difficult; blood should be allowed to clot and serum used if electrophoresis is to be performed.

ELECTROPHORETIC PATTERNS IN DISEASE (FIG. 16.2)

Some abnormal electrophoretic patterns are characteristic of a particular disorder or group of related disorders, while others indicate

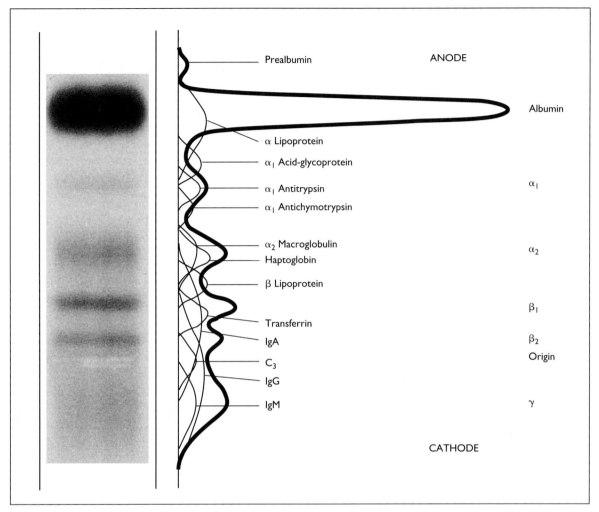

Fig. 16.1 The normal serum electrophoretic pattern. In this example the globulin has separated into β_1 and β_2 fractions. This finding is not invariable, especially in stored specimens.

nonspecific pathological processes. For example, the α_2 band which contains haptoglobin (p.**320**) may be reduced if there is *in vivo* haemolysis and split into two if *in vitro* haemolysis has occurred.

- Parallel *changes in all fractions* (not shown in Fig. 16.2). Reduction may occur in severe malnutrition, sometimes due to malabsorption, unless accompanied by infection and haemodilution. An increase may occur in haemoconcentration;
- *The acute-phase pattern.* Tissue damage of any kind triggers the sequence of biochem-

ical and cellular events associated with inflammation (p.**319**). The biochemical changes include stimulation of synthesis of the so-called *acute-phase proteins*, with a rise in the α_1- and α_2-globulin fractions. The plasma concentrations of these proteins reflect the activity of the inflammatory response and their presence is responsible for the rise in the erythrocyte sedimentation rate (ESR) and increased plasma viscosity characteristic of such a response.

- *Chronic inflammatory states.* In chronic inflammation the usual increase in immunoglobulin synthesis may be visible

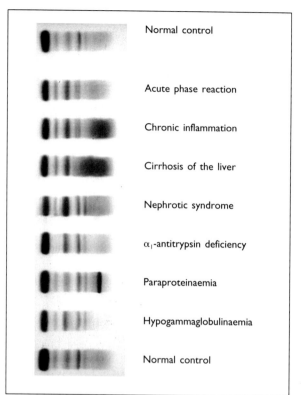

Normal control

Acute phase reaction

Chronic inflammation

Cirrhosis of the liver

Nephrotic syndrome

α_1-antitrypsin deficiency

Paraproteinaemia

Hypogammaglobulinaemia

Normal control

Fig. 16.2 Protein electrophoretic patterns in disease.

as a diffuse rise in γ-globulin. If there is an active inflammatory reaction the increased density in the γ-globulin region is associated with an increase in the α_1- and α_2-fractions of the acute phase response.

- *Cirrhosis of the liver.* The changes in the concentrations of plasma proteins in liver disease are considered more fully on p.**289**. They are usually 'nonspecific', but in cirrhosis a characteristic pattern is sometimes seen. Albumin and often α_1-globulin concentrations are reduced and the γ-globulin concentration markedly raised, with apparent fusion of the β and γ bands because of an increase in plasma IgA concentrations.
- *Nephrotic syndrome.* Plasma protein changes depend on the severity of the renal lesion (p.**332**). In early cases a low plasma albumin concentration may be the only abnormality, but the typical pattern in established cases is a reduced albumin,

α_1- and sometimes γ-globulin bands (Fig. 16.6; p.332) and an increase in α_2-globulin due to a relative or absolute increase in the high molecular-weight α_2-macroglobulin. If the syndrome is due to conditions such as systemic lupus erythematosus (SLE) the γ-globulin may be normal or raised.

- *α_1-antitrypsin deficiency.* The α_1-band consists almost entirely of α_1-antitrypsin and its absence or an obvious reduction in its density suggests α_1-antitrypsin deficiency (p.**326**). Occasionally α_1-antitrypsin variants may present with a split α_1 band.

Paraproteinaemia and hypogammaglobulinaemia are discussed in the sections on immunoglobulins (p.**327** and p.**325**). Although the changes in the electrophoretic pattern usually indicate disease, they are rarely pathognomonic.

Albumin

Albumin, with a molecular weight of about 65 000, is synthesized by the liver. It has a normal plasma biological half-life of about 20 days. About 60 per cent in the extracellular fluid is in the interstitial compartment. However, the *concentration* of albumin in the smaller intravascular compartment is much higher because of the relative impermeability of the blood vessel wall. This concentration gradient across the capillary membrane is important in maintaining plasma volume (p.**35**).

There are several inherited abnormalities of albumin synthesis:

- the *bisalbuminaemias,* in which two forms of albumin are present; these are curiosities only because there are usually no clinical consequences;
- *analbuminaemia* in which there is deficient synthesis of the protein. Clinical consequences are slight, and oedema, although present, is surprisingly mild.

An abnormally high plasma albumin concentration is found only artefactually in a sample taken with prolonged venous stasis (p.**424**) or after loss of protein-free fluid.

Causes of hypoalbuminaemia. A low plasma albumin concentration may be due to dilution or to redistribution. True albumin deficiency may be caused by a decreased rate of synthesis, or by an increased rate of catabolism or loss from the body.

Dilutional hypoalbuminaemia may, as in the case of total protein, result from:

- *artefactual changes* due to taking blood from the arm into which an infusion is flowing (p.**425**);
- *administration of an excess of protein-free fluid*;
- *fluid retention*, usually in oedematous states or during late pregnancy.

Redistribution of albumin from plasma into the interstitial fluid space results from:

- *recumbency*; plasma albumin concentrations may be five to 10 g/L lower in the recumbent than in the upright position because of the redistribution of fluid;
- *increased capillary membrane permeability*. This is the usual cause of the rapid fall in plasma concentration found in many circumstances, for example postoperatively and in most illnesses.

The slight fall in plasma albumin concentration found in mild illness may be due to a combination of the above two factors.

Decreased synthesis of albumin. Normally about four per cent of the body albumin is replaced each day. Hepatic impairment causes hypoalbuminaemia if the rate of synthesis of new amino acids is inadequate to replace those deaminated during metabolism; most of the amino nitrogen is then lost as urinary urea. Hypoalbuminaemia may therefore be due to:

- impairment of synthesis due to *chronic liver dysfunction*;
- *malnutrition* resulting in an inadequate supply of dietary nitrogen;
- *malabsorption* resulting in impaired absorption of dietary peptides and amino acids.

Increased catabolism of albumin. Catabolism, and therefore nitrogen loss, is increased in many illnesses. This may aggravate the hypoalbuminaemia due to other causes.

Increased loss of albumin from the body. Because of its relatively low molecular weight, significant amounts of albumin and other low molecular weight proteins are lost in conditions associated with increased membrane permeability. The plasma concentration of albumin is higher than that of the others and its loss is therefore more obvious. Protein loss occurs through:

- the glomeruli in the nephrotic syndrome (p.**17**);
- the skin because of extensive burns or skin diseases such as psoriasis; a large part of the interstitial fluid is subcutaneous;
- the intestinal wall in protein-losing enteropathy (p.**256**).

Protein loss in the nephrotic syndrome may be selective, with the loss of low molecular weight proteins, such as albumin only.

CONSEQUENCES OF HYPOALBUMINAEMIA

Fluid distribution. Albumin is quantitatively the most important protein contributing to the plasma colloid osmotic pressure (p.**35**). Oedema may occur in severe hypoalbuminaemia.

Binding functions. Albumin binds calcium, bilirubin, free fatty acids and a number of drugs such as salicylates, penicillin and sulphonamides. The albumin-bound fractions are physiologically and pharmacologically inactive. A marked reduction in plasma albumin, by reducing the binding capacity, may increase the plasma free concentration of those substances, not maintained by negative feedback control, and cause toxic effects if, for example, drugs are given in their usual dosage (p.**412**). Albumin-bound drugs may, if administered together, compete for binding sites, thus increasing free concentrations (p.**412**); an example of this is the simultaneous administration of salicylates and the anticoagulant warfarin, potentiating the effect of the latter.

*T*HE INFLAMMATORY RESPONSE AND THE IMMUNE SYSTEM

The body responds to tissue damage and to the presence of infecting organisms or other foreign substances by a complex, interrelated series of cellular and humoral responses. These act together to initiate and control the inflammatory reaction and so to remove damaged tissues and foreign substances. Defence mechanisms can be separated into two main groups:

- *the inflammatory response* which is non-specific and which depends on the changes in permeability of membranes, on humoral factors such as acute-phase reactants, complement or cytokines released in response to inflammation and on a phagocytic cellular response, dependent on the function of polymorphonuclear leucocytes and monocytes;
- *the immune response* in which cellular or humoral factors act on specific foreign organisms. It depends on the function of lymphocytes which can be differentiation into:

  B-lymphocytes, activated by antigens and by lymphokines. They develop into plasma cells in the bone marrow and synthesize and secrete immunoglobulins;

  T-lymphocytes, which, in the thymus, acquire a range of surface antigens that play a vital role in T-cell function after migration to other lymphoid tissue. These include cytotoxicity and delayed hypersensitivity. They also have a regulatory function as either helper or suppressor cells. Each group can be further subdivided using antibodies against the cell surface markers; this is known as cluster differentiation (CD).

The inflammatory response and the ability to kill foreign organisms may be impaired if there is deficiency of either cellular or humoral components.

A more detailed account of the cellular response will be found in textbooks of immunology.

The Inflammatory Response

ACUTE-PHASE PROTEINS

The non-specific changes in plasma protein concentrations, occurring in response to acute or chronic tissue damage, are caused by increased protein synthesis in the liver in response to peptide mediators or *cytokines*.

Cytokines regulate the immune and inflammatory responses. They are classified, depending on their principal biological functions, into groups such as interleukins (IL), interferons (IFN) and tumour necrosis factors (TNF). They activate receptors on adjacent cells (paracrine) or on the same cell (autocrine) but those involved in the inflammatory response, such as the interleukins (IL-1, IL-6) and TNF, affect distant (endocrine) organs. At the time of writing their measurement in plasma as markers of inflammation and tissue cell damage is still being evaluated.

The acute-phase reactants include:

- activators of other inflammatory pathways such as *C-reactive protein* (CRP), so-called because it reacts with the C-polysaccharide of *pneumococci*. This protein combines with bacterial polysaccharides or phospholipids released from damaged tissue to become an activator of the complement pathway; plasma concentrations of CRP rise rapidly in response to acute inflammation and its assay is particularly useful in the early detection of acute infection;

320 PROTEINS IN PLASMA AND URINE

- *inhibitors* such as α_1-antitrypsin, which control the inflammatory response and so minimize damage to host tissue;
- *scavengers* such as haptoglobin which binds haemoglobin released by local *in vivo* haemolysis during the inflammatory response.

The concentrations of plasma *fibrinogen* and of several *complement* components also increase. An acute-phase response increases blood viscosity and therefore the erythrocyte sedimentation rate (ESR). The plasma albumin concentration falls (p.**318**) and secondary decreases of complement and haptoglobin occur if they are used up excessively. Haptoglobin may be undetectable if much haemoglobin is released from red cells due to intravascular haemolysis or haemorrhage into tissues.

The non-specific nature of the response means that measurement of individual acute-phase proteins is rarely helpful as an aid to diagnosis. The demonstration of a rise in plasma CRP concentration is more sensitive and specific than measurement of the ESR and is most often raised in bacterial infections and in other acute inflammatory conditions. Plasma CRP concentrations are not usually increased in viral infections.

COMPLEMENT

The complement group of proteins are synthesized by macrophages or hepatocytes. Because of the presence of inhibitors they usually circulate in an inactive form. Sequential activation, with their use during the inflammatory process reduces their plasma concentrations, but in many instances this is compensated for by increased synthesis of acute-phase reactants. The products of activation attract phagocytes to the area of inflammation (*chemotaxis*) and, by increasing the permeability of the capillary wall to both cellular and chemical components, allows them to reach affected cells. Activation of the complete complement pathway on foreign

cell surfaces results in their lysis and, together with immunoglobulins, some of the complement components act as opsonins, which enhance phagocytosis.

Clinically the most important of the complement proteins is C_3. Two main pathways are concerned with its activation (Fig. 16.3). The names of these pathways reflect the order in which they were discovered, rather than their importance. Activation of either results in low plasma C_3 concentrations.

- *In the alternative pathway*, which is the more important of the two, C_3 is activated by IgA immune complexes and substances such as lipopolysaccharides and peptidoglycans in the walls of certain bacteria and viruses. C_{3b} is formed which in turn activates more C_3. Other products of C_{3b} cause vasodilation and cell lysis. The cyclical process is self-perpetuating and *plasma C_3 concentrations fall.* If the initial stimulus is removed, inhibitors, such as those formed in the acute-phase reaction, control the reaction and C_3 concentrations return to normal. The alternative pathway is most important in the absence of preformed antibodies.
- *In the classical pathway*, C_3 is activated by the products of a pathway initiated by the activation of C_1 usually by antigen-bound IgG or IgM (immune complexes), by protein within the cell walls of many strains of *Staphylococcus aureus*, or by CRP. C_4 (and C_2) are used during the resultant sequence of events, which also activates the alternative pathway via C_3; plasma C_3 and C_4 concentrations fall. Once the formation of immune complexes stops plasma C_3 and C_4 concentrations are restored.

In immune-complex disease, such as systemic lupus erythematosus (SLE) circulating immune complexes persist. The products of C_3, released by continued activation of the classical pathway, may damage blood vessels, joints and the kidneys. Both plasma C_3 and C_4 concentrations are low. Persistently low plasma C_3 concentrations may help to

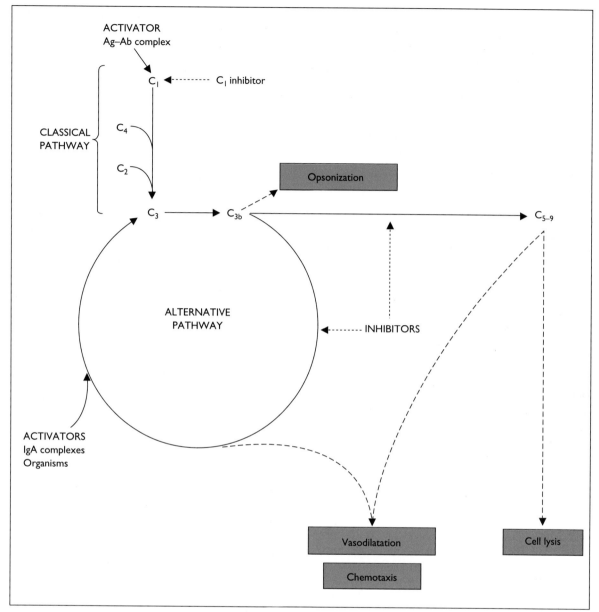

Fig. 16.3 The complement pathway, much simplified.

distinguish chronic mesangiocapillary glomerulonephritis, with a poor prognosis, from the less serious and self-limiting acute post-streptococcal glomerulonephritis, in which plasma C_3 concentrations return to normal within a few months.

This account is, of necessity, simplified. *Before requesting complement studies, contact the laboratory for advice.*

NORMAL CELLULAR RESPONSE TO INFECTION

Two types of phagocytic cells help to combat infection.

- *Polymorphonuclear neutrophil leucocytes* migrate into sites of acute inflammation and represent a non-specific first line of defence against *pyogenic bacteria*.

- *Mononuclear phagocytes* circulate in blood as monocytes. They migrate to sites of chronic inflammation where they develop into macrophages. Under T-cell control macrophages are activated and develop a greatly enhanced ability to phagocytose and digest pathogenic organisms.

The most important functions of T-cells in the inflammatory response are:

- initiation and maintenance of chronic cellular inflammatory responses to invading organisms;
- control of immune inflammation by providing helper and suppressor influences on other cells. B-cells need the co-operation of T-cells (helper cells) to make antibodies to complex antigens

T-cell modulation of inflammatory and immune responses is mediated by chemical messengers called lymphokines. T-cells also have a cytotoxic function directed towards destroying the body's own cells infected by intracellular pathogens such as viruses.

Immune Response

IMMUNOGLOBULINS

Immunoglobulins, synthesized by B lymphocytes, are incorporated into cell membranes, where they act as antigen receptors. On exposure to a specific antigen in the presence of T-helper cells these B lymphocytes proliferate and differentiate into plasma cells synthesizing and secreting immunoglobulins.

Structure

The basic immunoglobulin is a Y-shaped molecule depicted schematically in Fig. 16.4.

- Usually four polypeptide chains are linked by disulphide bonds. There are two heavy (H) and two light (L) chains in each unit. *The H chains* in a single unit are identical and determine the immunoglobulin *class* of the protein. H chains, γ, α, μ,

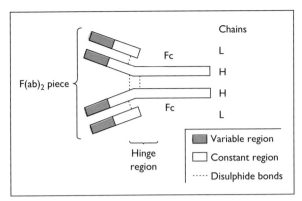

Fig. 16.4 Schematic representation of an immunoglobulin monomer.

δ and ϵ occur in IgG, IgA, IgM, IgD and IgE respectively.
The L chains are of two types, κ and λ. In a single molecule the L chains are of the same type, although the Ig class as a whole contains both types.

- There are two antigen-combining sites per monomer, together known as the $F(ab)_2$ piece. These lie at the ends of the arms of the Y; both H and L chains are necessary for full antibody activity. The amino acid composition of this part of the chain varies in different units (*variable region*). When the $F(ab)_2$ site combines with antigen, conformational changes are transmitted through the hinge region of the heavy chain (Fig. 16.4) and the Fc segment of the molecule becomes activated and reacts with Fc receptors on a number of immune cell types resulting in immune activation.
- The rest of the H and L chains is less variable (*constant region which includes the Fc segment*). The activated Fc segments of the H chains are responsible for such properties as the ability to bind complement or actively to cross the placental membrane. The H chains are associated with a variable amount of carbohydrate; IgM has the highest content.

Some immunoglobulin molecules contain more than one basic unit bound together by 'J' chains; for example, the IgM molecule

Table 16.1   Properties and functions of plasma immunoglobulins

	IgG	IgA	IgM	IgE	IgD
Molecular weight	160 000	160 000 (polymers occur)	1 000 000	200 000	190 000
Sedimentation coefficient	7S	7S	19S	8S	7S
% total plasma Ig	73	19	7	0.001	1
Complement activation	Yes	Yes (as complexes)	Yes	No	No
Placental transfer	Yes	No	No	No	No
Approx. mean normal adult concentration (g/L)	10	2.0	1.0	0.0003	0.03
Adult levels reached by:	3 to 5 years	15 years	9 months	~15 years	~15 years
Major function	Protects extravascular tissue spaces Secondary response to antigen Neutralizes toxins	Protects body surfaces as secretory IgA (11S)	Protects blood stream Primary response to antigen Lyses bacteria	Mast-cell bound antibodies of immediate hypersensitivity reactions	Not known

consists of five units. Because of the variation in size and therefore in density, the classes can be separated by ultracentrifugation. They are classified by their Svedberg coefficient (S), the S value of a protein increasing with increasing size.

The S values, together with the most important functions and properties of immunoglobulins are shown in Table 16.1.

Normal Immunoglobulin Response to Infection

In response to infection each plasma cell produces an immunoglobulin of a single class.

- **IgM** is synthesized first in response to particulate antigens such as blood-borne organisms. Because of their relatively large size they mostly remain in the vascular compartment. This, together with the speed of synthetic response, makes them the first line of defence amongst immunoglobulins against invading organisms. The fetus can synthesize IgM and high plasma concentrations at birth usually

indicate that there has been an intrauterine infection (p.**346**).
- **IgG** concentrations rise slightly later in response to soluble antigens such as bacterial toxins. Because of their relatively low molecular weight they can diffuse into the interstitial fluid and act against tissue infection. Within a few weeks of the initial infection raised plasma concentrations of all immunoglobulins may be demonstrated and may be detectable as a diffusely increased γ zone on the electrophoretic strip.
- **IgA** is synthesized predominantly submucosally and is present in intestinal and respiratory secretions, sweat, tears and colostrum. It is affected more than other immunoglobulins in diseases of the gastrointestinal and respiratory tracts. Secretory IgA is a dimer in which two subunits are joined by a peptide 'J' chain and has a 'secretory piece' synthesized by epithelial cells.

Infections, particularly if chronic, activate B lymphocytes and cause a *polyclonal*

Table 16.2 Some abnormalities of plasma immunoglobulins in disease

Predominant class of Ig increased	Examples of clinical conditions
IgG	Autoimmune diseases, such as SLE and chronic active hepatitis
IgA	Diseases of the intestinal tract, e.g. Crohn's disease Diseases of the respiratory tract, e.g. tuberculosis, bronchiectasis
IgM	Primary biliary cirrhosis Haemoprotozoan infections, such as malaria At birth indicating interuterine infections Viral hepatitis and some acute viral infections
IgG, IgA, IgM	Chronic bacterial infections, sarcoidosis, AIDS

immunoglobulin response. However, immunoglobulin estimation adds little to the observation of increased γ-globulin visible in the serum electrophoretic pattern. In certain conditions, some of which are listed in Table 16.2, one or more immunoglobulin class predominates. Although there is considerable overlap, individual immunoglobulin estimation may occasionally help in the diagnosis of some of these conditions.

Immunoglobulin Response to Allergy

IgE is synthesized by plasma cells beneath the mucosae of the gastrointestinal and respiratory tracts and in the lymphoid tissue of the nasopharynx. Circulating IgE is rapidly bound to cell surfaces, particularly those of mast cells and basophils; plasma concentrations are therefore very *low*. Combination of antigen with this cell-bound antibody stimulates cells to release biologically active mediators and accounts for such immediate hypersensitivity reactions as occur in hay fever, the severest form of hypersensitivity being anaphylactic shock.

Raised plasma IgE concentrations are found in several diseases with an *allergic* (atopic) component such as some cases of eczema, asthma due to allergens ('extrinsic') and parasitic infestation (Table 16.3).

The diagnosis of an allergic disorder is usually made from the history but skin testing and the measurement of plasma IgE concentrations may be needed. In skin testing a small drop of dilute allergen is injected subcutaneously; a positive 'wheal and flare' develops within a few minutes (immediate hypersensitivity). *In patients with a history of eczema or anaphylaxis this test is contraindicated* and plasma IgE may be assessed to detect specific allergens.

Deficiencies of Components of the Inflammatory Response and of Proteins of the Immune System

Deficiencies of the inflammatory or immune response of the host defence system may result in an increased risk of infection and

Table 16.3 Diseases associated with increased serum IgE

Allergic disease (Type I hypersensitivity)	'Extrinsic' asthma Hay fever Atopic eczema Urticaria-angioedema Anaphylaxis
Allergic disease arising secondary to immunodeficiency immunosuppression	Some genetic defects Other primary T cell deficiencies and AIDS
Direct response to infections	Mainly parasitic helminths In Britain consider Echinococcosis, Ascariasis and Toxocariasis

lack of immune regulation. Plasma immunoglobulins reflect only the humoral phase of the immune system; their measurement does not assess cellular immunity. *Normal plasma immunoglobulin concentrations do not exclude an immune deficiency state*; they may, in fact, be raised as in acquired immune deficiency syndrome (AIDS). As a general rule any patient with a severe, protracted, unusual or recurrent infection should be investigated for an underlying deficiency in defence mechanisms.

T-CELL DEFICIENCY

Patients with T-cell deficiency present with severe, protracted infections due to viruses, fungi or rarely detected organisms such as *Pneumocystis carinii* and *Cryptococcus*. It is important to identify T-cell deficiencies because administration of live vaccines and blood products are then strongly contraindicated. T-cell deficiency may be classified as:

- *secondary (acquired) deficiencies*, associated with metabolic disorders such as diabetes mellitus, malnutrition, drug abuse, autoimmunity, malignancy and immunosuppressive treatment or radiation. Secondary T-cell deficiency is relatively common, often mild and presents at any age.
- *primary (congenital) deficiencies*, which are *rare*, often severe and usually present soon after birth. They range from total or partial T-cell depletion or loss of function.

T-cells may be decreased in number or may function abnormally. The total lymphocyte count may be normal despite severe T-lymphopaenia, such as occurs in acquired deficiencies or malignancy as in chronic lymphocytic leukaemia. T-cell function may be assessed by determining cell-surface markers and therefore changes in the different T-cell subsets. Changes in the ratio of helper to suppressor cells occur in many conditions but are profound in AIDS in which the virus specifically affects the CD4 cell population (p.**319**).

IMMUNOGLOBULIN DEFICIENCY

A marked reduction in plasma immunoglobulin concentrations may be detectable as obvious hypogammaglobulinaemia in the serum electrophoretic pattern, but usually measurement of individual proteins is needed to make a diagnosis. The effects of deficiencies of individual immunoglobulins are related to their functions and distribution.

- *IgM deficiency* frequently predisposes to septicaemia.
- *IgG deficiency* may result in recurrent pyogenic infections of tissue spaces, especially in the lungs and skin, by toxin-producing organisms such as staphylococci and *streptococci*. Those susceptible may be identified by determining which of four IgG subclasses is deficient.
- *IgA* deficiency may be symptomless, or may be associated with recurrent, mild respiratory tract infections or intestinal diseases.

Primary immunoglobulin deficiency is less common than that secondary to other disease.

Several classifications have been proposed for these deficiencies and three groups will be discussed.

Transient immunoglobulin deficiency. In the newborn infant circulating IgG is derived from the mother by active placental transfer. Plasma concentrations decrease over the first three to six months of life and then gradually rise as endogenous IgG synthesis increases. In some infants onset of synthesis is delayed and 'physiological hypogammaglobulinaemia' may persist for several months.

Most of the IgG transfer across the placenta takes place in the last three months of pregnancy. Severe deficiency may therefore develop in very premature babies because the concentration of IgG derived from the mother falls before the endogenous concentration rises.

Primary immunoglobulin deficiency. Primary IgA deficiency in plasma, saliva and other secretions is relatively common, with an incidence of about 1 in 500 of the population. Most are symptom-free.

Several rare syndromes, usually familial, have been described. In *infantile sex-linked agammaglobulinaemia* (Bruton's disease), which occurs only in males, there is almost complete absence of B-cells and circulating immunoglobulins, while cellular (T-cell) immunity is normal. Other syndromes have varying degrees of immunoglobulin deficiency and impaired cellular immunity and can occur in either sex.

Secondary immunoglobulin deficiency. Low plasma immunoglobulin concentrations are commonest in patients with malignant disease, particularly of the haemopoietic and immune systems, and are often precipitated by chemo- or radiotherapy; they are an almost invariable finding in patients with myelomatosis. In severe protein-losing states, such as the nephrotic syndrome, low plasma immunoglobulin concentrations (especially of IgG) are partly due to the loss of relatively low molecular weight immunoglobulins and partly due to increased catabolism.

Deficiencies of Other Proteins of the Inflammatory Response

Other proteins involved in complement activation or as acute-phase reactants may be deficient in addition to immunoglobulins. The most clinically significant are discussed below.

COMPLEMENT DEFICIENCY

Inherited deficiencies of most of the proteins of the complement system have been described. They may be associated with repeated infection or immune-complex disease or may have no clinical consequences. Most are extremely rare.

In *hereditary angioneurotic oedema*, C_1 inhibitor (Fig. 16.3, p.**321**) is deficient or non-functioning. The condition is characterized by episodes of increased capillary permeability and consequent oedema of the subcutaneous

tissues and mucous membranes of the upper respiratory or gastrointestinal tract. Laryngeal oedema may be fatal. Plasma C_1 inhibitor concentration or activity can be measured.

α_1-ANTITRYPSIN DEFICIENCY

α_1-antitrypsin normally controls the proteolytic action of lysosomal enzymes from phagocytes (protease inhibitors; PI), and is an acute phase reactant. Plasma concentrations rise two to three days after trauma or acute infection.

There are more than 50 genetic variants of α_1-antitrypsin, inherited as autosomal codominant alleles. The most common allele is PIM with a genotype MM. At least seven of the phenotypes are associated with low functional plasma α_1-antitrypsin concentrations, the most important of which is PInull, associated with complete deficiency of the protein. Others include PIS and PIZ, in which protein accumulates in the liver because it cannot be secreted after synthesis and PIM duarte in which plasma concentrations of the protein may be normal but there is deficient functional activity.

α_1-antitrypsin deficiency may be suspected after serum electrophoresis if the α_1 band is much reduced, absent (Fig. 16.2, p.**317**) or split; the condition may present clinically with:

- *pulmonary disease*. The unopposed action of proteases from phagocytes in the lung may, by destroying elastic tissue, cause basal panlobular emphysema in adults, aged between 30 and 40 years, who are homozygous for the abnormal alleles; the condition may be exacerbated by cigarette smoking, air pollution or infection.
- *hepatic cirrhosis*, occurring in 10 to 20 per cent of subjects, such as those with PIZZ, in whom the protein cannot be secreted by hepatocytes; the condition may present as hepatitis in the neonatal period or as cirrhosis in children or young adults.

The diagnosis can usually be confirmed by demonstrating that the plasma α_1-antitrypsin concentration is low; the phenotype should then be identified. Blood relations should be investigated and all those with abnormal plasma concentrations should receive genetic counselling and be advised not to smoke.

B-cell Disorders

Each B-cell clone is highly specialized and synthesizes a single class and type of immunoglobulin. The normal B-cell response to an antigenic stimulation, such as infection, is synthesis of a range of different immunoglobulins by groups (clones) of cells. This is known as a *polyclonal response* and causes a diffuse hypergammaglobulinaemia in the electrophoretic pattern. If one of these cells proliferates to form a clone of like cells, a single protein will be produced in excess. This *monoclonal* proliferation of B cells is often, but not always, malignant.

PARAPROTEINAEMIA

The term 'paraprotein' refers to the appearance of an abnormal, narrow, dense band on the electrophoretic strip. It is found most commonly in the gamma but may be anywhere from the α_2 to the γ region (Fig. 16.5). A paraprotein can often be shown to be monoclonal.

Causes of paraproteinaemia. Although the presence of a paraprotein is strongly suggestive, it is not diagnostic of a malignant process. Paraproteins may be found in the following malignant conditions:

* *myelomatosis*, which accounts for most of the cases of malignant paraproteinaemia;
* *macroglobulinaemia* (Waldenström's macroglobulinaemia);
* *B-cell lymphomas*, including chronic lymphatic leukaemia.

Coexistent features very suggestive of malignancy of B-cells include:

* *immune paresis.* The synthesis of immunoglobulins from other clones of cells may be suppressed by the proliferation of a single clone. In such cases the band, other

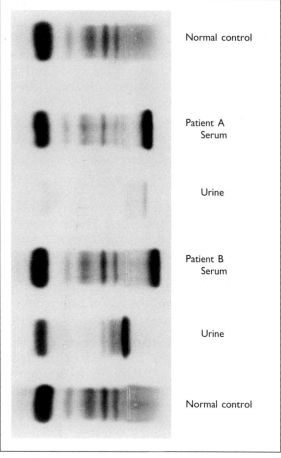

Fig. 16.5 Serum and urinary protein electrophoretic patterns in myelomatosis. Patient A with paraprotein and immune paresis in serum and BJP band in urine. Patient B with paraprotein and immune paresis in serum and with heavy BJP on the right and leakage of albumin and other low molecular-weight proteins (glomerular permeability) in urine.

than the narrow paraprotein, is reduced or absent and concentrations of the other immunoglobulins are also low (Fig. 16.5).
* *Bence-Jones protein* (BJP). BJP is usually, but not invariably or exclusively, found in the urine of patients with malignancy of B-cells (Fig. 16.5); it can also be found in the absence of malignant disease. It consists of free monoclonal light chains, or fragments of them, which have been synthesized much in excess of H-chains, implying a degree of dedifferentiation. Because of its relatively low molecular

weight (20 000 to 40 000) the protein is filtered at glomeruli and only accumulates in plasma if there is glomerular impairment or if it polymerizes. BJP may damage renal tubular cells and form large casts, producing the 'myeloma kidney'. It may also be a precursor for amyloid deposition in tissues.

THE CONSEQUENCES OF MALIGNANT B-CELL PROLIFERATION

Some of the clinical and laboratory findings are similar in all malignant B-cell tumours. Whether they occur depends on the concentration of paraprotein, the presence or absence of immune paresis and the presence of BJP. However, malignant tumours of B-cells can exist without all, or rarely any, of these findings.

Consequences of the presence of paraprotein. *Unless the concentration of paraprotein is very high these findings are not present.* Very high plasma concentrations, which are suggestive of malignancy, may be associated with a very high ESR and may cause:

- *in vivo* effects of increased plasma viscosity with sluggish blood flow in small vessels. This may result in *retinal-vein thrombosis* with impairment of vision, *cerebral thrombosis*, or even *peripheral gangrene* (*hyperviscosity syndrome*);
- an increased blood viscosity that may be noticeable during venepuncture; it may also be difficult to prepare blood films. Hyperviscosity is most common in macroglobulinaemia but may sometimes occur in myelomatosis;
- a high plasma total protein concentration despite a normal or low plasma albumin concentration;
- spurious hyponatraemia due to the space-occupying effect of the protein (pseudo-hyponatraemia; p.**38**).

Consequences of immune paresis. Because of the abnormal spectrum of immunoglobulins there may be increased susceptibility to infection.

Effects of Bence-Jones protein. Cases with large amounts of BJP are especially likely to be associated with:

- *renal glomerular dysfunction*, due to deposition of BJP in tubular cells;
- *amyloidosis*.

Other common findings in patients with malignant B-cell tumours are:

- *normochromic, normocytic anaemia*, a common presenting feature of any malignant disease;
- *small haemorrhages*, perhaps due to complexing of coagulation factors by the paraprotein;
- *Raynaud's phenomenon* if the paraprotein is a cryoglobulin (p.**329**).

β_2-**microglobulin** is a low molecular weight (11 800) protein that forms part of the HLA antigen on the surface of all nucleated cells. The protein is readily filtered by glomeruli and plasma concentrations are normally low. In myelomatosis, for example, the plasma β_2-microglobulin concentration is an index of the extent of the disease and of the prognosis. Occasionally raised plasma concentrations may occur in a number of haematological malignancies.

MYELOMATOSIS (MULTIPLE MYELOMA; PLASMA-CELL MYELOMA)

Myelomatosis is caused by the malignant proliferation of plasma cells throughout the bone marrow. The condition becomes increasingly frequent after the age of 50; it can occur before the age of 30 but is rare. The sex incidence is equal. The clinical features are due to:

- malignant proliferation of plasma cells;
- disordered immunoglobulin synthesis and/or secretion from the cell.

Malignant proliferation of plasma cells. Bone pain may be severe and is due to pressure from the proliferating cells. X-rays may show discrete *punched-out* areas of radiotranslucency, most frequently in the skull, vertebrae, ribs and pelvis. There may be generalized osteoporosis. Pathological fractures may occur. Histologically there is little osteoblastic activity around the lesion, which arises in the marrow rather than in the bone itself; consequently the plasma alkaline phosphatase activity is normal unless there is liver involvement in which case the raised level is of hepatic, not bony, origin. A normal plasma alkaline phosphatase activity in cases with bone lesions suggest myelomatosis rather than bony metastases (p.**306**). Hypercalcaemia may occur (p.**180**).

Disordered immunoglobulin synthesis. The immunoglobulin most frequently increased is IgG, less commonly IgA (about 2.5 : 1). Occasionally IgD, IgM or IgE are found, the last two being very rare. Bence-Jones protein may sometimes be present in plasma if renal failure is present. In about 20 per cent of cases, no paraprotein is detected in the plasma but BJP is detected in urine. Rarely, neither a paraprotein nor BJP can be found. In either case there is usually immune paresis. In IgD myelomatosis an increase in γ-globulin may not be detectable by routine electrophoresis. The paraprotein should be typed and the plasma concentration monitored to follow progress.

Bone marrow appearance. The proportion of plasma cells in the bone marrow is increased and many of these cells are atypical ('myeloma cells'). *Examination of a bone marrow aspirate must be carried out before myelomatosis is diagnosed or excluded.*

Soft tissue plasmacytoma. Rarely myeloma involves soft tissues, without marrow changes (*extramedullary* plasmacytoma). Although the protein abnormalities of myelomatosis are often found, the behaviour and prognosis of the two conditions are different. Spread of soft-tissue plasmacytoma is slow and tends to be local. Local excision of the solitary tumour is often effective.

WALDENSTRÖM'S MACROGLOBULINAEMIA

Waldenström's macroglobulinaemia is caused by a malignancy of B cells, with increased synthesis of IgM; the cells resemble lymphocytes rather than plasma cells. There is generalized lymphadenopathy. Like myelomatosis, macroglobulinaemia usually occurs in patients between 60 and 80 years, but unlike myelomatosis it is more common in men than in women. Symptoms of the 'hyperviscosity syndrome' are more common than in myelomatosis, probably because of the large size of the IgM molecule; skeletal manifestations are rare.

Laboratory findings and diagnosis include:

- IgM monoclonal paraprotein in the gamma region on protein electrophoresis. The serum IgA concentration is usually reduced, but that of IgG may be raised.
- the bone marrow aspirate or lymph node biopsy contains atypical lymphocytoid cells.

HEAVY-CHAIN DISEASE

The heavy-chain diseases are a rare group of disorders characterized by the presence of an abnormal protein in plasma or urine, identifiable as part of the H chain (α, γ or μ). The clinical picture is that of:

- intestinal lymphomatous lesions, with severe malabsorption (*α-chain disease*). The condition usually affects young adults of Mediterranean origin;
- generalized lymphadenopathy with recurrent infections in the elderly (*γ-chain disease*);
- chronic lymphatic leukaemia (*μ-chain disease*).

In some of these conditions a paraprotein may be detectable.

CRYOGLOBULINAEMIA

Cryoglobulins are proteins that precipitate when cooled below body temperature. They may be associated with diseases known to produce paraproteins. About half of them can be shown to consist of a monoclonal immunoglobulin (usually IgM or IgG). The patient usually presents with other symptoms of the underlying disease and the cryoglobulin is found during investigation. Occasionally, intravascular precipitation may occur at temperatures above 22°C and, if the concentration of protein is high, presenting symptoms and signs may be skin lesions such as purpura and *Raynaud's phenomenon*.

In some cases the protein is polyclonal and includes complement; these cases may be associated with immune-complex disease (p.**320**); occasionally no underlying abnormality can be found (*essential cryoglobulinaemia*).

PARAPROTEINAEMIA WITHOUT OBVIOUS CAUSE ('BENIGN' PARAPROTEINAEMIA)

If a paraprotein is found on electrophoresis, investigation for one of the diseases discussed above should be initiated. In up to 30 per cent of hospital cases, and probably more in the 'well population', no cause can be found. The condition, which may be transient, has been called 'benign' or 'essential' paraproteinaemia or monoclonal gammopathy of undetermined significance. The diagnosis should be made provisionally and the patients followed up; they may later develop obvious myelomatosis or macroglobulinaemia.

Proteins in Urine

The loss of most plasma proteins through the glomeruli is restricted by the size of the pores in, and by a negative charge on, the basement membrane that repel negatively-charged protein molecules. Alteration of either of these factors by glomerular disease may allow albumin and larger proteins to enter the filtrate. Low molecular weight proteins are filtered even under normal conditions; most are absorbed and metabolized by tubular cells. Normal subjects excrete up to 0.08 g of protein a day in the urine, amounts undetectable by usual screening tests. Proteinuria of more than 0.15 g a day almost always indicates disease.

Significant proteinuria may be due to renal disease or, more rarely, may occur because large amounts of low molecular weight proteins are circulating and therefore being filtered. *Blood and pus in the urine give positive tests for protein.*

RENAL PROTEINURIA

Glomerular proteinuria is due to increased glomerular permeability, as in the *nephrotic syndrome*. Albumin is usually the predominant protein in the urine.

'Orthostatic (postural) proteinuria'. Proteinuria is usually more severe in the upright than in the prone position. The term 'orthostatic' or 'postural' has been applied to proteinuria, often severe, which disappears at night. It appears to be glomerular in origin and is commonest in adolescents and young adults. Although it is often harmless, evidence of renal disease may occur after some years.

Microalbuminuria. Sensitive immunological assays have shown the normal daily excretion of albumin to be less than 0.05 g. Patients with diabetes mellitus who excrete more than this, but whose total urinary protein excretion is 'normal', are said to have microalbuminuria and to be at greater risk of developing progressive renal disease than those whose albumin excretion is normal. The incidence of this complication may be reduced by more stringent control of plasma glucose concentrations and blood pressure (p.**207**). One must question whether seeking microalbuminuria is of any further help.

Tubular proteinuria may be due to renal tubular damage from any cause, especially pyelonephritis. If glomerular permeability is normal proteinuria is usually less than 1 g a day and consists mainly of low molecular weight globulins. Low molecular weight α- and β-globulins are sensitive markers of renal tubular damage. However, because the β_2-microglobulins in urine are unstable, other proteins, such as retinal binding protein, are better indicators of tubular damage.

PROTEINURIA WITH NORMAL RENAL FUNCTION

Proteinuria can be due to production of *Bence-Jones protein*, to severe haemolysis with *haemoglobinuria*, or to severe muscle damage with *myoglobinuria*. In the latter two cases the urine may be red or brown in colour.

Bence-Jones proteinuria can be inferred by comparison of urinary and serum electrophoretic patterns (Fig. 16.5; p.**327**) and by immunochemical assays. BJP is the only protein of a molecular weight lower than albumin likely to be found in significant amounts in unconcentrated urine in the absence of haemoglobinuria or myoglobinuria. The presence of a band in urine, which is denser than that of albumin, especially if not present in the serum, is suggestive of BJP.

Apparent proteinuria has occasionally been found because the patient has added egg white or animal blood to the urine.

NEPHROTIC SYNDROME

An established case of nephrotic syndrome is characterized by proteinuria, hypoalbuminaemia, oedema and hyperlipidaemia. The clinical condition is caused by increased glomerular permeability, resulting in a daily urinary protein loss of, by definition, more than 5 g. There may be hypertension and evidence of other impaired renal function. The syndrome may be caused by:

- *primary renal disease*:
  most types of glomerulonephritis, usually due to deposition of circulating immune complexes in the glomeruli in about 80 per cent of cases. In children 'minimal change' glomerulonephritis is the most common cause;
- *secondary renal disease associated with*:
  diabetes mellitus;
  amyloidosis;
  systemic lupus erythematosus (SLE) (due to deposition of immune complexes);
  malaria due to *P. malariae* (due to immune complexes);
  inferior vena caval or renal-vein thrombosis;
- *drugs and toxins*:
  gold, penicillamine.

LABORATORY FINDINGS

Protein abnormalities. *Proteinuria* in the nephrotic syndrome ranges from 5 to 50 g a day. The relative proportion of different proteins lost is an index of the severity of the glomerular lesion. In mild cases albumin (MW 65 000) and transferrin (MW about 80 000) are the predominant urinary proteins but α_1-antitrypsin (MW 50 000) is also present. With increasing glomerular permeability larger proteins, such as IgG (MW 160 000), appear.

The serum electrophoretic picture depends on the severity of the renal lesion. In early cases a low plasma albumin concentration may be the only abnormality, but the typical pattern includes reduced albumin, α_1- and γ-globulin bands, with an increase in α_2-globulin because of an increase in the high molecular weight α_2-macroglobulin (Fig. 16.6). The γ-globulin may be normal or raised. *Urinary electrophoresis* gives some idea of the severity of the glomerular lesion.

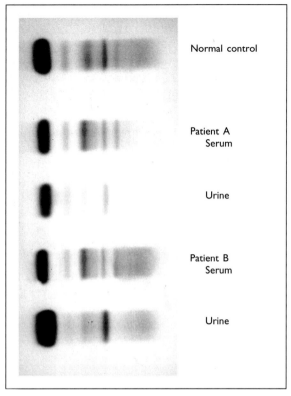

Normal control

Patient A
Serum

Urine

Patient B
Serum

Urine

Fig. 16.6 Serum and urinary protein electrophoretic patterns from patients with the nephrotic syndrome. Patient A has selective glomerular proteinuria and Patient B non-selective proteinuria.

The differential protein clearance is a more precise measure of the selectivity of the lesion. The clearance of a low molecular weight protein, such as transferrin or albumin, is compared with that of a larger one, such as IgG. The result is usually expressed as a ratio, obviating the need for timed urine collections. A ratio of IgG to transferrin or albumin clearance of less than 0.2 indicates high selectivity (predominant loss of small molecules) and has a more favourable prognosis than when the ratio is higher; such cases usually respond well to steroid or cyclophosphamide therapy.

The consequences of the protein abnormalities are:

- *oedema* caused by a fall in the intravascular colloid osmotic pressure, due to hypoalbuminaemia (p.**35**);
- *reduction in the concentration of protein-bound substances* due to loss of carrier proteins. It is important not to misinterpret low plasma *total* concentrations of calcium, thyroxine, cortisol and iron.

Lipoprotein abnormalities. In mild cases plasma LDL concentrations increase, with consequent *hypercholesterolaemia* probably due to the increased rate of protein synthesis, including that of apoB lipoprotein, in the liver. In more severe cases a rise in plasma VLDL (triglycerides) may cause plasma turbidity. Fatty casts may be detectable in the urine.

Renal function tests. In the early stages glomerular permeability is high and the plasma urea and creatinine concentrations are normal. Later enough glomerular dysfunction may develop to cause uraemia. At this stage, protein loss is reduced and plasma concentrations of protein and lipid may revert to normal. In the presence of uraemia this does *not* indicate recovery.

The student should read the indications for protein estimation on p334.

Summary

1. Albumin is the specific plasma protein most often measured. Its functions include control of fluid distribution between plasma and the extracellular compartment and binding and consequent inactivation of many endogenous and exogenous substances.

2. Groups of proteins may be separated by electrophoresis. In normal serum at least five bands can be seen: albumin and α_1-,

α_2-, β- and γ-globulins. In plasma, fibrinogen is also present.

3. Electrophoretic patterns that suggest a specific clinical cause may be found in paraproteinaemias, hypogammaglobulinaemia, α_1-antitrypsin deficiency, the nephrotic syndrome and some cases of cirrhosis of the liver.

4. The 'acute-phase' reaction occurs in many inflammatory states and in tissue damage. It is characterized by increased density of the α_1 and α_2 bands on electrophoresis.

5. Measurement of specific acute-phase proteins, such as CRP, is occasionally helpful in monitoring inflammatory disease. The plasma concentration of the C_3 fraction of complement may fall in such disease.

6. The immune response is dependent on functioning lymphocytes; the cellular component is mediated through the T-cells and the humoral response (immunoglobulins) through the B-cells.

7. The immunoglobulins, complement and other acute-phase proteins act together in the presence of invading organisms.

8. The immunoglobulins (Ig) are a group of proteins that are structurally related. Five classes are described. The most important ones are IgG, IgA and IgM.

9. The functions and properties of the immunoglobulin classes and their response to antigenic stimuli differ. Estimation of serum IgG, IgA and IgM concentrations may be helpful in a few circumstances.

10. Immunoglobulin deficiencies, which may be primary or secondary and may involve one or all immunoglobulin classes, are only one aspect of immunological deficiency. *Normal serum immunoglobulin concentrations do not exclude immunological deficiency;* serum concentrations may be raised in some cases of T-cell deficiency.

11. A paraprotein is a narrow band, most commonly found in the γ-globulin region of the electrophoretic strip. It usually consists of monoclonal immunoglobulins and almost always, but not invariably, indicates malignant proliferation of B cells.

12. Paraproteins are most commonly associated with myelomatosis. Myelomatosis presents clinically in a variety of ways, reflecting bone marrow replacement and abnormal plasma protein concentrations. The laboratory diagnosis is made by bone marrow examination, and by finding protein abnormalities in serum and/or urine.

13. Bence Jones protein (usually found only in urine) consists of monoclonal free light chains. Its presence usually indicates malignancy of B cells.

14. Cryoglobulins are abnormal proteins that precipitate when cooled below body temperature. They may cause symptoms on exposure to cold. They may occur in any of the diseases associated with paraproteinaemia.

Proteinuria

1. Proteinuria may be due to glomerular or tubular disease. Glomerular proteinuria is the commoner form; massive proteinuria is always of glomerular origin.

2. Proteinuria may occur in spite of normal renal function if abnormally large amounts of low molecular weight proteins are being produced.

3. The nephrotic syndrome is characterized by proteinuria of at least 5 g a day, with a low serum albumin concentration, oedema and hyperlipidaemia. The proteinuria is glomerular in type. The severity of the lesion may be assessed by differential protein clearances.

*B*LOOD SAMPLING FOR PROTEIN ESTIMATIONS

Blood for protein estimations, including those for immunoglobulins, should be taken with a *minimum of stasis,* otherwise falsely high results may be obtained. Special preservatives are needed.

- *Electrophoresis* should be performed on serum from clotted blood, because the presence of fibrinogen may mask, or be interpreted as, an abnormal band or protein.
- *Samples for complement estimations* must be taken and processed so as to minimize *in vitro* activation. *It is essential to contact your laboratory for details before taking the blood.*
- *Blood for cryoglobulin* measurement should be collected in a syringe *warmed to 37°C, and should be maintained at this temperature until it has been tested.* Failure to observe this precaution may result in false negative findings, because the cryoprecipitate is incorporated into the blood clot on cooling.

Indications for Protein Estimations

Before making a request, some assessment should be made as to whether the result of the estimation will aid diagnosis or treatment. The following are the more common indications for protein estimation.

To assess changes in hydration. Changes in plasma *total protein or albumin* concentrations over short periods of time are almost certainly due to changes in hydration, or to changes in capillary permeability (p.**318**).

To evaluate apparently abnormal concentrations or changes in concentrations of a protein bound substance. Plasma albumin estimation must always accompany that of total calcium (p.**172**). If changes in this or other protein-bound substances parallel those of albumin they are probably due to changes in protein concentrations.

To investigate oedema. Very low plasma *albumin* concentrations, in the presence of oedema suggest that hypoalbuminaemia is the cause. Conditions causing severe hypoalbuminaemia include the nephrotic syndrome and hepatic cirrhosis, both of which have typical serum electrophoretic patterns. The diagnosis of nephrotic syndrome depends on finding gross proteinuria. If oedema is due to causes other than hypoalbuminaemia, dilution leads to a fall in the albumin concentration *and all other protein fractions.*

To investigate suspected immune complex disease. The electrophoretic pattern may show a diffuse rise in γ-globulin in immune-complex disease. *It must be remembered that this finding may be due to a number of other types of disease.* Plasma C_3 determination is indicated if immune-complex disease is suspected. The *plasma concentration will be low* if such disease is in an active phase; if it is high it suggests another cause for tissue damage.

To investigate the cause of recurrent infection. Serum immunoglobulin concentrations should be measured as part of the assessment of the adequacy of the immune system. Note that these tests assess only *humoral* immunity. Serum electrophoresis may indicate the cause of low immunoglobulin concentrations (for example, there may be a protein-loss pattern (p.**315**) or a paraprotein).

The investigation of T-cell dysfunction is beyond the scope of this text and the reader is advised to consult textbooks on immunology.

To investigate suspected myelomatosis or macroglobulinaemia. *Electrophoresis* should be carried out on *serum* to detect a paraprotein, and on *urine* to detect Bence-Jones protein. The diagnosis of myelomatosis must be confirmed by microscopic inspection of a bone marrow aspirate or biopsy.

Plasma immunoglobulin concentrations should be measured to assess the degree of immune paresis.

TESTING FOR URINARY PROTEIN

Several rapid screening tests are in routine use. There are two limitations of screening tests.

- The tests were developed to detect albumin and may be negative in the presence of other proteins, such as BJP.
- Because the test depends on protein *concentrations*, very dilute urine may give negative results despite significant proteinuria.

It is *essential* that the sample should be *fresh*.

Albustix. The test area of the reagent strip is impregnated with an indicator, tetrabromphenol blue, buffered to pH 3. At this pH it is yellow in the absence of protein. Because protein forms a complex with the dye, stabilizing it in the blue form, it is green or bluish-green if protein is present. The colour after testing is compared with the colour chart provided, which indicates the approximate protein concentration. The strips should be kept in the screwtop bottles, in a cool place. The instructions on the container should be carefully followed. False positive results occur:

- if the specimen is contaminated with vaginal or urethral secretions;
- in strongly alkaline (infected or stale) urine, when buffering capacity is exceeded. A green colour in this case is a reflection of the alkaline pH;
- if the urine container is contaminated with disinfectants such as chlorhexidine.

False negative results occur if acid has been added to the urine as a preservative (for example, for the estimation of urinary calcium).

Clinical Chemistry of the Newborn

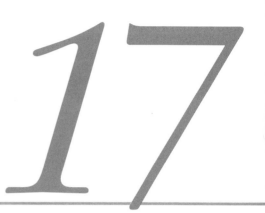

17

The survival rate of very small premature infants has increased because of improved specialized medical and nursing techniques for treating the newborn. However, these advantages must be weighed against the fact that such infants may suffer serious short- and long-term effects.

Diseases occurring during the newborn period can be divided into two main groups:

- those of infants born before term, in whom immaturity contributes to the severity of the disease;
- those of ill, full-term infants.

The commonest disorders in both groups are perinatal asphyxia, the respiratory distress syndrome and infection.

With the exception of some tests for the investigation of inborn errors of metabolism, the same biochemical investigations are used to diagnose and monitor diseases during the neonatal period as in adults. Requesting is inevitably less selective because of the non-specificity of the presenting clinical signs and the inability of the infant to give a history; by contrast, the number of investigations that can be performed may be limited by the small volume of the samples. Because the blood volume of a premature infant weighing 1 kg is about 90 ml, compared with about 5 litres in a 70 kg adult, only a small amount of blood can be taken without causing volume depletion or anaemia. Venous (or arterial) samples, although sometimes difficult to obtain, are preferable to capillary ones, since the latter are more prone to contamination from the interstitial and cellular fluids. *Before requesting tests on small samples the clinician should contact the laboratory to discuss the tests needed in order of priority.*

Interpretation of results is influenced by the different reference ranges at different ages; these are particularly difficult to define during the premature newborn period. Some of these, such as the relatively high plasma alkaline phosphatase activity found during childhood, are discussed in other chapters; some will be mentioned here.

Many disorders of infancy and childhood are described in the relevant chapters, including some inborn errors of metabolism in Chapter 18. In this chapter only those disorders that affect the newborn infant will be discussed.

Renal Function

By the 36th week of gestation the kidneys have a full complement of nephrons but renal function is not fully developed until the age of about two. Glomerular function develops more rapidly than that of the tubules.

The glomerular filtration rate (GFR) doubles during the first two weeks of life because of an increase in, and redistribution of, renal blood flow. The GFR, *related to surface area*, reaches adult values by about six months of age.

- *The plasma creatinine concentration*, which is inversely related to GFR, is higher at birth than in the adult. It decreases rapidly at first, the fall being slower in preterm infants, and then rises before reaching adult values, allowing for the surface area, by about six months.
- *The plasma urea concentration* is low in newborn infants compared with that in adults despite the relatively low GFR; the high anabolic rate results in more nitrogen being incorporated into protein rather than into urea than in adults. Plasma urea concentrations fluctuate markedly with varying nutritional states, metabolic rates and states of hydration.

Neither the plasma urea nor creatinine concentration is a very sensitive indicator of renal function in this age group unless these tests are performed serially. Renal function is often difficult to assess in the newborn period.

Although the control of antidiuretic hormone (ADH) and aldosterone secretion is well developed, even in premature infants, the kidneys cannot respond fully to these hormones; the resultant picture is similar to that of renal dysfunction in adults but in the newborn it is due to renal immaturity rather than disease.

- *Renal concentrating capacity* is lower in the newborn than in the adult; the maximum urinary osmolality that can be achieved in response to water deprivation, even if stimulated by exogenous ADH, is between 500 and 700 mmol/kg. The countercurrent mechanism is relatively inefficient, partly because the loops of Henle do not penetrate as deeply into the renal medulla as in the adult and partly due to the relatively low rate of urea production and therefore excretion. Because reabsorption of urea from the collecting ducts contributes to the interstitial medullary osmolality, so facilitating water reabsorption in response to ADH (p.**29**), renal concentrating ability may rise if urea production is increased when a high protein diet is given.
- *Renal conservation of sodium* is inefficient in premature infants, despite relatively high plasma renin activities and aldosterone concentrations compared to adults, because of immature renal tubular function. Excretion of a sodium load is impaired, perhaps because of the low GFR. Sodium balance should be carefully controlled, bearing in mind the very low total body sodium content at this age.

The hydrogen ion secretory capacity is relatively less than in adults. The urinary phosphate concentration, important for renal buffering in older children and in adults, may be low, especially if dietary phosphate intake is inadequate; formation of ammonia by tubular cells (p.**87**) is also inefficient. The resultant inability to fully 'reabsorb' all the filtered bicarbonate and to regenerate enough to replace that used in buffering may contribute to the relatively low neonatal plasma bicarbonate concentration, compared to that in older children and adults.

Renal function in newborn infants can maintain basic homeostasis but may not be able to respond adequately to illness or other stresses. It is often difficult to determine if there is renal impairment because of the unsatisfactory nature of renal function tests at this age. A plasma urea concentration above about 8 mmol/L suggests retention due to glomerular impairment, whether parenchymal or prerenal in origin, especially if the urinary output can be shown to be low. Management depends to a large extent on clinical criteria.

Water and Electrolytes

WATER

About 80 per cent of the weight of an infant of less than 1 kg consists of water, compared with about 60 per cent of that of an adult; the relative amount of water is related more to the proportion of fat to lean tissue than to total body weight. Relatively more is probably in the extracellular than in the intracellular compartment at birth. During the first week of life the extracellular fluid compartment contracts; urinary loss may account for the relatively high total amount of sodium excreted by preterm infants and does not necessarily indicate a disturbance in sodium homeostasis.

'Insensible' water loss is proportionately much higher in infants than in adults because:

- the ratio of surface area to body volume is high;
- there is very little subcutaneous fat;
- more fluid is lost through the skin because the epidermis is not fully developed before about the 28th week of gestation;
- there is a high metabolic and respiratory rate.

Daily fluid requirements are therefore up to five times higher per kg body weight than in adults.

SODIUM

The total body sodium content of a newborn infant of 1 kg is less than 100 mmol, compared with about 3000 mmol in the adult. A premature infant may need up to

6 mmol/kg of sodium a day because of the high losses and a normal full-term infant about 2 to 4 mmol/kg compared to about 1.5 mmol/kg in an adult.

The total body sodium and the plasma sodium concentration (and therefore osmolality) may fluctuate because renal function is immature. The newborn infant, unlike fully conscious children and adults, is unable to make its need for water clear and it is difficult for the doctor accurately to assess requirements. Rapid changes in extracellular osmolality due to inappropriate intake of water cause significant shifts of water between the intra- and extracellular compartments; signs varying from listlessness to convulsions, or even coma, may be caused by changes in cerebral hydration. The plasma sodium concentration should be monitored to ensure that the *proportion* of sodium to water is correct.

Hyponatraemia is a common finding. As in adults it may either be dilutional or due to high renal loss with inappropriate replacement with fluid of low sodium concentration. Causes include:

- prolonged maternal infusion of oxytocin ('Syntocinon') in five per cent glucose, or other hypo-osmolal fluid, to induce labour (p.**49**). Oxytocin has an antidiuretic action similar to that of ADH and may cause dilutional hyponatraemia in both mother and infant;
- inappropriate ADH secretion:
    following postpartum intracranial haemorrhage;
    in severe pulmonary disease, such as the respiratory distress syndrome (hyaline membrane disease) or pneumonia.
- infusion of water in excess of sodium, either as five per cent glucose or as hypo-osmolal sodium solutions;
- acute renal disease, especially if hypo-osmolal fluid is given to a child with glomerular dysfunction;
- diuretic treatment, particularly in premature infants.

The urinary sodium concentration must, as always, be interpreted with caution, especially in premature infants.

Clinical signs of hyponatraemia are related to the rate of fall of the plasma sodium concentration, and therefore of the plasma osmolality, rather than to the actual concentration and may be associated with hypotension, drowsiness and convulsions.

Congenital adrenal hyperplasia (p.**128**) must always be considered as a possible cause of hyponatraemia at this age.

Hypernatraemia develops if water loss exceeds that of sodium, or if excess of sodium relative to water is infused or fed.

If replacement is inadequate the high 'insensible' water loss, aggravated by impaired urinary water retention, may cause rapid extracellular fluid depletion with hypotension and, if water depletion is predominant, hypernatraemia. This is particularly likely if 'insensible' loss is increased through the:

- *intestine* if there is diarrhoea;
- *lungs* if the patient is hyperventilating, for example due to pneumonia;
- *skin*, for example due to sweating caused by pyrexia or to phototherapy for jaundice (p.**343**).

Infants given sodium bicarbonate are even more likely than adults to develop hypernatraemia because the addition of a given amount of extra sodium increases the very low extracellular sodium content proportionally more than if it were diluted in a larger pool, as it is in adults; this tendency is aggravated by impaired renal excretion.

POTASSIUM

The total body potassium of a newborn infant of 1 kg is less than 100 mmol, compared to about 3000 mmol in an adult. A normal full-term infant requires about 2 to 4 mmol/kg of potassium a day, compared to about 1.0 mmol/kg in an adult, to replace losses.

As in the adult, artefactual causes of abnormal plasma potassium concentrations must be excluded. Pseudohyperkalaemia is especially likely if capillary samples are used, because tissue cells may be damaged if the skin is squeezed. It may also be due to *in vitro* haemolysis, or to withdrawal of blood from a cannula through which a potassium solution is being infused; pseudohypokalaemia may, of course, result if the infused fluid is potassium-free.

Hypokalaemia may be caused by increased loss due to diarrhoea or diuretic treatment.

Hyperkalaemia. Since only about two per cent of the very low total body potassium is in the extravascular compartment, overzealous potassium treatment can easily cause hyperkalaemia. Other common causes include glomerular dysfunction and tissue damage due to hypoxia.

Hyperkalaemia is better tolerated than in adults, particularly in premature infants. Plasma concentrations of up to 8 mmol/L only need urgent treatment if there are significant changes in the electrocardiogram.

Perinatal Asphyxia

Renal complications and disturbances of electrolyte balance are especially likely to develop in infants with perinatal asphyxia.

Cerebral oedema or haemorrhage may stimulate ADH secretion, causing *oliguria and a dilutional hyponatraemia* with hypo-osmolality, accompanied by a *high urinary sodium concentration due to plasma volume expansion* (p.**49**).

The hypotension occurring during asphyxia may reduce renal blood flow enough to cause acute oliguric renal failure (acute tubular necrosis). In addition to the oliguria and hyponatraemia, there will be *uraemia* and *hyperkalaemia*, with proteinuria and often haematuria.

Hydrogen Ion Homeostasis

The plasma $T\text{CO}_2$ (bicarbonate) concentration is normally about 3 mmol/L lower in

newborn infants than in adults. This is partly due to renal immaturity and partly to the low concentration of urinary buffers (p.**339**); both these factors impair bicarbonate 'reabsorption' and regeneration. However, the plasma concentrations must be interpreted with caution as they are likely to be artefactually low in very small samples (p.**102**).

Disturbances of hydrogen ion homeostasis are common in newborn infants.

METABOLIC ACIDOSIS

Causes of metabolic acidosis include:

- *renal dysfunction*;
- *lactic acidosis* due to:
    tissue hypoxia resulting from poor tissue perfusion due to hypotension and the low $P\text{O}_2$ accompanying asphyxia or sepsis;
    some inborn errors of metabolism, such as glucose-6-phosphatase deficiency (p.**214**).
- *inborn errors of amino acid or organic acid metabolism.*

Unless the cause is obvious inherited disorders of intermediary metabolism should be considered. Simple screening tests (Table 17.1) may give the clue, but, whether they are positive or negative, further tests must be carried out, if necessary in a specialist centre.

MIXED RESPIRATORY AND METABOLIC ACIDOSIS

Respiratory distress may be caused by:

- *pulmonary disorders*, such as:
    respiratory distress syndrome;
    pneumonia;
    meconium aspiration during birth.
- *non-pulmonary disorders*, such as:
    congenital heart disease and patent ductus arteriosus;
    acute blood loss;
    metabolic acidosis.

The commonest cause in the preterm infants is the *respiratory distress syndrome* (RDS). Its incidence is inversely related to the

Table 17.1 Screening tests for inborn errors of metabolism in the neonatal period

	Test	Remark
May suggest disorder	Blood pH, P_{CO_2}, P_{O_2}	Detects hydrogen ion disturbances, and type
Possible disorder or group		
Congenital adrenal hyperplasia	Plasma $Na^+\downarrow, K^+\uparrow$	Nonspecific finding
		Cause must be confirmed
Renal tubular acidosis	Plasma $T_{CO_2}\downarrow$, $Cl^-\uparrow$	More commonly acquired, or due to other inborn error than congenital
Disorders of amino acid metabolism	Plasma and urinary amino acids	
Urea cycle disorders	Plasma urea $\downarrow$, ammonia $\uparrow$	Unable to form urea from ammonia
	Urinary amino acids, orotic acid	Specific amino acids high in some forms
Disorders of organic acid metabolism	Urinary organic acids, ketones	
Disorders of carbohydrate metabolism	Plasma glucose $\downarrow$	Non-specific finding
	Urinary reducing substances, ketones, sugar chromatography	Suspected disorder must be confirmed and typed

gestational age of the infant at birth (p.**143**). It is due to immaturity of the enzymes responsible for intrauterine synthesis of pulmonary surfactant, which maintains the patency of the alveoli. Surfactant synthesis begins at about the 20th week of gestation and increases rapidly after about the 34th week following maturation of alveolar cells.

The condition presents with pulmonary collapse (atelectasis); secondary lung infections are common. The blood P_{CO_2} is high, causing respiratory acidosis. The low blood P_{O_2} and reduced blood flow due to hypotension cause tissue hypoxia with lactic acidosis; renal dysfunction may aggravate the metabolic acidosis. The combination of respiratory and metabolic components may cause severe acidosis, with a blood pH well below 7.0.

The infant may benefit from administration of surfactant, given through an endotracheal tube, and from positive pressure ventilation, which help to expand the lungs and correct blood gas abnormalities. If these treatments are successful, the improved general condition increases tissue perfusion, correcting the lactic acidosis and improving renal function.

The P_{O_2} and P_{CO_2} of cutaneous capillary blood can be monitored continuously using electrodes placed on the skin. These bring the capillary P_{O_2} and P_{CO_2} to near arterial levels by heating the skin to about 44°C and so increasing cutaneous blood flow. The electrodes must be repositioned every four hours to prevent local burns and need to be recalibrated frequently. In case of litigation results of transcutaneous monitoring may not be legally acceptable as evidence. P_{O_2} may also be assessed using pulse oximetry, a method which does not require calibration during use. *Transcutaneous blood gas monitoring supplements, but does not replace, arterial blood gas analysis.*

Bilirubin Metabolism

Bilirubin metabolism is discussed in Chapter 14.

Proportionally more unconjugated bilirubin reaches the liver in the newborn infant than in the adult because:

- *the red cell half-life is shorter*, the blood haemoglobin concentration falls rapidly during the first week of life, even in normal infants;
- *delayed clamping of the umbilical cord* may significantly increase red cell mass;
- *bruises* may occur during birth, and resorption of haemoglobin breakdown products from these increases the plasma bilirubin concentration.

The mature liver can conjugate very large amounts of bilirubin and jaundice due to increased bilirubin production is rarely severe in adults. In the newborn, even at term, the conjugating process is not fully developed and even a marginally increased load causes jaundice.

'Physiological jaundice' (unconjugated hyperbilirubinaemia) is defined as mild jaundice *not present at birth*, which develops during the first few days and continues during the first week of life, and for which there is no obvious pathological reason. Such jaundice is very common in normal newborn infants, the incidence being inversely related to the gestational age at birth.

UNCONJUGATED HYPERBILIRUBINAEMIA

Plasma unconjugated bilirubin concentrations may be very high in premature infants because of hepatic immaturity. If the bilirubin concentration exceeds the albumin-binding capacity the unbound, fat-soluble unconjugated bilirubin may cross cell membranes and be deposited in the brain, causing *kernicterus* (p.**283**). This is a serious complication, which may cause permanent brain damage or death.

The risk of kernicterus is increased:

- the more premature the infant;
- if the plasma unconjugated bilirubin concentration is rising rapidly, perhaps due to haemolysis;
- if the bilirubin-binding capacity is low, due to:
  hypoalbuminaemia;
  displacement of bilirubin from albumin by some drugs;
  displacement of bilirubin from albumin by hydrogen ions in acidosis due to hypoxia or other serious illness.

Jaundice during the first 24 hours of life is more likely to be pathological than physiological. Causes include:

- *maternofetal rhesus or ABO blood group incompatibility*; this is particularly likely in infants born to multiparous mothers, who may have developed antibodies during previous pregnancies;
- *inherited erythrocyte abnormalities* associated with haemolysis, such as glucose-6-phosphate dehydrogenase deficiency or hereditary spherocytosis;
- *interuterine infections*, which affect the liver, such as syphilis, rubella or toxoplasmosis.

Bilirubin should be measured in blood taken from the umbilical cord of all infants known to be at risk for one of the above reasons; blood group typing and Coombs' testing for red cell antibodies can also be performed on cord blood.

Management. If the plasma bilirubin concentration is rising rapidly or exceeds about 340 µmol/L (20 mg/dl) in full-term infants exchange transfusion may be needed. This 'action level' may be significantly lower in the preterm infant. Biochemical complications of exchange transfusions are usually due to the anticoagulant used in the infused blood, and are transitory. They include:

- hyperkalaemia;
- hypocalcaemia;
- metabolic acidosis;
- hypoglycaemia.

Bilirubin is destroyed by ultraviolet light and lesser degrees of unconjugated hyperbilirubinaemia may be treated by phototherapy. Water loss from the skin may be high and fluid balance must be carefully monitored.

Prolonged unconjugated hyperbilirubinaemia, not in itself requiring treatment, may accompany chronic infections such as that of cytomegalovirus, or with *hypothyroidism*. It is more common in *breast-fed infants* than in those given formula feeds: the reason for this is unknown.

CONJUGATED HYPERBILIRUBINAEMIA

Impaired excretion of bilirubin which has been conjugated in hepatocytes may be due to:

Table 17.2 Some causes of neonatal hypoglycaemia discussed in Chapter 10 (p.**214**)

Age	Cause of hypoglycaemia
Newborn period	Infants of diabetic mothers
	Erythroblastosis fetalis
	islet cell hyperplasia
	Intrauterine malnutrition
	prematurity and small for dates infants
Early infancy	Inborn errors of metabolism
	glycogen storage disease (GSD type I)
	hereditary fructose intolerance
Later infancy	Idiopathic hypoglycaemia
	nesidioblastosis (p.**215**)
	Leucine sensitivity (p.**215**)
	Ketotic hypoglycaemia (p.**215**)
	infants usually small for dates at birth

- *congenital biliary atresia* (*Byler's disease*); it is important to make this diagnosis early because some forms may be amenable to surgical treatment;
- *biliary obstruction* by pressure on the bile ducts by, for example, extrabiliary tumours.

OTHER CAUSES OF JAUNDICE IN THE NEWBORN PERIOD

Neonatal hepatitis rarely presents clinically until after the first week of life. Causes include intrauterine infection with organisms such as cytomegalovirus and rubella.

Metabolic causes of jaundice include galactosaemia (p.**290**) and α_1-antitrypsin deficiency (p.**326**). It may also be associated with parenteral nutrition.

Other *inherited abnormalities* associated with jaundice include the Dubin-Johnson syndrome (p.**292**).

INVESTIGATION OF JAUNDICE IN THE NEWBORN PERIOD

The same investigations are used as in adults, but the different reference ranges must be allowed for. Plasma transaminase activities are up to twice the upper limit of the adult reference range during the first three months of life and falls to adult levels by the age of about one year. The plasma total alkaline phosphatase activity is higher in infancy and during childhood because of the contribution from actively growing bone; it falls to adult levels after the pubertal growth spurt (p.**306**).

Glucose Metabolism

Causes of hypoglycaemia in the newborn period, discussed on p.**214**, are shown in Table 17.2. Hepatic glycogen stores increase about threefold, and adipose tissue (another source of energy) is laid down during the last 10 weeks of pregnancy. Very premature infants therefore have little liver glycogen and are especially prone to hypoglycaemia. Full-term infants may become hypoglycaemic if initially adequate stores are drawn on more rapidly than normal, for example during perinatal asphyxia.

Plasma glucose concentrations as low as 1.7 mmol/L (about 30 mg/dl) during the first 72 hours of life in the premature infant, or 2.2 mmol/L (about 40 mg/dl) during the later neonatal period, may not be associated with any clinical signs. When such signs do occur they include tremors, apnoeic attacks and convulsions. However, impaired neurological development has been reported if the plasma glucose concentration repeatedly falls to below 2.2 mmol/L despite the absence of clinical signs. It is now recommended that the plasma glucose concentration be maintained above 2.2 mmol/L in at risk patients.

Calcium, Phosphate and Magnesium Metabolism

Calcium metabolism in adults is discussed in Chapter 9.

Calcium with phosphate are actively transported across the placenta; total and free-ionized calcium concentrations are higher in fetal than in maternal plasma. 25-hydroxyvitamin D, but not its active metabolite 1,25-dihyroxyvitamin D nor parathyroid hormone (PTH), can pass placental membranes. Calcium and phosphate accumulate rapidly only between the 30th and 36th week of fetal life; a very premature infant may become calcium and phosphate deficient when feeds are not supplemented.

During intrauterine life the relatively high maternally derived fetal plasma free-ionized calcium concentration suppresses PTH release from the fetus' own parathyroid glands. The glands may take time to recover after birth and there may be transient hypoparathyroidism. Plasma total and free-ionized calcium concentrations fall by up to 30 per cent immediately after birth, but, in the normal infant, spontaneously regain adult concentrations within about three days; this fall rarely needs to be treated.

The reference range for plasma total calcium concentration in the newborn period is wider than that for adults. Plasma phosphate concentrations are higher in actively growing infants and in children compared to adults.

Neonatal hypocalcaemia. Hypocalcaemia during the first two weeks of life can be divided into two groups.

- *Hypocalcaemia of early onset* occurs during the first three days of life and is commonest:
    in low birthweight, preterm infants for the reasons given above;
    following perinatal asphyxia;
    in infants of diabetic mothers.

    It may also occur if the mother was hypercalcaemic during pregnancy, for example due to primary hyperparathyroidism; the maternal hypercalcaemia is reflected in the fetus, and the suppressed fetal parathyroid glands may take some time to recover. This condition is a more severe form of the 'physiological' condition described above.
- *Hypocalcaemia of late onset* is less common than it used to be. It usually followed the use of high phosphate-containing feeds.

RICKETS OF PREMATURITY

Bone demineralization (osteopenia) is common in small preterm infants and often resolves spontaneously before obvious clinical features of rickets develop. The plasma alkaline phosphatase activity may rise to more than six times the upper adult reference limit, the plasma calcium concentrations are usually low normal and those of phosphate low.

Rickets of prematurity usually becomes clinically evident between the fourth and 12th weeks of life, and occurs more frequently in very premature, low birth-weight infants than in infants of older gestational age at birth. Longitudinal growth slows, and the decalcification of the bones predisposes to pathological fractures; in severe cases respiration is impaired by the soft ribs.

X-ray changes may be minimal or absent in early cases. In more advanced disease the classical radiological changes appear at the ends of long bones.

Rickets of prematurity may be due to:

- *calcium and phosphate depletion*. If an infant is born prematurely unsupplemented breast milk may not contain enough of these minerals to replace that which should have accumulated *in utero* during the last 10 weeks of gestation. Phosphate depletion is probably the commonest cause and is indicated by a very low plasma phosphate concentration, compared to the appropriate reference range, and a low urinary phosphate excretion. Glomerular dysfunction reduces phosphate excretion even without deficiency (p.**175**), and the diagnosis must not be made on the basis of this finding alone;
- *maternal vitamin D deficiency during pregnancy, or in the infant after birth*. In very premature infants such deficiency may be due to low activity of the renal 1α-hydroxylase needed to convert 25-hydroxyvitamin D to the active 1,25-dihydroxvitamin D (p.**175**). Whatever the cause of 1,25-dihydroxvitamin D deficiency, calcium absorption may be impaired. In such cases the urinary

phosphate excretion will be inappropriately high due to secondary hyperparathyroidism, provided that renal glomerular function is normal;

- *drugs*, such as frusemide (furosemide), which increase urinary calcium loss;
- *renal tubular disorders* of phosphate reabsorption which may cause phosphate depletion (p.**184**). In such cases the plasma calcium concentration is usually normal, but may even be high because it cannot be deposited in bone without phosphate.

Treatment. Vitamin D and calcium and phosphate supplementation may be monitored by measuring serial plasma alkaline phosphatase activities. Despite successful treatment these may continue to rise for several weeks, when bone is being actively laid down, before falling once the bone is adequately calcified.

Many premature infants are given prophylactic vitamin D supplementation. This is unlikely to prevent rickets unless accompanied by an adequate calcium and phosphate intake.

Hypercalcaemia in the newborn period. Hypercalcaemia is less common than hypocalcaemia at this age. It may be associated with phosphate depletion and hypophosphataemia because calcium cannot be deposited in bone without phosphate and because hypophosphataemia enhances 1α-hydroxylase activity and therefore the formation of the active vitamin D metabolite (p.175). After treatment with phosphorus the plasma calcium concentration may fall rapidly enough to cause clinical symptoms.

Idiopathic hypercalcaemia may occur in full-term infants receiving inappropriately high-dose vitamin D prophylaxis.

Magnesium

Hypomagnesaemia often accompanies hypocalcaemia and may be caused by dietary deficiency, or by increased intestinal or urinary loss. Low plasma magnesium concen-

trations may impair the release and action of PTH and so delay correction of plasma calcium concentrations.

Hypomagnesaemia should be considered if the infant has convulsions despite normocalcaemia.

Plasma Proteins

At birth, the relative concentrations of individual plasma proteins differ from those found in adults. That of total protein is about 12 g/L lower than in adults but that of albumin only slightly lower; as always the latter may fall during illness. The acute-phase proteins (p.**319**), reflected in the α- and β-globulins in the electrophoretic pattern, reach adult concentrations by about six months, but are affected by illness, again as they are in adults.

The immunoglobulin pattern differs significantly from that of adults. During normal pregnancy, placental transfer of maternal IgG leads to a gradual increase in fetal plasma concentrations of these immunoglobulins. After birth maternally derived IgG is degraded and endogenous immunoglobulin synthesis starts. Adult concentrations of plasma IgM are reached by about nine months, IgG by between three to five years and IgA only by the age of 15 (Table 16.1; p.**313**).

Measurement of plasma immunoglobulin concentrations may be indicated if an immune-deficiency state, whether primary, secondary or transient, is suspected (p.**325**). It may also help to detect infection, whether it occurred during the intrauterine period or has developed after birth. Results must be compared with age-matched reference ranges, allowance being made for both the time since conception (gestational age) and age since birth (postnatal age).

A high plasma IgM concentration in blood obtained from the umbilical cord, or within the first four weeks of life, may indicate intrauterine or neonatal infections such as syphilis, rubella, toxoplasmosis or cytomegalovirus. Allowance must be made for the normal rise in plasma IgM which starts after about six weeks of postnatal age.

Specific inborn errors, such as α_1-antitrypsin deficiency, may be diagnosed by measuring the appropriate plasma protein.

Neonatal Thyroid Function

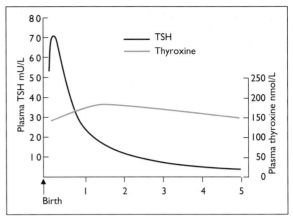

Fig. 17.1 An example of changes in plasma total thyroxine and TSH concentrations in a full-term infant during the first five days after birth.

The fetal hypothalamic–pituitary–thyroid axis develops independently of maternal hormones.

Immediately after birth plasma TSH concentrations rise rapidly, probably in response to the stress of birth, to about 15 times the upper adult reference limit. They reach a peak within the first hour before falling, rapidly at first, during the next week. Plasma total thyroxine concentrations peak within the first 24 hours and then fall gradually (Fig. 17.1). Screening tests for neonatal congenital hypothyroidism should be delayed for about a week after birth to allow the plasma TSH concentration to stabilize (p.**353**).

There is a similar pattern of secretion in healthy preterm infants, but the peak concentrations of both hormones are lower. This reduced response is even more marked in ill preterm infants, in whom it may be very difficult to interpret results of thyroid function tests; plasma total thyroxine concentrations are low, those of TSH 'normal' and of thyroxine-binding globulin normal or low. This pattern resembles that in ill adults. Treatment with thyroxine is usually not indicated.

The incidence and diagnosis of neonatal hypothyroidism is discussed on p.**164**. Thyroid function tests should be repeated in infants found to have a positive screening tests at a week after birth; if the diagnosis is confirmed thyroid replacement should be started immediately. Thyroid function should be reassessed, after withdrawal of treatment, at the age of one year because neonatal hypothyroidism is sometimes transient. Results of screening tests may be misleading in ill, premature infants and may need to be repeated before discharge from hospital.

Hypothyroidism may be suspected clinically, for example, because of failure to thrive or persistent jaundice. In such cases thyroid function should be fully investigated.

Summary

1. In preterm infants immaturity contributes to the pathogenesis of disease.
2. Biochemical results in infants and children must be interpreted using matched sex and age reference ranges.
3. 'Insensible' water loss is much higher in newborn infants than in adults.
4. Renal glomerular function may be difficult to assess by measuring plasma urea or creatinine concentrations.

5. A mixed respiratory and metabolic acidosis, usually due to the respiratory distress syndrome, is relatively common in preterm infants.

6. 'Physiological' jaundice is very common in newborn infants. Severe jaundice, needing treatment, occurs in premature neonates and those with maternofetal blood group incompatibility.

7. Hypoglycaemia is common in preterm infants because of inadequate glycogen stores.

8. Metabolic bone disease, including rickets, may occur in very small preterm infants.

9. Plasma IgM concentrations measured in blood taken from the umbilical cord may help to diagnose infections that have developed *in utero*.

10. Thyroid function tests may be particularly difficult to interpret in very premature and ill infants.

Inborn Errors of Metabolism

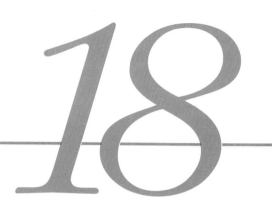

The inherited characteristics of an individual are determined by about 50 000 gene pairs, arranged on 23 pairs of chromosomes, one of each pair coming from the father and one from the mother. Genotype diversity is introduced by random selection and recombination during meiosis, as well as by occasional mutation. These genetic variants may, at one extreme, be incompatible with life, or at the other, produce biochemical differences detectable only by special techniques, if at all. Between the two extremes there are many variations that produce functional abnormalities.

Genetic disorders fall into three main categories.

- *Chromosomal disorders* due to the absence, or abnormal arrangement, of chromosomes affecting many genes and therefore many gene products. Examples include Down's syndrome (trisomy for chromosome 21) and Klinefelter's syndrome (47,XXY).
- *Multifactorial disorders* due to the interaction of multiple genes with environmental or other exogenous factors, such as diabetes mellitus.
- *Monogenic disorders* due to an abnormality of a single gene which is the primary determinant of the disorder and which is inherited in a predictable pattern, such as phenylketonuria.

GENERAL PRINCIPLES

Genes, located on chromosomes, comprise a sequence of bases on deoxyribonucleic acid (DNA) and code for the synthesis of proteins through the medium of ribonucleic acid (RNA) in its 'messenger' form (messenger RNA). All nucleated cells contain an identical complement of genes but only about one per cent is expressed.

In disorders of single genes (monogenic) the abnormalities may be of:

- *a structural gene*, with production of an *abnormal protein*; in this case all the biochemical abnormalities can be explained by defective synthesis of a single peptide;
- *a controlling (enhancing) gene* which, by altering the rate at which one or more structural genes function, affects the *amounts* of one or more structurally normal peptides.

In most of the examples discussed in this chapter the affected protein is an enzyme, but in other conditions it may, for example, be a receptor, a transport or a structural protein, a peptide hormone, an immunoglobulin or a coagulation factor. However, in many inherited disorders the abnormal protein is not yet known and the defect is only recognized by its characteristic clinical presentation.

Patterns of Inheritance

Every inherited characteristic is governed by a pair of genes on homologous chromosomes, one gene being received from each parent. Different genes governing the same characteristic are called *alleles*. If an individual has two identical alleles he is *homozygous* for that gene or inherited characteristic; if he has two different alleles he is *heterozygous*. Genes may be carried on the *autosomes* (similar in both sexes) or on the *sex chromosomes* (X and Y); the patterns of inheritance differ.

AUTOSOMAL INHERITANCE

If one parent (Parent 1 in the example below) is heterozygous for an abnormal gene (*A*) and the other parent is homozygous for the normal gene (N), the possible combination in the offspring are shown in the square.

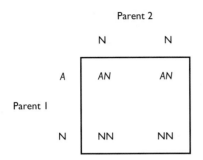

On a statistical basis, half the offspring will be heterozygous (*AN*) for gene A, like Parent 1. None will be homozygous for the abnormal gene (*AA*).

If both parents are heterozygous (*AN*), a quarter of the offspring will be homozygous (*AA*) and half heterozygous (*AN*).

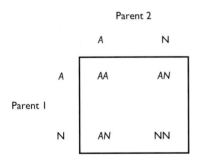

If one parent is homozygous (*AA*) and the other normal (NN) all the offspring will be heterozygous.

The metabolic consequences of an abnormal gene depend on the effectiveness of that gene compared with the normal one.

Autosomal dominant inheritance. Dominant abnormal genes affect both heterozygotes (*AN*) and homozygotes (*AA*), although homozygotes may be more severely affected. In the first example, Parent 1 (*AN*) and half the offspring, and in the second example both parents and three out of four of the offspring (*AA* and *AN*) will be affected. Characteristically, if there is autosomal dominant inheritance:

- every affected individual has at least one affected parent;
- offspring in successive generations are affected;
- clinically normal offspring are not carriers of the abnormal gene;
- statistically, three in four children are affected if both parents are heterozygous.

Autosomal recessive inheritance. Recessive abnormal genes only affect homozygous offspring (*AA*). In the first example neither parent nor the offspring will be affected and in the second example both parents will appear normal, but statistically one in four of the offspring will be affected. Therefore, in autosomal recessive inheritance:

- heterozygous parents are not clinically affected;
- clinical consequences may miss offspring in succeeding generations;
- clinically normal children may be heterozygous and therefore may be carriers of the abnormal gene;
- statistically, one in four children of heterozygous parents are clinically affected.

Disorders inherited as a recessive trait have a lower expression frequency in affected families than dominant disorders, but tend to be more severe.

SEX-LINKED INHERITANCE

Some abnormal genes are carried only on the sex, almost always the X, chromosomes.

X-linked recessive inheritance. Women have two X chromosomes and men one X and one Y. In X-linked recessive inheritance an abnormal X chromosome (*Xa*) is latent when combined with a normal X, but active when combined with a Y, chromosome. If the mother carries *Xa* she will appear to be normal but statistically half her sons will be affected (*YXa*). Half her daughters will be carriers (*XXa*) but all her daughters will be clinically unaffected.

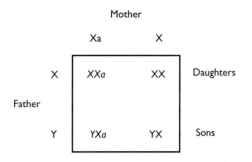

If the father is affected and the mother carries two normal genes none of the sons will be affected, but all the daughters will be carriers.

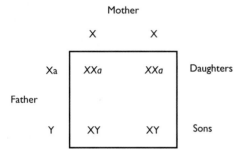

Inherited disease manifesting in male offspring and carried by females is typical of X-linked inheritance. The female is only clinically affected in the extremely rare circumstance when she is homozygous for the abnormal gene. This will only occur if she inherited the abnormal genes from an affected father and a carrier mother.

Haemophilia is the classical example of an X-linked recessive disorder.

X-linked dominant inheritance. In this type of inheritance both *XXa* women and *YXa* men are affected. An example of this very rare type of disorder is familial hypophosphataemia (p.**184**).

MULTIPLE ALLELES

Occasionally there may be several alleles governing the same characteristic. Different pair combinations may then produce different disease patterns such as, for example, some of the haemoglobinopathies, or the variant may only be detectable by biochemical testing, such as, for example, some of the plasma protein variants.

The rules outlined above may not apply in all cases, because new mutations can occur at any time and may produce dominant disorders in unaffected families.

The terms 'dominant' and 'recessive' are relative. A dominant gene may fail to manifest itself (*incomplete penetrance*) and may therefore appear to skip a generation. A gene may vary in its *degree of expression*, and therefore in the degree of abnormality that it produces. A recessive gene, which produces disease only in homozygotes (*AA*), may be detectable by laboratory tests in clinically unaffected heterozygotes.

Possible Metabolic Consequences

As stated above, although monogenic disorders may involve any peptide, they are usually most obvious if there is an enzyme abnormality.

Deficiency of a single enzyme in a metabolic pathway may produce its effects in several ways. Suppose that substance A is acted on by enzyme X to produce substance B, and that substance C is on an alternative pathway.

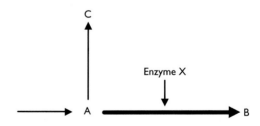

The consequences of a deficiency of X may be due to:

- *deficiency of the products of the enzyme reaction* (B), for example:
  cortisol deficiency in congenital adrenal hyperplasia (p.**128**);
  hypoglycaemia of some disorders of glycogen breakdown (glycogenoses).
- *accumulation of the substance acted on by the enzyme* (A), for example:

phenylalanine in phenylketonuria (p.**357**); galactose in galactosaemia (p.**290**).

- *diversion through an alternative pathway.* Some product(s) of the latter (C) may accumulate and produce effects, for example:

  congenital adrenal hyperplasia when accumulation of androgens causes virilization (p.**128**).

The effects of the last two types of abnormality will be aggravated if the whole metabolic pathway is controlled by negative feedback from the final product. For example, in congenital adrenal hyperplasia cortisol deficiency reduces negative feedback, so increasing the rate of steroid synthesis and therefore the accumulation of androgens, causing virilization in the female.

The clinical effects of some inborn errors of metabolism may be modified by, or depend entirely on, physiological or environmental factors. For example, iron loss occurs during menstruation and pregnancy; women with idiopathic haemochromatosis accumulate iron less rapidly than men with the same condition and they rarely present with clinical features before the menopause. Patients with cholinesterase variants develop symptoms only if the muscle relaxant suxamethonium is given (p.**311**).

Clinical Importance of Inborn Errors of Metabolism

The recognition of many inborn errors of metabolism is only of academic interest because the abnormality produces no clinical effects. In others, it may be important to make a diagnosis, even though no effective treatment is yet available, so that genetic counselling can be undertaken and, if termination is acceptable, prenatal diagnosis offered during subsequent pregnancies.

There is a group of diseases in which recognition in early infancy is of great importance because *treatment may prevent irreversible clinical consequences or death*. Some of the more important of these are:

- phenylketonuria (p.**357**);
- galactosaemia (p.**290**);
- maple syrup urine disease (p.**359**).

Other conditions should be sought *in the blood relatives of affected patients*, either because further ill effects may be prevented, or because a precipitating factor should be avoided. Examples include:

- familial hypercholesterolaemia (p.**234**);
- cholinesterase abnormalities (p.**311**);
- glucose-6-phosphate dehydrogenase deficiency (p.**363**);
- acute porphyrias (p.**384**);
- cystinuria (p.**360**);
- haemochromatosis (p.**382**);
- Wilson's disease (p.**361**).

Some inherited disorders that can be treated *symptomatically*, for examples are:

- hereditary nephrogenic diabetes insipidus (p.**47**);
- congenital disaccharidase deficiency (p.**255**);
- Hartnup disease (p.**360**).

Finally, some inborn errors are completely, or almost completely, harmless. They are important because they produce *effects that may lead to misdiagnosis or that may alarm the patient*. Examples are:

- renal glycosuria (p.**205**);
- alkaptonuria (p.**358**);
- Gilbert's disease (p.**292**).

Screening for Inborn Errors of Metabolism

SCREENING NEWBORN INFANTS

Many countries have instituted programmes for screening all newborn infants for certain inherited metabolic disorders. The criteria should depend on the following characteristics of the disorder or of the test.

- The disease should not be clinically apparent at the time of screening and should have a relatively high incidence in the population screened.
- The disease should be treatable; it must be possible to obtain the result of the screening test before irreversible damage is likely to have occurred.
- The screening test should be simple and reliable and the cost of the programme should ideally be, at least partly, offset by the cost-savings resulting from early treatment. For example, such treatment may sometimes eliminate the need for prolonged institutional care.

Not all these criteria are necessarily fulfilled in all screening programmes. Some commonly used programmes screen for:

- phenylketonuria (PKU);
- congenital hypothyroidism (CH). In the majority of cases there is an absence of the thyroid gland rather than an inherited disorder of thyroxine synthesis;
- galactosaemia;
- cystic fibrosis (CF).

Screening for PKU and CH is carried out in most affluent countries but, at the time of writing, unselective screening for other disorders remains controversial.

Screening tests in Europe are usually performed on blood from a heel prick collected on filter paper at between the third and fifth day after birth; this is easy to transport to the laboratory. The timing of sample collection is important if false results are to be avoided. Substances on the metabolic pathway before the enzyme block, such as galactose in galactosaemia, only accumulate once the infant starts ingesting the precursor, in this case milk or milk products.

Although analysis of DNA by molecular biological techniques, for example in circulating mononuclear cells, may sometimes directly identify an abnormal gene, such methods are, at the time of writing, still at an experimental stage and are not yet suited to unselective screening programmes. There are, for example, more than 200 different mutations associated with cystic fibrosis. Identification of the commonest would identify only about 70 per cent of cases. Such procedures are usually limited to screening infants or fetuses of heterozygote parents in whom the precise mutation has previously been identified (p.**253**).

A positive result of a screening test should be confirmed by quantitative analysis or by identifying the enzyme defect. Many abnormalities are transient and do not necessarily indicate the presence of an inborn error. Therefore despite a second positive test the individual should be reassessed after a period of time. For example, for an infant with congenital hypothyroidism, thyroid function tests should be repeated at the age of one year, after temporarily withdrawing treatment.

PRENATAL SCREENING

Prenatal screening of high-risk groups only may be performed for some disorders in order to:

- plan the appropriate place and method of delivery for the well-being of the infant;
- offer termination, if the diagnosis is made early enough and if it is available and acceptable.

Prenatal screening for inherited metabolic disorders is most commonly done by demonstrating the metabolic defect in cultured fetal fibroblasts obtained by amniocentesis early in the second, or by chorionic villus sampling during the first, trimester. Examples of those groups in whom such screening may be indicated are:

- *women with a previously affected infant*;
- *ethnic groups thought to have a relatively high incidence of the carrier state*, such as of Tay-Sach's disease in Ashkenazi Jews. In these high risk populations screening is often performed before conception enabling genetic advice and prenatal diagnosis to be offered to couples who are carriers.

Table 18.1 Some clinical findings suggestive of an inborn error of metabolism

Early	hypoglycaemia
	metabolic acidosis
	failure to thrive
	vomiting
	fits or spasticity
	hepatosplenomegaly
	prolonged jaundice
	a peculiar smell, or staining, of the nappies
Late	retarded mental development
	refractory rickets
	renal calculi

If, as in cystic fibrosis, the gene defect of the parent of an affected infant is known, there may be a case for selective screening of subsequent pregnancies using molecular biological techniques.

Prenatal screening for congenital or chromosomal abnormalities may be performed by measuring the concentration of α-fetoprotein in maternal serum between 14 and 18 weeks of pregnancy. This may be used to detect:

- *fetal neural tube defects,* when serum concentrations are increased (p.**142**);

- *Down's syndrome,* when serum concentrations are low. The diagnostic efficiency can be increased by simultaneously measuring human β-choriogonadotropin concentrations (β-HCG), the maternal concentration of which is increased during the first trimester of pregnancies affected by Down's syndrome. The results of the investigations are interpreted allowing for the gestational age of the fetus and the statistically established risk associated with maternal age.

When to Suspect an Inborn Error of Metabolism

The possibility of an inherited metabolic defect should be considered if there are bizarre and inexplicable clinical features (Table 18.1) or abnormal laboratory findings in infancy or early childhood, especially if more than one infant in the family has been affected. The older the infant the more specific the symptoms may be.

LABORATORY DIAGNOSIS OF INBORN ERRORS OF METABOLISM

Disorders may present in the neonatal period with non-specific findings and the disease may progress rapidly; a screening policy must be standardized. Screening tests should be interpreted with caution and a *suspected diagnosis confirmed by more specific techniques in a laboratory specializing in such disorders.*

Inborn errors presenting acutely are usually due to an enzyme abnormality. This may be demonstrated:

- *indirectly* by detecting a high concentration of the substance normally metabolized

by the enzyme, or a low concentration of the product;
- *directly* by demonstrating a low enzyme activity in the appropriate tissue or blood cells. These assays may only be available at special centres. If possible all cases should be confirmed in this way.

Examples of indirect screening methods include:

- estimation of plasma ammonia concentration to test for disorders of the urea cycle, in which it accumulates because it cannot be converted to urea as efficiently as normal;

- chromatography of plasma and urine for amino acids for detection of disorders of amino acid metabolism;
- detection of organic acids in urine in disorders of branched-chain amino acid metabolism and organic acidurias.

If the clinical signs and symptoms are strongly suggestive of a particular disorder, specific measurements, such as those of urinary glycosaminoglycan excretion and white cell enzymes characteristic of mucopolysaccharidoses (p.**361**), may be used.

Aminoaciduria. Amino acids are usually filtered by the glomeruli and reach the proximal tubules at concentrations equal to those in plasma and are almost completely reabsorbed as they pass through this part of the nephron. Aminoaciduria may therefore be of two types:

- *overflow aminoaciduria* in which, because of *raised plasma concentrations*, amino acids reach the proximal tubules at concentrations higher than the reabsorptive capacity of the cells;
- *renal aminoaciduria* in which *plasma concentrations are low* because of urinary loss due to defective tubular reabsorption.

Aminoaciduria may also be subdivided according to the pattern of excreted amino acids.

- *Specific aminoaciduria* is due to increased excretion of either a single amino acid, or a group of chemically related amino acids. It may be overflow or renal in type.
- *Nonspecific aminoaciduria*, in which there is increased excretion of a number of unrelated amino acids, is almost always due to an acquired disorder. It may be overflow in type, as in severe hepatic disease when impaired deamination of amino acids causes raised plasma concentrations; more commonly renal aminoaciduria results from non-specific proximal tubular damage (p.**19**), and other substances that are usually almost completely reabsorbed by the proximal tubule are also lost (phosphoglucoaminoaciduria; the Fanconi syndrome). If it

occurs due to an inborn error of metabolism it is rarely a direct result of the genetic defect, but more commonly secondary to tubular damage caused by deposition of the substance not metabolized normally, such as copper in Wilson's disease.

Organic aciduria. Those organic acids derived from the metabolism of amino acids, carbohydrates and lipids are often detectable in the urine; others accumulate if there is an enzyme deficiency in a specific metabolic pathway. These disorders, known as *organic acidurias, are individually extremely rare*, but collectively have an incidence of about one in 12 000 births, similar to that of PKU (p.**357**). They may present in the neonatal period with life-threatening metabolic acidosis, vomiting and hypotonia or in early infancy with failure to thrive, a Reye-like syndrome (p.**290**) and convulsions associated with profound hypoglycaemia. They may also be a cause of sudden infant death (SID).

Diagnosis is suggested by the clinical findings and supported by initial tests demonstrating a metabolic acidosis, with or without ketosis. It is confirmed by measuring urinary organic acid excretion and subsequent enzyme analysis. These should only be performed in specialized laboratories.

Principles of Treatment of Inborn Errors of Metabolism

Some inborn errors can be treated by:

- *limiting the dietary intake* of precursors in the affected metabolic pathway, such as phenylalanine in phenylketonuria or lactose in galactosaemia;
- *supplying the missing metabolic product*, such as cortisol in congenital adrenal hyperplasia;
- *removing or reducing the accumulated product*, such as ammonia in urea cycle disorders.

Experimental treatments may be tried for some disorders with hopeless prognoses; one is enzyme replacement by bone marrow transplantation, but the results have been disappointing. Insertion of the missing or defective gene is being attempted for such disorders as adenosine deaminase deficiency and cystic fibrosis. However, for many disorders there is, at the time of writing, still no treatment unless they respond to one of the measures listed above.

Diseases Due to Inborn Errors of Metabolism

Only a very few of the known inborn errors of metabolism will be discussed. The choice must be biased by what the author feels to be important; others might disagree. A fuller, but not complete list of the more important disorders is given on p.**362**, with the mode of inheritance when known, included. Many of these conditions are mentioned briefly in the relevant chapters.

Disorders of Amino Acid Metabolism

Most disorders of amino acid metabolism are characterized by raised plasma concentrations of one or more amino acids, with overflow aminoaciduria.

Disorders of Aromatic Amino Acid Metabolism

The main metabolic pathway for aromatic amino acids is outlined in Fig. 18.1, which also indicates the known enzyme defects. Tyrosine, normally produced from phenylalanine, is the precursor of several important substances, inherited disorders of which are considered briefly.

PHENYLKETONURIA

Phenylketonuria is an autosomal recessive disorder caused by an abnormality of the *phenylalanine hydroxylase* system. This is the enzyme most commonly affected, but in about three per cent of cases those responsible for synthesis of the cofactor, tetrahydrobiopterin, are abnormal. Therefore several different inherited deficiencies may have very similar biochemical and clinical consequences. Because phenylalanine cannot be converted to tyrosine it accumulates in plasma and is excreted in the urine with its metabolites, such as phenylpyruvic acid; the disease acquired its name from the detection of the latter 'phenylketone' in the urine.

The clinical features include:

- *irritability, feeding problems, vomiting* and *fits* during the first few weeks of life;
- *mental retardation* developing at between four and six months, with psychomotor irritability;
- often generalized eczema;
- a tendency to reduced melanin formation because of reduced production of tyrosine. Many patients are *pale-skinned, fair-haired* and *blue-eyed*.

Diagnosis. The phenylalanine concentration may be measured in blood taken from a heel prick. The microbiological Guthrie test is only suitable for mass screening and should be performed about four days after birth when

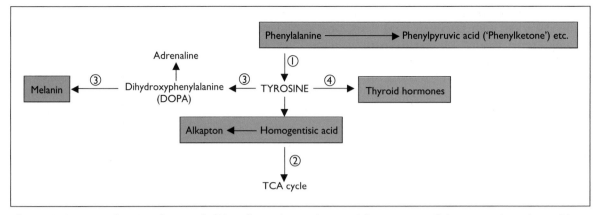

Fig. 18.1 Diagram showing the metabolism of tyrosine and some inborn errors of the aromatic amino acid pathway. Substances highlighted may be present in abnormal amounts in certain inborn errors of metabolism.
1 phenylalanine hydroxylase   phenylketonuria, PKU
2 homogentisic acid oxidase   alkaptonuria
3 tyrosinase   albinism
4 thyroid enzymes   thyroid dyshormonogenesis

the infant is taking milk. In the newborn and especially in premature infants the enzyme system may not be fully developed and false positive results are likely if the test is performed too early. If a positive result is found the test should be repeated later, to allow time for development of the enzyme. Concentrations may be raised in conditions other than phenylketonuria. Measurement of plasma tyrosine concentrations may identify other causes of false positive results; plasma concentrations do not rise in phenylketonuria but are high in many of the other conditions.

Heterozygotes may be clinically normal, but can be detected by biochemical tests.

A variant, persistent hyperphenylalaninaemia, without mental retardation has been described.

Infants who are exposed *in utero* to the high phenylalanine concentrations of undiagnosed or poorly controlled phenylketonuric mothers may be mentally retarded, although they themselves do not have detectable phenylketonuria (*maternal phenylketonuric syndrome*).

Management. The aim of management is to lower plasma phenylalanine concentrations by giving a low phenylalanine diet. Such treatment is difficult, expensive and tedious for both the patient and the parents, and should be monitored carefully, especially if the patient is planning to conceive or is pregnant. It is now recommended that, in proven cases, dietary restriction should be lifelong.

Deficiency of phenylalanine, an essential amino acid, has deleterious effects which include an impaired growth rate, eczema and mental retardation. Some of these problems can be overcome by supplementing the diet with the immediate metabolic product of phenylalanine metabolism, tyrosine; tyrosine is not usually an essential amino acid, but becomes so if it cannot be produced from phenylalanine.

There is no effective treatment for the form of hyperphenylalaninaemia caused by cofactor deficiency.

ALKAPTONURIA

Alkaptonuria is an autosomal recessive disorder due to a deficiency of *homogentisic acid oxidase*. Homogentisic acid accumulates in tissues and blood, and is passed in the urine. Oxidation and polymerization of homogentisic acid produces the pigment *alkapton* in much the same way as polymerization of DOPA (Fig. 18.1) produces melanin. Deposition of alkapton in cartilages, with consequent darkening, is called *ochronosis*, and results in visible darkening of the cartilages of the ears and often arthritis in later life. Conversion of homogentisic acid to alkapton is accelerated in alkaline conditions, and the most obvious abnormality in alkaptonuria is *darkening of the urine as it becomes more alkaline on standing*; however, this finding may not always be present. If it is, the condition is often first noticed by the mother, who is worried by the black nappies which become even blacker when washed in alkaline detergents.

The condition is compatible with a normal life span despite the tendency for patients to develop arthritis in later life.

Homogentisic acid, a reducing substance, reacts with Clinitest tablets (p.**222**).

ALBINISM

A deficiency of *tyrosinase* in melanocytes causes one form of albinism; it is inherited as a autosomal recessive disorder. Pigmentation of the skin, hair and iris is reduced and the eyes may appear pink. Reduced pigmentation of the iris causes photosensitivity and decreased skin pigmentation is associated with an increased incidence of skin cancer. The tyrosinase involved in catecholamine synthesis is a different isoenzyme, controlled by a different gene; consequently adrenaline metabolism is normal.

Disorders of Other Amino Acids

MAPLE SYRUP URINE DISEASE

In maple syrup urine disease (MSUD), which is inherited as an autosomal recessive condition, there is deficient decarboxylation of the oxoacids resulting from deamination of the three *branched-chain amino acids*, leucine, isoleucine and valine. These amino acids accumulate in the plasma and are excreted in the urine with their corresponding oxoacids. The smell of the urine is like that of maple syrup giving the condition its name.

The disease presents during the first week of life and, if not treated, severe neurological lesions develop which cause death within a few weeks or months. If a diet low in branched-chain amino acids is given normal development seems possible.

Diagnosis is made by demonstrating raised concentrations of branched-chain amino acids in plasma and urine. It may be confirmed by demonstrating the enzyme defect in leucocytes.

HISTIDINAEMIA

Histidinaemia is associated with deficiency of *histidinase*, an enzyme needed for normal histidine metabolism, and is probably inherited as an autosomal recessive trait. About half the described cases have mental retardation and speech defects, but the other half seem to be normal. Results of dietary treatment are inconclusive.

Diagnosis is made by demonstrating raised plasma levels of histidine, and by finding histidine and a metabolite, imidazole pyruvic acid, in the urine.

Like phenylpyruvic acid, imidazole pyruvic acid reacts with Phenistix.

Inherited Disorders of Transport Mechanisms

Groups of chemically similar substances are often transported by shared or interrelated pathways. Such group-specific mechanisms usually affect transport across all cell membranes and defects often involve both the renal tubules and intestinal mucosa. Inborn errors of the following amino acid group pathways have been identified:

- the *dibasic* amino acids (with two amino groups), cystine, ornithine, arginine and lysine (*cystinuria*); COAL is a useful mnemonic;
- many *neutral* amino acids (with one amino and one carboxyl group) (*Hartnup disease*);
- the *imino* acids, proline and hydroxyproline, which probably share a pathway with glycine (*familial iminoglycinuria*).

CYSTINURIA

Cystinuria is due to an autosomal recessive inherited abnormality of tubular reabsorption, with excessive urinary excretion, of the dibasic amino acids, cystine, ornithine, arginine and lysine. A similar transport defect has been demonstrated in the intestinal mucosa, but although dibasic amino acid absorption is reduced, deficiencies do not occur because they can be synthesized in the body. Cystine is relatively insoluble and, because of the high urinary concentrations in homozygotes, may precipitate and form calculi in the renal tract. In heterozygotes increased excretion can be demonstrated, but concentrations. are rarely high enough to cause precipitation.

Diagnosis of cystinuria is made by demonstrating excessive urinary excretion of the characteristic amino acids. All these must be identified to distinguish the stone-forming homozygotes from the heterozygous condition, cystine-lysinuria, and from cystinuria occurring as part of a generalized aminoaciduria.

Management of cystinuria aims to prevent calculi formation by reducing urinary concentration. The patient should drink plenty of fluid *day and night.* Alkalinizing the urine increases the solubility of cystine. If these measures prove inadequate D-penicillamine may be given; this forms a chelate, which is more soluble than cystine alone.

CYSTINOSIS

This is a very rare but serious disorder of cystine metabolism, characterized by intracellular accumulation and storage of cystine in many tissues. It must be distinguished from cystinuria, a relatively harmless condition. Renal tubular damage by cystine causes the Fanconi syndrome. Aminoaciduria is nonspecific and of renal origin. Affected individuals die young.

HARTNUP DISEASE

Hartnup disease, named after the first patient described, is a rare autosomal recessive disorder in which there are renal and intestinal transport defects involving neutral amino acids.

Most, if not all, the clinical manifestations can be ascribed to reduced intestinal absorption and increased urinary loss of *tryptophan.* This amino acid is normally partly converted to nicotinamide, the conversion being especially important if dietary intake of nicotinamide is marginal (p.**397**). The clinical features of Hartnup disease are intermittent and resemble those of pellagra, namely:

- a red scaly rash on exposed areas of skin;
- reversible cerebellar ataxia;
- mental confusion of variable degree.

In spite of the generalized defect of amino acid absorption there is no evidence of protein malnutrition; this may be because intact peptides can be absorbed by a different pathway.

Excessive amounts of *indole* compounds, originating from bacterial action on unabsorbed tryptophan, are absorbed from the gut and excreted in the urine.

Diagnosis of homozygotes is made by demonstrating the characteristic amino acid pattern in the urine.

FAMILIAL IMINOGLYCINURIA

Increased urinary excretion of the imino acids, proline and hydroxyproline, and of glycine, despite normal plasma concentrations, is due to a transport defect for these three compounds. It is inherited as an autosomal recessive trait. The condition is apparently harmless, but must be differentiated from other more serious causes of iminoglycinuria, such as the defect of proline metabolism, hyperprolinaemia.

Storage Defects

A variety of disorders affects the degradation and/or excretion of metabolic products. Some, such as the glycogen storage disorders (p.**214**) and the mucopolysaccharidoses, present in infancy and childhood; in others, such as haemochromatosis (p.**382**) the abnormal accumulation only becomes severe enough to cause clinical features by adult life.

THE MUCOPOLYSACCHARIDOSES (MPS)

These rare conditions are caused by defects of any of the several enzymes that hydrolyse mucopolysaccharides (glycosaminoglycans), which therefore accumulate in tissues such as the liver, spleen, eyes, central nervous system, cartilage and bone.

- *Hurler's syndrome (MPS I H)* is the least rare, and is inherited as an autosomal recessive disorder. Patients present in infancy or early childhood with the characteristic coarse features of 'gargoylism', short stature, mental retardation and clouding of the cornea. They usually die young of cardiorespiratory disease. *Scheie's syndrome (MPS I S)* is difficult to distinguish clinically from Hurler's syndrome at the time of diagnosis, but has a much better prognosis; there is little mental retardation.
- *Hunter's syndrome (MPS II)*, in contrast to all the other mucopolysaccharidoses, is inherited as a sex-linked recessive trait.

The mucopolysaccharidoses can initially be diagnosed biochemically by demonstrating increased urinary excretion of sulphated glycosaminoglycans, such as dermatan, heparan and keratan sulphates, the excretion pattern being characteristic of each syndrome. The diagnosis should be confirmed by direct enzyme assay.

There is, as yet, no proven effective treatment.

WILSON'S DISEASE

Some plasma copper is loosely bound to albumin, but most is incorporated in the protein *caeruloplasmin*. Copper is excreted mainly in bile. There are two defects of copper metabolism in Wilson's disease:

- *impaired biliary excretion* leads to *deposition in the liver*;
- *deficiency of caeruloplasmin* results in *low plasma copper concentrations*; most is in a loosely bound form and is therefore deposited in tissues; more than normal is filtered at the glomeruli and *urinary copper excretion is increased*.

Excessive deposition of copper in the basal ganglia of the brain, and in the liver, renal tubules and eyes, produces:

- *neurological symptoms* due to degeneration of the basal ganglia;
- *liver damage* leading to cirrhosis;
- *renal tubular damage* with any or all of the associated biochemical features, including aminoaciduria (Fanconi syndrome);
- *Kayser-Fleischer rings* at the edges of the cornea due to deposition of copper in Desçemet's membranes.

Diagnosis: Most patients have low plasma caeruloplasmin and copper concentrations and high urinary copper excretion.

Low plasma caeruloplasmin concentrations may also occur during the first few months of life, due to malnutrition, and in the nephrotic syndrome due to urinary loss.

Raised plasma concentrations are found in active liver disease, in women taking oral contraceptives, during the last trimester of pregnancy and non-specifically when there is tissue damage due for example to inflammation or neoplasia. These may account for the rare finding of 'normal' plasma caeruloplasmin concentrations in patients with Wilson's disease.

Histological examination with the demonstration of an increased copper content of a liver biopsy specimen is essential to confirm the diagnosis.

The clinical condition has a recessive mode of inheritance, but reduced plasma caeruloplasmin concentrations may be demonstrable in heterozygotes. The distinction between pre-symptomatic homozygotes and heterozygotes is important because the former can be treated.

Treatment with copper-chelating agents such as D-penicillamine may reduce tissue copper concentrations.

Table 18.2 Some inborn errors of metabolism and their mode of inheritance

	Inheritance	Page		Inheritance	Page
1. Disorders of cellular transport			Combined hyperlipidaemia	R	234
Most of these are recognized as renal tubular transport			Plasma LCAT deficiency	R	236
defects, and in some, defective intestinal transport can also			**5. Disorders of lysosomal metabolism**		
be demonstrated			Mucopolysaccharidoses		
			Hurler's syndrome (MPS I H)	R	361
Amino and imino acids			Hunter's syndrome (MPS II)	X-linked R	361
Dibasic amino acids. Cystinuria	R	360	Gaucher's disease	R	308
Neutral amino acids. Hartnup disease	R	360	**6. Abnormalities of plasma proteins**		
Familial iminoglycinuria	R	360	Immunoglobulin deficiencies	–	325
Glucose			Carrier protein abnormalities		
Renal glycosuria	D	205	Transferrin deficiency	?R	382
Water (failure to respond to ADH)			Thyroxine-binding globulin		
Hereditary nephrogenic diabetes			deficiency	X-linked	161
insipidus	X-linked R	47	Cholinesterase variants	R	311
Potassium (all cells)			α_1-antitrypsin deficiency	–	326
Familial periodic paralysis	D	64	Bisalbuminaemia	D	317
Calcium (failure to respond to PTH)			Analbuminaemia	R	317
Pseudohypoparathyroidism	X-linked D	183	**7. Disorders of metal metabolism**		
Phosphate			Haemochromatosis	R	382
Familial hypophosphataemia	X-linked D	184	Wilson's disease	R	361
Hydrogen ion			**8. Erythrocyte abnormalities**		
Renal tubular acidoses	D	93	(see haematology textbooks)		
Bilirubin (liver cells)			Haemoglobinopathies	–	
Congenital hyperbilirubinaemias			Glucose-6-phosphate dehydrogenase		
Crigler–Najjar syndrome Type I	R	292	deficiency	X-linked	363
Crigler–Najjar syndrome Type II	D	292	NADP methaemoglobin reductase		
Dubin–Johnson syndrome	R	292	deficiency	R	
Gilbert's disease	D	292	**9. Disorders of porphyrin metabolism**		
Rotor syndrome	R	292	Porphyrias	–	383
2. Disorders of amino and imino acid metabolism			**10. Disorders of steroid metabolism**		
Aromatic amino acids			Congenital adrenal hyperplasia	All R	128
Phenylketonuria	R	357	**11. Disorders of purine metabolism**		
Alkaptonuria	R	358	Primary hyperuricaemia	?	370
Albinism	R	359	Xanthinuria	R	371
Thyroid dyshormonogenesis	All R	164	Lesch-Nyhan syndrome	X-linked R	371
Sulphur amino acids			**12. Disorders of digestion**		
Cystinosis	R	360	Disaccharidase deficiencies	R	255
Homocystinuria	R		Cystic fibrosis	R	253
Branched-chain amino acids			**13. Disorders of oxalate metabolism**		
Maple syrup urine disease	R	359	Primary hyperoxaluria	R	22
Histidinaemia	R	359	**14. Disorders precipitated by drugs**		
3. Disorders of carbohydrate metabolism			Suxamethonium sensitivity	R	311
Glycogenoses	R	214	Slow inactivation of isoniazid	R	363
Galactosaemia	R	290	Phenytoin toxicity	D	363
Hereditary fructose intolerance	R	215	Glucose-6-phosphate dehydrogenase		
Essential fructosuria	R	221	deficiency	X-linked	363
Diabetes mellitus	?	206	Malignant hyperpyrexia	D	363
4. Disorders of lipid metabolism					
Familial hypercholesterolaemia	R	234			

This list of inborn errors of metabolism is far from complete. It is meant for reference only and the student should not attempt to learn it. Most of the abnormalities have been discussed in this book, and a page reference is given. Where it is known, the mode of inheritance is stated, unless the heading applies to a group of diseases of different modes of inheritance.

D = autosomal dominant, R = autosomal recessive, X-linked D = X-linked dominant, X-linked R = X-linked recessive.

Drugs and Inherited Metabolic Disorders

The variation in individual response to drugs may partly be due to genetic variation. There are a number of well-defined inherited disorders that are aggravated by, or which only become apparent after, administration of certain drugs. These disorders may be classified into two groups.

DISORDERS RESULTING FROM DEFICIENT METABOLISM OF A DRUG

The muscle relaxant, suxamethonium (succinyl choline; 'scoline') normally has a very brief action because it is rapidly broken down by plasma cholinesterase. In *suxamethonium sensitivity* (p.**311**) a cholinesterase variant of low biological activity impairs breakdown of the drug, and prolonged postoperative respiratory paralysis may result ('scoline apnoea').

Two other inherited disorders are characterized by defective metabolism of the drugs *isoniazid* and *phenytoin*. In both toxic effects occur more frequently, and at lower dosages, than in normal individuals.

DISORDERS RESULTING FROM AN ABNORMAL RESPONSE TO A DRUG

Deficiency of *glucose-6-phosphate dehydrogenase* (G-6-PD) may cause haemolytic anaemia, and is relatively common in such ethnic groups as those of Mediterranean origin. This enzyme catalyses the first step in the hexose monophosphate pathway and is needed for the formation of NADP, which is probably essential for the maintenance of intact red cell membranes. Numerous variants of G-6-PD deficiency have been described. Haemolysis may be precipitated by certain antimalarial drugs, such as primaquine, and by sulphonamides and vitamin K analogues.

In the inherited *hepatic porphyrias* (p.**384**) acute attacks may be precipitated by several drugs, particularly barbiturates.

Some people react to general anaesthetics (most commonly halothane with suxamethonium) with a rapidly rising temperature, muscular rigidity and acidosis (*malignant hyperpyrexia*); most of them die as a result. Many, but not all, susceptible subjects in affected families have a high plasma creatine kinase activity.

This short section should remind readers of the possibility of an inborn error when an abnormal reaction to a drug is encountered.

Summary

1. Inborn errors of metabolism are genetic diseases, most presenting with early clinical symptoms due to abnormalities of enzyme synthesis.
2. Inborn errors of metabolism may produce no clinical disadvantage, may only produce them under certain circumstances or, at the other extreme, may produce severe disorders incompatible with life.
3. Recognition of some inherited abnormalities is only of academic interest. Diagnosis is important if the condition is serious but treatable, if precipitating factors can be avoided, if confusion with other diseases is possible or if genetic counselling is considered.
4. Inheritance may be autosomal or sex-linked, dominant or recessive. In diseases producing severe clinical effects inheritance is most often autosomal recessive; they are most common in the offspring of consanguineous marriages.
5. In many cases in which the clinical disease is inherited as a recessive trait lesser degrees of abnormality can be detected by laboratory testing.

Purine and Urate Metabolism

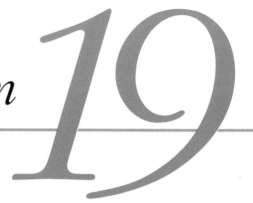

19

*N*ORMAL URATE METABOLISM

Urate is the end-product of purine metabolism in primates, including man. In most other mammals it is further metabolized to the more water soluble allantoin. It is because of the poor solubility of urates that man is prone to such clinical effects of hyperuricaemia, as gout and renal damage. The purines adenine and guanine are constituents of both types of nucleic acid (DNA and RNA). The purines used by the body for nucleic acid synthesis may be derived from the breakdown of ingested nucleic acid, mostly taken in cell-rich meat, or they may be synthesized *de novo* from small molecules.

SYNTHESIS OF PURINES

The purine synthetic pathway involves the incorporation of many small molecules into the relatively complex purine ring. The upper part of Fig. 19.1 summarizes some of the more important synthetic steps. The following stages should especially be noted.

- The first step in purine synthesis is condensation of pyrophosphate with phosphoribose to form phosphoribose diphosphate (phosphoribosyl pyrophosphate; PRPP).
- The amino group of glutamine is incorporated into the ribose phosphate molecule and pyrophosphate (PP) is released. Amidophosphoribosyl transferase catalyses this *rate-limiting* or controlling step. The enzyme is subject to feedback inhibition by increasing concentrations of purine nucleotides; thus the rate of synthesis is slowed when its products increase. The control of this rate-limiting step may be impaired in primary gout.
- Glycine is added to phosphoribosylamine. By using labelled glycine it has been shown that the rate of purine synthesis is increased in primary gout. In Fig. 19.1 the atoms in the glycine molecule have been numbered to correspond with those in the purine and urate molecules, and the heavy

lines further indicate the final position of the amino acid in these molecules.

After many further steps purine ribonucleotides (purine ribose phosphates) are formed which, as previously mentioned, control the second step in the synthetic pathway–the formation of phosphoribosylamine. Ribose phosphate is split off, thereby releasing the purines. Some cytotoxic drugs inhibit various stages of the pathway, so preventing DNA formation and cell growth.

FATE OF PURINES

Purines synthesized in the body, those derived from the diet, and those liberated by endogenous catabolism of nucleic acids may be:

- *oxidized to urate* (lower part of Fig. 19.1). Some adenine is oxidized to hypoxanthine, which is further oxidized to xanthine. Guanine can also form xanthine. Xanthine, in turn, is oxidized to form urate. The oxidation of both hypoxanthine and xanthine is catalysed by *xanthine oxidase* in the liver. Thus the formation of urate from purines depends on xanthine oxidase activity: gout may be treated using an inhibitor of this enzyme (allopurinol);
- *reused for nucleic acid synthesis.* Some xanthine, hypoxanthine and guanine can be resynthesized to purine nucleotides by pathways involving, among other enzymes, hypoxanthine-guanine phosphoribosyl transferase (HGPRT) and adenine phosphoribosyl transferase (APRT).

Excretion of urate. Urate is filtered through the glomeruli and most is reabsorbed from the proximal tubular lumina. More than 80 per cent of that in formed urine is derived from more distal tubular secretion.

Urinary excretion is slightly lower in males than in females; this may contribute to the higher incidence of hyperuricaemia in men.

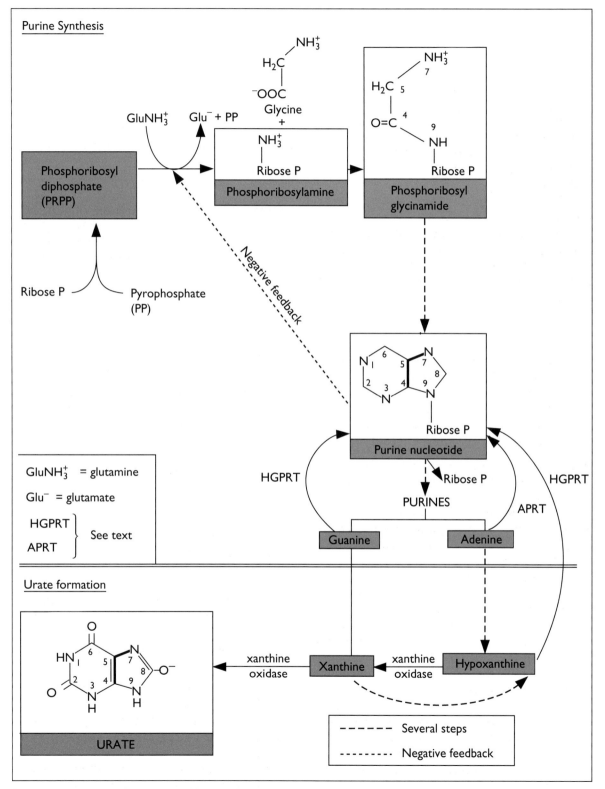

Fig. 19.1 Summary of purine synthesis and breakdown, showing the steps of clinical importance.

Renal secretion may be enhanced by urico-suric drugs, which block tubular urate reabsorption. Tubular secretion of urates is inhibited by organic acids, such as lactic and oxo-acids, and by thiazide diuretics.

Seventy-five per cent of urate leaving the body is in urine. The remaining 25 per cent passes into the intestinal lumen, where it is broken down by intestinal bacteria, the process being known as *uricolysis*.

HYPERURICAEMIA

Causes of Hyperuricaemia

Hyperuricaemia may be due to a familial primary abnormality of purine metabolism or be secondary to a variety of other conditions. It may be asymptomatic, or may be associated with the clinical syndrome of gout.

Factors that may contribute to hyperuricaemia, summarized in Fig 19.2, are:

- *increased rate of urate formation* (step 1): increased synthesis of purines (step 2); increased intake of purines (step 3); increased turnover of nucleic acids.
- *reduced rate of excretion* (step 5).

Increased synthesis, due to impaired feedback control, is probably the most important mechanism causing primary hyperuricaemia whereas abnormalities of the other three steps are causes of secondary hyperuricaemia.

DANGERS OF HYPERURICAEMIA

Urate is poorly soluble in plasma. At plasma pH most urate is ionized at position 8 of the purine ring (Fig. 19.1). This anionic group is associated with the predominant extracellular cation, sodium. Unequivocally high urate concentrations, even if symptomless, should be treated because the relatively insoluble monosodium urate may, like calcium, precipitate in tissues. This precipitation may be caused by a variety of local factors of which the most important are probably pH and trauma. If it takes place in the kidney it may cause renal damage. Ionization of uric acid decreases as the pH falls, and it therefore becomes less soluble; at a urinary pH below about 6 uric acid may form renal calculi.

Crystallization in *joints*, especially those of the feet, produces the classical picture of gout first recorded by Hippocrates in 469 BC. Urate precipitation at these sites causes an inflammatory response with leucocytic infiltration and it is thought that lactic acid production by these cells causes a local fall in pH: this converts urate to uric acid, which is less soluble than urate, and a vicious circle is set up in which further precipitation, and therefore further inflammation, occurs. In *acute attacks* of gouty arthritis local factors are more important than the *plasma urate concentration*, which is usually *normal* during the attack.

Precipitation may occur in subcutaneous tissues, especially of the ears, and in the olecranon and patellar bursae and tendons. Such deposits are called *gouty tophi*.

A potentially serious effect of hyperuricaemia is precipitation of urate in the kidneys, causing progressive renal damage. For this reason it has been recommended that even asymptomatic cases should be treated if the plasma urate concentration is consistently higher than 0.6 mmol/L (10 mg/dl).

Secondary Hyperuricaemia (Fig. 19.2)

High plasma urate concentrations may be secondary to:

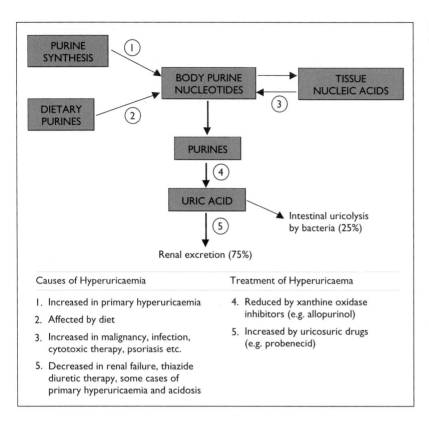

Fig. 19.2 Origin and fate of urate in normal subjects.

increased turnover of nucleic acids:

- *in rapidly growing malignant tissue,* especially in leukaemias, lymphomas and polycythaemia rubra vera;
- *in psoriasis,* when turnover of skin cells is increased;
- *following increased tissue breakdown:*
  after treatment of large malignant tumours by radiotherapy or cytotoxic drugs. This can cause massive, sudden release of urate, which may crystallize in and block renal tubules causing acute oliguric renal dysfunction. During such treatment allopurinol should be given and, if glomerular function is not impaired, fluid intake kept high;
  due to trauma including that of surgery; endogenous urate release is increased;
  during starvation or stringent dieting. The patient's own tissues may be used as an energy source with increased urate release. Starvation may be associated with mild ketoacidosis and protein catabolism releases acidic amino acid residues (p.**80**). The acidosis, by inhibiting secretion of urate, may aggravate the hyperuricaemia. During complete fasting plasma concentrations may exceed 0.9 mmol/L (15 mg/dl).

reduced excretion of urate due to:

- *renal glomerular dysfunction.* Before the diagnosis of primary hyperuricaemia is made, the plasma concentration of urea and/or creatinine should be assayed on the same specimen as urate, to exclude renal dysfunction as a cause. It may be difficult to decide which abnormality is the primary one because hyperuricaemia can cause renal dysfunction. As a rough guide the plasma urate concentration would be expected to be about 0.6 mmol/L (10 mg/dl) due to glomerular retention alone at a plasma urea concentration of about 50 mmol/L (300 mg/dl); if it is much higher than this hyperuricaemia is probably the primary cause of the renal dysfunction. Clinical gout is rare in the secondary hyperuricaemia of renal disease;

- *thiazide diuretics*. Although hyperuricaemia is relatively common during diuretic treatment, clinical gout is a rare complication. It may, however, be precipitated in those patients with a gouty tendency;
- *prolonged metabolic acidosis*;
- *low doses of salicylates*.

Hyperuricaemia associated with:

- *hypercalcaemia*. For unknown reasons hyperuricaemia, and even clinical gout, are relatively common in patients with hypercalcaemia from any cause, and in patients with recurrent renal calculi, even when not associated with hypercalcaemia;
- *glucose-6-phosphatase deficiency* (p.**214**). The tendency to hyperuricaemia in these patients may be related directly to the inability to convert glucose-6-phosphate (G-6-P) to glucose. More G-6-P is available for metabolism through intracellular pathways, including:
    the pentose-phosphate pathway, thus increasing ribose phosphate (phosphoribose) synthesis. This may accelerate the first step in purine synthesis, with consequent urate overproduction;
    glycolysis, thus increasing lactic acid production (p.**203**). Lactic acid may reduce renal urate excretion.

Primary Hyperuricaemia and Gout

FAMILIAL INCIDENCE

In AD 150 Galen said that gout was due to 'debauchery, intemperance and an hereditary trait'. As we shall see, 'intemperance' may aggravate the condition. The striking familial incidence of hyperuricaemia confirms that there is probably an 'hereditary trait', but in this respect we know little more than Galen; the mode of inheritance, like that of diabetes mellitus, is still not fully established.

SEX AND AGE INCIDENCE

Primary hyperuricaemia and gout are very rare in children and rare in women of child-bearing age. The higher incidence in males cannot be due to sex-linked inheritance because the syndrome can be transmitted by males. Plasma urate concentrations are low in children and rise in both sexes at puberty, more so in males than females. Women become more prone to hyperuricaemia and gout in the post-menopausal period (compare plasma cholesterol and iron concentrations). It may be that renal excretion of urate is affected by sex-hormone levels.

PRECIPITATING FACTORS

The classical image of the gouty subject is the red-faced, good-living, hard drinking squire depicted in novels and paintings of the 18th century. Two factors probably account for the high incidence of clinical gout in this type of subject.

- *Alcohol* has been shown to decrease renal excretion of urate. This may be because it increases lactic acid production, which inhibits urate secretion.
- *A high meat diet* contains a relatively high proportion of purines.

Neither of these factors is likely to precipitate gout in a normal person, but, like thiazide diuretics, may do so in a subject with a hyperuricaemic tendency.

BIOCHEMICAL DEFECTS IN PRIMARY HYPERURICAEMIA

Purine synthesis is increased in about 25 per cent of cases of primary hyperuricaemia due to overactivity of amidophosphoribosyl transferase which controls the formation of phosphoribosylamine (p.**366**).

Reduced renal tubular secretion of urate has also been demonstrated in other cases of primary hyperuricaemia. Many subjects may have both increased synthesis and decreased excretion.

PRINCIPLES OF TREATMENT OF PRIMARY HYPERURICAEMIA (FIG. 19.2)

Treatment may be based on:

- *reducing dietary purine intake.* This treatment is not very effective by itself;
- *increasing renal excretion of urate with uricosuric drugs*, such as probenecid and salicylates in large doses. These drugs are very effective if renal function is normal, but are useless if there is renal glomerular dysfunction. Fluid intake must be kept high. Low doses of most uricosuric drugs reduce urate secretion;
- *reducing urate production* by using drugs that *inhibit xanthine oxidase activity*, such as *allopurinol* (hydroxypyrazolopyrimidine), which is structurally similar to hypoxanthine, so acting as a competitive inhibitor of the enzyme. *De novo* synthesis may also be decreased by this drug;
- *colchicine*, which has an anti-inflammatory effect in acute gouty arthritis but does not affect urate metabolism.

JUVENILE HYPERURICAEMIA (LESCH–NYHAN SYNDROME)

This is an *exceedingly* rare X-linked, recessively inherited disorder of urate metabolism caused by a reduced activity of *hypoxanthine-guanine phosphoribosyl transferase* (HGPRT). Severe hyperuricaemia occurs in young male children. Hypoxanthine and other purines cannot be recycled to form purine nucleotides, and probably produce more urate. The syndrome is associated with mental deficiency, a tendency to self-mutilation, aggressive behaviour, athetosis and spastic paraplegia.

Pseudogout

Pseudogout is not a disorder of purine metabolism although the clinical prresentation is similar to that of gout. Calcium pyrophosphate precipitates in joint cavities, and calcification of cartilages is demonstrable radiologically. The plasma urate concentration is normal. The crystals of calcium pyrophosphate may be identified in joint fluid using a polarizing microscope.

*H*YPOURICAEMIA

Hypouricaemia, unless the result of treatment of hyperuricaemia with, for example allopurinol, is rare. It is an unimportant finding associated with proximal renal tubular damage, in which reabsorption of urate is reduced. It is also an unimportant finding in some patients receiving parenteral nutrition.

Xanthinuria is a very rare inborn error of purine metabolism, inherited as an autosomal recessive disorder, in which there is a deficiency of xanthine oxidase in the liver. Purine breakdown stops at the xanthine-hypoxanthine stage, and plasma and urinary urate concentrations are very low. Increased xanthine excretion may lead to formation of xanthine stones: this does not occur during treatment of gout with xanthine oxidase inhibitors, perhaps because the drugs also inhibit purine synthesis.

Summary

1. Urate is the end-product of purine metabolism.
2. Hyperuricaemia may result from:
   - an increased rate of nucleic acid turnover (malignancy, tissue damage, starvation);
   - an increased rate of synthesis of purines (primary gout);
   - a reduced rate of renal excretion of urate (glomerular dysfunction, thiazide diuretics, acidosis).
3. Hyperuricaemia may be aggravated by:
   - high purine diets;
   - acidosis or a high alcohol intake.
4. Primary hyperuricaemia and gout have a familial incidence. Both are rare in women of child-bearing age.
5. Severe hyperuricaemia may cause renal damage and should be treated even if asymptomatic.
6. Hypouricaemia is rare and usually unimportant. It occurs in the very rare inborn error, xanthinuria.

Haem Metabolism: Iron and the Porphyrias

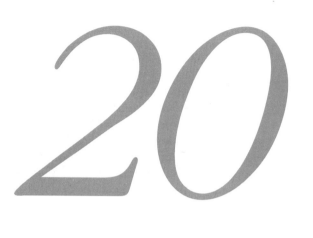

Haem Metabolism

Haem is synthesized in most tissues of the body. In bone marrow it is incorporated into haemoglobin, an iron-containing pigment that carries oxygen from the lungs to tissues, and in muscle into myoglobin which binds oxygen and provides a local reservoir of the gas. In other cells it is used for the synthesis of cytochromes and related compounds. The cytochromes are constituents of the electron transport chain which harnesses the energy of metabolic processes. The liver is quantitatively the largest nonerythropoietic haem-producing organ.

All haem pigments contain iron; the oxygen-carrying ability of the haem molecule depends on the presence of ferrous iron (Fe^{2+}), the form present in both haemoglobin and oxyhaemoglobin.

BIOSYNTHESIS OF HAEM AND HAEMOGLOBIN

The main steps in the synthesis of haem are outlined below and in Fig. 20.1. Each step is controlled by a specific enzyme.

- *5-aminolaevulinate* (*ALA*) is formed by condensation of glycine and succinate. The reaction requires pyridoxal phosphate and is catalysed by *ALA synthase*. This is the rate-limiting step in the synthetic pathway and is regulated by feedback inhibition by haem.
- Two molecules of ALA condense to form a monopyrrole, *porphobilinogen* (*PBG*).
- Four molecules of PBG combine to form a tetrapyrrole ring, *uroporphyrinogen* (Fig. 20.2). Two isomers are formed, I and III. The major pathway involves the III isomer.
- Haem is formed by the successive production of coproporphyrinogen and protoporphyrin, followed by incorporation of ferrous iron (Fe^{2+}) into the centre of the ring.
- Haemoglobin consists of four haem molecules, covalently linked to four (two pairs) of polypeptide chains. Inherited

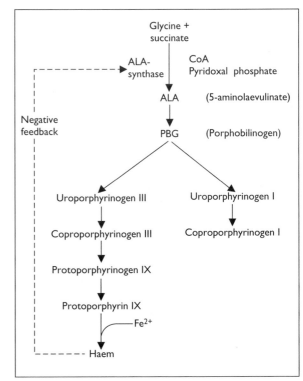

Fig. 20.1 Biosynthesis of haem.

disorders of haemoglobin (haemoglobinopathies) and of red cell synthesis are beyond the scope of this text; a textbook of haematology should be consulted.

EXCRETION OF HAEM PRECURSORS

Intermediates on the haem pathway, in excess of those used, are excreted in either urine or faeces.

- *The porphyrin precursors ALA, PBG and uroporphyrinogen* are water-soluble and appear in the *urine*. They are colourless, but PBG may spontaneously oxidize to form uroporphyrin when exposed to air and light. Porphyrinogens also oxidize spontaneously to the corresponding porphyrins, which are dark red and which

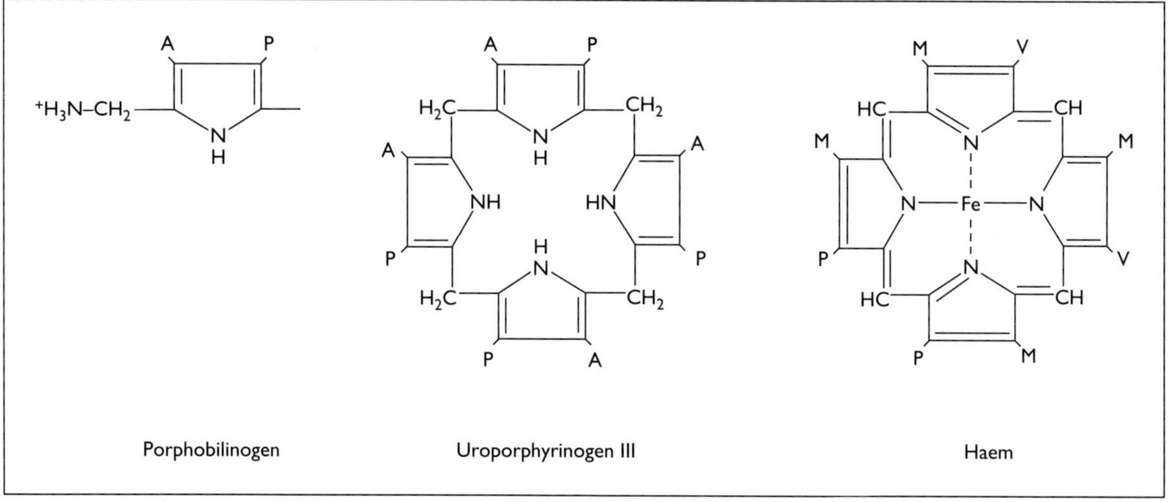

Fig. 20.2 Porphobilinogen, the tetrapyrrole uroporphyrinogen III which incorporates four porphobilinogen units and haemoglobin. Uroporphyrinogen I differs only in the order of the side-chains on one of the rings. (Side-chains: A = acetate; M = methyl; P = propionate; V = vinyl).

fluoresce in ultraviolet light. A urine specimen containing large amounts of porphyrinogens or their precursors will gradually darken if left standing.

- *Protoporphyrin* is excreted in bile and appears in the *faeces* whereas coproporphyrin(ogen) may be excreted by either route.

HAEMOGLOBIN AND RELATED COMPOUNDS

When haemoglobin incorporates oxygen to form oxyhaemoglobin, the spatial arrangement of the haem complexes is altered in such a way as to facilitate further oxygen uptake (p.98). Other compounds related to haemoglobin may sometimes be formed and some of these may hinder the oxygen carrying capacity.

- *Myoglobin,* the single haem-polypeptide complex is normally present in muscle. Plasma concentrations may rise if skeletal or myocardial muscle cells are damaged. Because of its small size, it is rapidly cleared by the kidneys. Increased filtrate levels may cause renal damage.
- *Carboxyhaemoglobin* is cherry-red in colour and is formed when carbon monoxide (CO) binds to haemoglobin or displaces oxygen from oxyhaemoglobin; haemoglobin have a greater affinity for CO than for oxygen. This occurs in carbon monoxide poisoning. Once CO is removed from inspired air, oxyhaemoglobin is reformed. Consciousness is not lost until about half the oxyhaemoglobin has been replaced by the carboxy form.
- *Methaemoglobin* is haemoglobin in which iron is in the ferric (Fe^{3+}) form (haemin); therefore it cannot carry oxygen. It is brown and is normally present in very low plasma concentrations; these may be increased by drugs, such as phenacetin and sulphonamides. Symptoms of methaemoglobinaemia are due to hypoxia, which causes cyanosis and an increased respiratory rate.

- *Methaemalbumin* is brown. It is formed when haem combines with plasma albumin in such conditions as severe intravascular haemolysis or acute haemorrhagic pancreatitis when haemoglobin has been converted to haemin in the abdominal cavity and absorbed. The haemoglobin-binding capacity of haptoglobin (p.**320**) has then been exceeded.
- *Sulphaemoglobin* is similar to methaemoglobin but contains sulphur; unlike methaemoglobin, it cannot be reconverted to haemoglobin *in vivo*. It remains in intact red blood cells. Methaemoglobinaemia-producing drugs cause sulphaemoglobinaemia if hydrogen sulphide is present, usually in the gut.

Metabolism of Haem

Red blood cells are broken down by the reticuloendothelial system, mainly in the spleen. The released haemoglobin is split into the peptide chain, globin, which enters the general protein pool, and haem. The ring of the latter is split, a process catalysed by haem oxidase to form a linear molecule, biliverdin. Released iron is reused and biliverdin reduced to lipid-soluble bilirubin. The metabolism of bilirubin is discussed in Chapter 14.

Iron Metabolism

DISTRIBUTION OF IRON IN THE BODY

Between 50 to 70 mmol (3 to 4 g) of iron are distributed between body compartments. The control of iron distribution is poorly understood but there is considerable interchange between stores and plasma.

Free iron is toxic. In normal subjects it is all protein-bound; in plasma it is bound to transferrin, in the stores to protein in ferritin and haemosiderin, and in erythrocytes it is incorporated into haemoglobin.

- About 70 per cent of the total iron is circulating in *erythrocyte haemoglobin*.
- Up to 25 per cent of the body iron is stored in the *reticuloendothelial system*, in the liver, spleen and bone marrow; bone marrow iron is drawn on for haemoglobin synthesis. Iron is stored as protein complexes, *ferritin* and *haemosiderin*. Ferritin iron is more easily released from protein than that in haemosiderin. Haemosiderin, probably an aggregate of ferritin, can be seen by light microscopy in unstained tissue preparations.

Ferritin and haemosiderin, but not haem iron, stain with potassium ferrocyanide ('Prussian blue reaction') and this staining characteristic may be used to assess the size of iron stores.

Iron deficiency only becomes haematologically evident when *no stainable iron* is detectable in the reticuloendothelial cells in bone marrow films.

Iron overload is likely when, because reticuloendothelial storage capacity is exceeded, *stainable iron is demonstrable in parenchymal cells in liver* biopsy specimens.

Histological assessment is more reliable for detecting iron deficiency than overload (p.**382**).

- *Only about 50–70 μmol (3 to 4 mg), or about 0.1 per cent of the total body iron, is circulating in plasma*, all bound to transferrin; this fraction is measured in plasma iron assays.
- The rest of the body iron is incorporated into myoglobin, cytochromes and iron-containing enzymes.

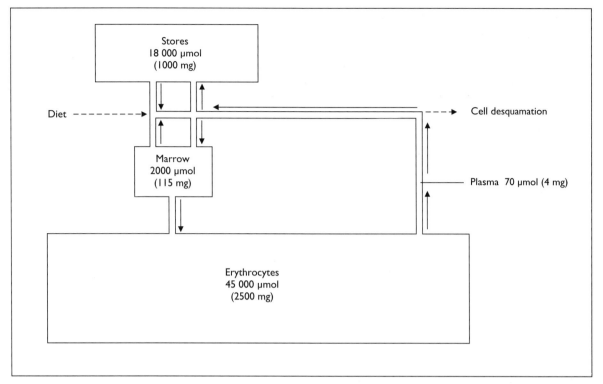

Fig. 20.3 Body iron compartments.

Iron can only cross cell membranes by active transport in the ferrous (Fe^{2+}) form; it is in this reduced state in both oxyhaemoglobin and 'reduced' haemoglobin. It is in the ferric (Fe^{3+}) form in ferritin and haemosiderin and when bound to transferrin.

IRON ABSORPTION

The control of body iron content depends upon control of absorption by an active process in the upper small intestine. Within the intestinal cell some of the iron combines with the protein *apoferritin* to form ferritin, which, as elsewhere in the body, is a storage compound.

Normally about 18 µmol (1 mg) of iron is absorbed each day and this just replaces loss. This amounts to about 10 per cent of that taken in the diet, although the proportion depends to some extent on the type of food. *Once in the body, iron is in a virtually closed system* (Fig. 20.3).

Iron absorption seems to be influenced by any or all of the following factors:

- oxygen tension in the intestinal cells;
- marrow erythropoietic activity;
- the size of the body iron stores.

Iron absorption is also increased in many non-iron deficiency anaemias.

- Most normal women taking an adequate diet probably absorb slightly more iron than men and so replace their higher losses in menstrual blood and during pregnancy.
- Iron requirements for growth during childhood and adolescence are similar to, or slightly higher than, those of menstruating women and can be met by increased absorption from a normal diet.

Table 20.1 Comparison of iron losses in men and menstruating and pregnant women

	Source of loss	Extra loss	Daily extra loss	Daily total loss
Men and non-menstruating women	Desquamation	–	–	18 µmol (1 mg)
Menstruating women (mean value)	Desquamation + menstruation	290 µmol (16 mg)/month	9 µmol (0.5 mg)	27 µmol (1.5 mg)
Pregnancy	Desquamation + loss to fetus and in placenta	7000 µmol (380 mg)/9 months	27 µmol (1.5 mg)	45 µmol (2.5 mg)
Male blood donors	Desquamation + 1 unit of blood	4500 µmol (250 mg)/4 months	36 µmol (2.0 mg)	54 µmol (3.0 mg)

IRON EXCRETION

There is probably no control of iron excretion; loss from the body may depend on the ferritin iron content of cells lost by desquamation, mostly into the intestinal tract and from the skin. The total daily loss by these routes is about 18 µmol (1 mg). Urinary loss is negligible, reflecting the fact that all circulating iron is protein-bound.

The comparison of iron losses between men and menstruating and pregnant women is shown in Table 20.1. Normal iron loss is so small, and normal iron stores are so large, that it would take about three years to become iron-deficient on a completely iron-free diet. Of course, this period is much shorter if there is any abnormal blood loss.

IRON TRANSPORT IN PLASMA

Iron is transported in the plasma in the ferric form, attached to the specific binding protein, *transferrin*, at a concentration of about 18 µmol/L (100 mg/dl). Transferrin is normally capable of binding about 54 µmol/L (300 mg/dl) of iron and is therefore about a third saturated. Transferrin-bound iron is carried to stores and to bone marrow cells and in the latter some iron passes directly into developing erythrocytes to form haemoglobin.

Factors Affecting Plasma Iron Concentration

Plasma iron estimation is often requested, but is rarely of clinical value, and results are often, sometimes dangerously, misinterpreted. The plasma iron concentration is likely to be a poor index of the total body content because only a very small proportion is in this compartment; it has no function, except as a protein-bound transport fraction. *The concentration is not tightly controlled, and varies greatly, even under physiological conditions.*

PHYSIOLOGICAL FACTORS AFFECTING PLASMA IRON CONCENTRATION

The causes of physiological changes in plasma iron concentrations are not well understood, but alterations can be very rapid and almost certainly represent shifts between plasma and stores, not changes in total body iron. The following factors are known to affect plasma concentrations within a population:

- *Sex and age differences.* Plasma iron concentrations, like those of haemoglobin and the erythrocyte count, are higher in men than in women, probably for hormonal reasons. The difference is first evident at puberty, before significant menstrual loss has occurred, and disappears at the menopause. Androgens tend to increase the plasma iron concentration and oestrogens to lower it.

- *Pregnancy and oral contraceptives.* In the first few weeks of pregnancy the plasma iron may rise to concentrations similar to those found in men. A similar rise occurs in women taking some oral contraceptives.

Variations within a individual, which can cause changes of 100 per cent or more, include:

- *random variations.* Day-to-day variations may be as much as three-fold and usually overshadow cyclical changes. They may be associated with physical or mental stress, but more usually no cause can be found;
- *circadian (diurnal) rhythm.* The plasma iron concentration is higher in the morning than in the evening. If subjects are kept awake at night this difference is less marked; it is reversed in night workers;
- *monthly variations in women.* The plasma iron may reach very low concentrations just before or during the menstrual period. The reduction is probably due to hormonal factors rather than blood loss.

PATHOLOGICAL FACTORS AFFECTING PLASMA IRON CONCENTRATION

Iron deficiency and iron overload usually cause low and high plasma iron concentrations respectively.

- *Iron deficiency* is associated with a *hypochromic, microcytic anaemia* and with reduced amounts of stainable bone marrow iron. Plasma ferritin concentrations are usually, but not always, low.
- *Iron overload* is associated with increased amounts of stainable iron in liver biopsy specimens and plasma ferritin concentrations are high.

Other pathological factors that may affect plasma iron concentrations include:

- *any acute or chronic illness*, even a bad cold, causing a fall in plasma iron concentration. Chronic conditions such as malignancy, renal disease, rheumatoid arthritis and chronic infections are often associated with *normochromic, normocytic anaemia.* Iron stores and plasma ferritin concentrations are normal or even increased; *the anaemia does not respond to iron therapy.* Iron deficiency may be superimposed on the anaemia of chronic illness especially if drugs are being taken that cause gastrointestinal bleeding; plasma ferritin concentrations are then variable. The finding of hypochromic erythrocytes is the most sensitive index of this complication. *Low plasma iron concentrations occur whether or not there is any iron deficiency;*
- *disorders in which the marrow cannot use iron*, either because it is hypoplastic, or because some other essential erythropoietic factor, such as vitamin B_{12} or folate, is deficient; plasma iron concentrations are often high. Blood and marrow films may show a typical picture, but, for example, in pyridoxine-responsive anaemia (p.**274**) and in thalassaemia, the findings in the blood film may resemble those of iron deficiency; in the last two conditions the presence of stainable marrow iron stores excludes the diagnosis of iron deficiency;
- *haemolytic anaemia.* The plasma iron concentration may be high during a haemolytic episode as iron, liberated from the destroyed erythrocytes, enters the plasma; it is usually normal during the quiescent periods when the iron enters the reticuloendothelial system. Marrow iron stores and plasma ferritin concentrations are usually increased in chronic haemolytic conditions;
- *acute liver disease.* Disruption of hepatocytes may release ferritin iron into the blood stream and cause a transient rise in the plasma iron concentration. Cirrhosis may be associated with a similar finding, perhaps due to increased iron absorption and intake.

Transferrin and Total Iron-binding Capacity (TIBC)

Plasma iron concentrations alone give no information about the state of iron stores. In rare situations in which doubt remains after haematological investigation, diagnostic precision may sometimes be improved by measuring *both* the plasma transferrin and iron concentrations. *It is completely uninformative to estimate only the plasma iron concentration.*

If plasma transferrin assay is not available its concentration can be assessed by adding an excess of inorganic iron to the plasma, any not bound to protein being removed, usually with an exchange resin. The concentration of iron remaining is assayed and the result expressed as the total iron-binding capacity (TIBC). This is usually a valid measure of the transferrin concentration. In rare circumstances, of which the most common is severe liver disease, plasma ferritin concentrations are high enough to bind significant amounts of iron and results of iron-binding capacity measurements are then misleading as an assessment of the transferrin concentration.

PHYSIOLOGICAL CHANGES IN THE PLASMA TRANSFERRIN CONCENTRATION

The plasma transferrin concentration is less labile than that of iron. However, it rises:

- after about the 28th week of *pregnancy even if iron stores are normal*;
- in women taking some *oral contraceptive preparations*;
- in any patient treated with *oestrogens*.

PATHOLOGICAL CHANGES IN THE PLASMA TRANSFERRIN CONCENTRATION

Plasma transferrin concentration and TIBC:

- *rise in iron deficiency* and *fall in iron overload*;

- *fall* in those *chronic illnesses* associated with low plasma iron concentrations;
- are unchanged in acute illness;
- may be *very low in the nephrotic syndrome*, associated with a low plasma iron concentration, because the relatively low molecular weight transferrin is lost in the urine together with iron.

Thus the low plasma iron concentration of uncomplicated iron deficiency is associated with a high transferrin concentration and TIBC; that of non-iron deficiency is associated with low concentrations.

If iron deficiency coexists with the anaemia of chronic illness the opposing effects of the two conditions on the transferrin concentration make it difficult to interpret transferrin, as well as plasma iron, concentrations.

Ferritin

Circulating ferritin is usually in equilibrium with that in stores. However, it is an 'acute phase' protein (p.**319**) and its synthesis is increased in many inflammatory conditions.

The normal plasma ferritin concentration is about 100 µg/L. A *plasma concentration below about 10 µg/L almost certainly indicates iron deficiency*, although the assay is rarely necessary to make the diagnosis. Results can be misleading if there is coexistent inflammatory disease, since accelerated synthesis may lead to normal or even high plasma concentrations despite very low iron stores. In this situation results of plasma iron and transferrin assays are also difficult to interpret; haematological parameters remain the most reliable diagnostic indicators of iron deficiency.

High concentrations of plasma ferritin always occur in significant iron overload, but may also be due to:

- inflammatory conditions;
- malignant disease;
- liver disease.

Table 20.2   Biochemical findings associated with plasma iron abnormalities

	Plasma concentrations			Marrow stores
	Iron	Transferrin	Ferritin	
Low iron concentration				
Before menstruation	↓	Normal	Normal	Normal
Iron deficiency	↓	↑	Usually ↓	Absent or ↓↓
Acute illness	↓	Normal	Normal or ↑	Normal
Chronic illness	↓	↓	Normal or ↑	Usually ↑
High iron concentration				
Early pregnancy	↑*	Normal	Normal	Normal
Late pregnancy or oral contraceptives	variable	↑	Normal	Normal
Iron overload	↑	↓	↑	Usually ↑
Liver disease	↑	↓	↑	May be ↑
Impaired marrow utilization	↑	Normal or ↓	↑	↑
Haemolysis	↑	Normal or ↓ (acute)	↑ (chronic)	↑ (chronic)

* = to male concentrations.

Thus the *finding of a normal or low plasma ferritin concentration almost certainly excludes the diagnosis of iron overload, but a high one does not necessarily confirm it.*

The laboratory findings in conditions which may affect plasma iron concentrations are summarized in Table 20.2.

The student should read the section on 'Investigation of anaemia' on p389.

Iron Therapy

Because the body iron content is determined by control of absorption, rather than excretion, parenteral iron therapy, which by-passes absorption, and repeated blood transfusions, which contains about 4.5 mmol (250 mg) of iron per unit, may cause iron overload. In anaemias other than those due to iron deficiency, stores are normal or even increased; *parenteral iron should only be given if the diagnosis of iron deficiency is beyond doubt, and even then the oral route is preferable.* Repeated blood transfusions may be needed to correct severe non-iron

deficiency anaemia, for example if the marrow is hypoplastic, but the danger of overload should be remembered.

Iron absorption is stimulated by anaemia even if iron stores are increased. Treatment of non-iron deficient anaemia with oral iron supplements is not only ineffective, but can lead to iron overload; this is especially likely in haemolytic anaemia in which the iron released from destroyed erythrocytes remains in the body.

The control of absorption is inefficient and overload has been reported in a non-anaemic woman who continued to take large amounts of oral iron for many years against medical advice.

Iron therapy is potentially dangerous and should be prescribed only when iron deficiency is proven.

Iron Overload

As emphasized on p.**378**, the only route of iron loss is cell desquamation. Iron absorbed from the gastrointestinal tract or administered parenterally in excess of daily loss accumulates in body stores. If such 'positive balance' is maintained over long periods, iron stores may exceed 350 mmol (20 g) (about five times the normal amount).

CAUSES OF IRON OVERLOAD

Increased intestinal absorption:

- idiopathic haemochromatosis;
- anaemia with increased, but ineffective, erythropoiesis;
- liver disease (rare cause);
- dietary excess;
- inappropriate oral therapy.

Parenteral administration:

- multiple blood transfusions;
- inappropriate parenteral iron therapy.

A very rare cause of iron overload is an inherited deficiency of transferrin.

CONSEQUENCES OF IRON OVERLOAD

The effect of the accumulated iron depends on its distribution in the body. This, in turn, is influenced partly by the route of entry. Two main patterns are seen at postmortem or in biopsy specimens.

- *Parenchymal iron overload* occurs in idiopathic haemochromatosis and in patients with ineffective erythropoiesis. Iron accumulates in the parenchymal cells of the liver, pancreas, heart and other organs. There is usually associated functional disturbance or tissue damage.
- *Reticuloendothelial iron overload* is seen after excessive parenteral administration of iron or multiple blood transfusions. The iron accumulates initially in the reticuloendothelial cells of the liver, spleen and bone marrow. There are few harmful effects but, under certain circumstances (p.**383**), the distribution may change so that parenchymal damage occurs.

In dietary iron overload both hepatic reticuloendothelial and parenchymal overload may occur, associated with scurvy and osteoporosis (p.**383**). Whatever the cause of *massive* iron overload, there may be parenchymal accumulation and tissue damage.

- *Haemosiderosis* is a histological definition. An increase in iron stores as haemosiderin can be seen. It does not necessarily mean that there is an increase in total body iron; for example, in many types of anaemia there is reduced haemoglobin iron (less haemoglobin) but increased storage iron.
- *Haemochromatosis* describes the clinical disorder due to parenchymal iron-induced damage.

SYNDROMES OF IRON OVERLOAD

Idiopathic haemochromatosis is an autosomal recessive disorder (p.**291**) in which increased intestinal absorption of iron over many years produces large iron stores of parenchymal distribution. It presents, usually in middle age, as cirrhosis of the liver with diabetes mellitus, hypogonadism and greyish skin pigmentation due to melanin, not iron. The disorder occurs more commonly in men, partly because of the protective effect of menstrual blood loss in women. Factors such as alcohol abuse may hasten the accumulation of iron and the development of liver damage. Consequently it may be difficult to distinguish between idiopathic haemochromatosis and alcoholic cirrhosis. The diagnosis of idiopathic haemochromatosis must be followed by investigation of other members of the family and treatment of those in whom increased iron stores are found.

Treatment of iron overload. The excess iron is usually removed from patients by weekly venesection until the haemoglobin concentration falls. Each unit of blood removes about 4.5 mmol (250 mg) of iron.

Anaemia and iron overload. Several types of anaemia may be associated with iron overload. In some, such as hypoplastic anaemia and the anaemia of chronic renal failure, the cause is multiple blood transfusions; the iron initially accumulates in the reticuloendothelial system. If overload is massive (over 100 units of blood), deposition may occur in parenchymal cells with the development of secondary haemochromatosis.

In anaemias characterized by erythroid marrow hyperplasia, but with ineffective erythropoiesis, such as thalassaemia major and sideroblastic anaemia, there is, in addition, increased absorption of iron. Haemochromatosis develops at a lower transfusion load than in hypoplastic anaemia.

Treatment of iron overload of anaemia. This can obviously not be treated by venesection. The tendency for transfusion further to aggravate iron overload can be minimized by giving the iron-chelating agent, desferrioxamine, each time; this can be excreted in the urine with any nonhaemoglobin iron.

Dietary iron overload. Increased iron absorption due to excessive intake is rare. One well-described form is, however, relatively common in the rural black population of southern Africa. The source is beer brewed in iron containers. Usually the excess is confined to the reticuloendothelial system and the liver (both portal tracts and parenchymal cells), and there is no tissue damage. In a small number of cases deposition in the parenchymal cells of other organs occurs and the clinical picture may resemble that of primary haemochromatosis; it may be distinguished by the high concentration of iron in the reticuloendothelial system seen in the bone marrow and spleen (at autopsy).

Scurvy and osteoporosis may occur in this form of iron overload. The ascorbate deficiency may be due to its irreversible oxidation in the presence of excessive amounts of iron, and osteoporosis sometimes accompanies scurvy. Ascorbate deficiency also interferes with normal mobilization of iron from the reticuloendothelial cells; plasma iron concentrations may be low and the response to chelating agents poor, despite iron overload.

*The student should read the section on 'Investigation of suspected iron overload' on p***390***.*

Disorders of Haem Synthesis: the Porphyrias

The porphyrias are a rare group of disorders, usually inherited, of haem synthesis, resulting from a deficiency of one of the enzymes on the haem synthetic pathway (p.**374**). Haem production is therefore impaired but *reduced feedback inhibition of ALA synthase, the rate limiting step, may maintain adequate haem levels at the expense of overproduction of porphyrins or their precursors.*

The symptoms of porphyria correlate well with the biochemical abnormalities.

Neurological disturbances, such as *peripheral neuropathy, abdominal pain,* or both in a serious acute attack, occur only in those porphyrias in which the precursors, *ALA and PBG*, are produced in excess. It is not known whether the neurological damage is due to haem deficiency in the nervous system or to a direct toxic effect of ALA or PBG.

Skin lesions, varying from mild *photosensitivity* to severe blistering, occur when *porphyrins* are produced in excess. The lesions typically occur in the exposed areas where sunlight activates porphyrins in the skin to release energy that damages tissue.

Many different forms of porphyria have been described. Although most are uncommon and some are very rare, it is important to recognize them and to investigate relatives of known cases. For example, drugs that may precipitate acute attacks, sometimes with fatal consequences, must be avoided in the inherited hepatic porphyrias. It is equally important not to confuse the commoner, secondary causes of abnormal porphyrin excretion with true porphyrias.

Porphyrias are usually classified according to whether the main site of porphyrin accumulation is in the liver or the erythropoietic system although this does not necessarily mean that the enzyme defect is confined to that system. The main porphyrias are:

- *hepatic porphyrias*
   acute intermittent porphyria ⎫ acute
   hereditary coproporphyria ⎬ porphyrias
   porphyria variegata ⎭
   porphyria cutanea tarda:
      genetic predisposition;
      acquired.

- *erythropoietic porphyrias*
   congenital erythropoietic porphyria;
   protoporphyria.

The major clinical and biochemical features are outlined in Table 20.3 and discussed briefly below.

The Acute Hepatic Porphyrias

- Acute intermittent porphyria.
- Hereditary coproporphyria.
- Porphyria variegata.

These three *dominantly* inherited disorders have latent and acute phases. The symptoms and biochemical abnormalities of the latent phases differ and reflect the nature of the enzyme defect. In the acute phases, however, the biochemical and clinical pictures characteristic of excessive ALA and PBG production, associated with neurological and abdominal symptoms, develop. The similarities and differences are best explained by referring to a simplified scheme of the haem synthetic pathway (Fig. 20.1; p.**374**).

Table 20.3 The major clinical and biochemical features of the porphyrias

	Hepatic porphyrias				Porphyrias involving the erythropoietic system	
	Acute intermittent porphyria	Porphyria variegata	Hereditary copro-porphyria	Porphyria cutanea tarda	Congenital erythropoietic porphyria	Proto-porphyria
	Acute Latent	Acute Latent	Acute Latent			
Clinical features						
Abdominal and neurological symptoms	+ −	+ −	+ −	−	−	−
Skin lesions	− −	+ +	Rarely Rarely	+	+	+
Biochemical abnormalities						
Urine PBG and ALA	+ +	+ −	+ −	−	−	−
Urine porphyrins	+ −	+ −	+ −	+	+	−
Faecal porphyrins	− −	+ +	+ +	−	+	+
	Acute attacks are precipitated by many drugs (for instance barbiturates, oestrogens, sulphonamides)			Symptoms may be relieved by venesection	Erythrocyte porphyrins increased	

LATENT PHASE

The enzyme defect tends to reduce haem levels, which in turn increase ALA synthase activity by a decrease in negative feedback inhibition. Increased ALA synthase activity has been demonstrated in all the porphyrias. Haem levels are maintained at the expense of accumulation and excretion of the substance immediately before the block. The main biochemical abnormalities are predictable (Fig. 20.4). In:

- acute *intermittent porphyria,* there is increased *urinary ALA and PBG* excretion although it may not be detectable in all patients; the latent phase is usually asymptomatic;
- *hereditary coproporphyria,* there is increased *faecal coproporphyrin* excretion; the increase in porphyrins may produce skin lesions but less commonly than in porphyria variegata;
- *porphyria variegata,* there is increased *faecal protoporphyrin* excretion; the increase in porphyrins may produce skin lesions.

Diagnosis of latent porphyria. It is essential to investigate the blood relatives of any patient with porphyria. Screening tests for excess urinary PBG and ALA are inadequate to diagnose latent acute intermittent porphyria, and even quantitative estimation may fail to detect all carriers. The activity of the enzyme, porphobilinogen deaminase, should be measured in erythrocytes, the most easily available cells.

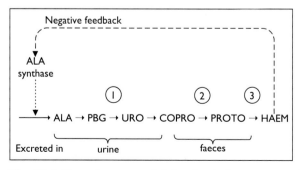

Fig. 20.4 Sites of enzyme deficiencies in:1. acute intermittent porphyria; 2. hereditary coproporphyria; 3. porphyria variegata.

ACUTE PHASE

ALA synthase activity may be further increased by a number of drugs, particularly barbiturates, oestrogens, sulphonamides and griseofulvin, and by acute illness; this may be a direct effect or may be due to an increased demand for haem. It results in a marked increase in ALA and PBG production. In acute intermittent porphyria this increase is due to the block imposed by an inherited deficiency of *porphobilinogen deaminase*; in hepatic coproporphyria and porphyria variegata, this enzyme becomes rate-limiting and is unable to respond normally to the increased demand. *The increase in urinary ALA and PBG is the hallmark of the acute porphyric attack* and, in hereditary coproporphyria and porphyria variegata, is superimposed on all the other biochemical abnormalities. The accelerated activity of the pathway and the spontaneous conversion of the precursors to porphyrin leads to increased urinary porphyrin excretion.

Acute attacks occur only in a small proportion of patients exposed to the provoking agents. They occur usually only after puberty and are commoner in women than men. Colicky abdominal pain, due to involvement of the autonomic nervous system, and neurological symptoms ranging from peripheral neuritis to quadriplegia are usually the presenting features. Death may result from respiratory paralysis.

The acute attack closely resembles serious acute intra-abdominal conditions and, if the diagnosis is not made, the patient may be subjected to surgery with the use of a barbiturate anaesthetic; barbiturates and the stress of operation may aggravate the condition.

Porphyria Cutanea Tarda

In patients with porphyria cutanea tarda the skin is unduly sensitive to minor trauma, particularly in sun-exposed areas; the commonest presenting feature is blistering on the backs of the hands. Less commonly the lesions appear on the face. Increased facial hair and hyperpigmentation occur in chronic cases. *Acute attacks do not occur.*

The basic defect is an inability to convert uroporphyrinogen to coproporphyrinogen due to a deficiency of uroporphyrinogen decarboxylase. This may be a dominantly inherited disorder, but most cases are sporadic. Factors that produce clinical disease, possibly by aggravating an underlying genetic deficiency, include alcohol abuse, iron overload or high-dose oestrogen therapy. Symptoms improve when the offending substance is withdrawn. Some liver toxins such as hexachlorbenzene directly inhibit the activity of the enzyme.

The impaired conversion leads to an accumulation of uroporphyrinogen and porphyrins intermediate between it and coproporphyrinogen. These deposit in the skin and are excreted in the urine in increased amounts. Faecal porphyrins are not increased but the abnormal pattern of intermediate porphyrins may be detected by chromatography; this finding is of diagnostic value.

It is important not to confuse this disorder with the coproporphyrinuria of liver disease (see below).

Erythropoietic Porphyrias

Two rare inherited disorders are associated with accumulation of porphyrins in erythrocytes. Acute porphyric attacks do not occur and ALA and PBG excretion are normal.

Congenital erythropoietic porphyria, unlike all the other porphyrias discussed, is inherited as a *recessive* characteristic. Usually from infancy onwards blood erythrocyte and plasma uroporphyrin I concentrations are very high and there is severe *photosensitivity*. Porphyrins are also deposited in bones and teeth, which fluoresce in ultraviolet light; the teeth may be brownish-pink in colour. Hirsutism, especially of the face, also occurs and there is haemolytic anaemia.

Urinary porphyrin concentrations are grossly increased, and faecal levels less so.

Protoporphyria. This is a *dominantly* inherited disorder in which *protoporphyrin concentrations are increased in erythrocytes and faeces.* There is mild photosensitivity, and hepatocellular damage may lead to liver failure.

Other Causes of Excessive Porphyrin Excretion

Porphyria is not the only cause of disordered porphyrin metabolism and positive screening tests *must be confirmed* by quantitative analysis, with identification of the porphyrin. Three causes must be considered.

- **Lead poisoning** inhibits several of the enzymes involved in haem synthesis and eventually causes anaemia. The urine contains increased amounts of ALA (an early and sensitive test), and coproporphyrin. Some of the symptoms of lead poisoning, such as abdominal pain, are similar to those of the acute porphyric attack, and may cause difficulty in diagnosis. PBG excretion, however, is not usually increased.

- **Liver disease** may increase urinary coproporphyrin levels, possibly because of decreased biliary excretion. This is probably the commonest cause of porphyrinuria. Occasionally there is mild photosensitivity (in porphyria cutanea tarda the more severe skin lesions are due to uroporphyrin excess).

- **Ulcerative lesions of the upper gastrointestinal tract** may produce raised levels of faecal porphyrin by degradation of haemoglobin. If there is bleeding from the lower part of the tract the blood reaches the rectum before there is time for conversion; this may help roughly to localize the site of bleeding.

Summary

Haem

1. Haem is incorporated into haemoglobin, myoglobin and the cytochromes.
2. Haem pigments may be detected in plasma or urine in a number of disorders.

Iron

1. Iron is essential for the oxygen carrying capacity of haemoglobin and myoglobin.
2. There is no significant iron excretion. Body stores are determined by control of absorption. Parenteral iron therapy should be given with care.
3. Anaemia, even if not due to iron deficiency, increases absorption. Prolonged oral iron therapy should only be given if iron deficiency is proven.
4. Plasma iron concentrations vary considerably for physiological reasons and fall in many cases of non-iron deficiency anaemia. They give no information about the size of body iron stores.
5. Plasma iron is transported bound to transferrin. Transferrin concentrations may be measured directly, or indirectly as the total iron-binding capacity (TIBC) of the plasma.
6. The plasma transferrin concentration rises in iron deficiency and falls in iron overload.
7. The plasma transferrin concentration falls in many cases of non-iron deficiency anaemia associated with a low plasma iron concentration. A low plasma iron with a high transferrin concentration is more suggestive of iron deficiency than a low plasma iron concentration alone.

8. Plasma ferritin concentrations are affected by the state of iron stores and by an increased rate of synthesis in inflammatory states. A very low plasma ferritin concentration almost certainly confirms the diagnosis of iron deficiency, but a normal or high one does not exclude it. A normal or low plasma ferritin concentration almost certainly excludes a diagnosis of iron overload, but a high one does not necessarily confirm it.
9. The factors governing the distribution of excessive iron are not fully understood. A feature common to all forms of parenchymal overload is a high percentage saturation of transferrin.
10. Iron overload may be the result of excessive intestinal absorption or of parenteral iron administration, usually as blood. The distribution of iron in the body differs in the various forms of iron overload.
11. Iron overload can be demonstrated by the response to repeated venesection or to chelating agents. The diagnosis of idiopathic haemochromatosis should only be made if massive iron overload is present.

The Porphyrias

1. Porphyrins are byproducts of haem synthesis. 5-aminolaevulinate (ALA) and porphobilinogen (PBG) are precursors.
2. The porphyrias are diseases associated with disturbed porphyrin metabolism. Most are inherited.
3. Acute attacks, with abdominal or neurological symptoms, are a feature of the inherited hepatic porphyrias. Such attacks are potentially fatal and may be provoked by a

number of drugs. The diagnosis of porphyria in the acute phase depends on the demonstration of ALA and PBG in the urine.

4. The diagnosis of inherited porphyria must be followed by investigation of all blood relatives to detect asymptomatic cases. Screening tests may be negative in some types and quantitative estimations are necessary. Both urine and faeces should be examined.

5. Other causes of abnormal porphyrin excretion are lead poisoning, liver disease and upper gastrointestinal bleeding.

6. The very rare erythropoietic porphyrias cause excessive accumulation of porphyrin in erythrocytes.

INVESTIGATION OF HAEM PIGMENTS

Haem pigments can be differentiated by their characteristic absorption spectra and by the changes in wavelength absorption in response to reducing agents; some can be quantitated by specific tests. For a more detailed account the reader should consult a textbook on techniques in clinical biochemistry.

INVESTIGATION OF DISORDERS OF IRON METABOLISM

Investigation of Anaemia

Anaemia may be due either to iron deficiency or, more commonly, to a variety of other conditions, sometimes associated with high iron stores. The subject of the diagnosis of anaemia is covered more fully in textbooks of haematology. However, so that we may see the value of chemical estimations in perspective, it is worth considering the order in which anaemia may usefully be investigated.

1. The clinical impression of anaemia should be confirmed by blood *haemoglobin* estimation. Iron deficiency can, however, exist with haemoglobin concentrations within the reference range.
2. The *mean corpuscular haemoglobin (MCH)* and *mean corpuscular volume (MCV)* should be noted and, if necessary, a blood film examined. Iron deficiency anaemia is hypochromic and microcytic in type, and these findings may be evident before the haemoglobin concentration has fallen below the reference range. Normochromic, normocytic anaemia is a non-specific finding, usually associated with other chronic disease; it is associated with iron deficiency only if there has been very recent blood loss. Typical appearances of other types of anaemia may be seen on the blood film.

   In most cases of anaemia consideration of these findings, together with the clinical picture, will elucidate the cause. Anaemias such as those due to thalassaemia or of the pyridoxine-responsive type, although rare, are most likely to confuse the picture, since they too are hypochromic, but are not due to iron deficiency.
3. A *bone marrow film* may be needed to confirm a diagnosis of, for example, megaloblastic anaemia. If such a film is available, staining with potassium ferrocyanide may indicate the state of the iron stores.
4. In the rare cases in which the diagnosis is not yet clear, and if a bone marrow aspiration is felt to be unjustified, biochemical investigations may occasionally help. *Plasma iron estimation without an assessment of transferrin concentration is uninformative.* An unequivocally low plasma ferritin concentration confirms iron deficiency, but a normal or high one should not be assumed to exclude it.

   If a patient *with proven iron deficiency* shows no response to oral iron treatment within a few weeks he is probably not taking the tablets; normal coloured, rather than black, faeces, detectable if necessary by rectal examination, confirms this suspicion. If iron has been taken malabsorption, usually as part of a general absorption defect, is a possible explanation of a poor response.

Investigation of Suspected Iron Overload

Initial tests. *Plasma iron, percentage saturation of transferrin and plasma ferritin* should be measured. The plasma iron concentration is almost invariably high in idiopathic haemochromatosis, often above 36 μmol/L (100 mg/dl). This is associated with a reduced plasma transferrin concentration and TIBC and the *percentage saturation* is usually over 80 per cent, and is often 100 per cent. In the presence of infection or malignancy, however, the plasma iron concentration and percentage saturation may be lower than expected; the plasma transferrin concentration remains low.

Plasma ferritin concentrations are high in most patients with iron overload (whether reticuloendothelial or parenchymal). Only a few families with idiopathic haemochromatosis despite normal plasma ferritin concentrations have been described. Raised plasma concentrations may also occur in many hepatic diseases, including cirrhosis.

If all these values are normal it is unlikely that the patient has iron overload.

Demonstration of increased iron stores. The diagnosis of iron overload can only be made after proof has been obtained of increased iron stores.

Response to venesection. The lack of response of patients to a therapeutic course of venesection offers the most convincing proof of increased iron stores, albeit retrospectively. In a subject with normal iron stores removal of a unit of blood (4.5 mmol or 250 mg of iron), repeated weekly, produces a rapid fall in plasma iron, soon followed by iron-deficiency anaemia. In patients with idiopathic haemochromatosis however, 350 mmol (20 g) or more of iron may be removed in this way before evidence of iron deficiency develops.

Liver biopsy specimens contain large amounts of stainable iron, which may be mainly in parenchymal or mainly in reticuloendothelial cells. Chemical estimation of iron is more reliable than histochemical evaluation.

Bone marrow iron content is usually *normal in haemochromatosis*, in which overload is predominantly parenchymal, but may be greatly increased in reticuloendothelial overload. A similar loading of the reticuloendothelial cells is found when there is deficient use of marrow iron for haemoglobin synthesis, as in many haematological, neoplastic and chronic inflammatory diseases.

Family studies. Relatives of patients found to have haemochromatosis should be investigated. Estimations of plasma iron and percentage saturation of transferrin are the most sensitive tests. Plasma ferritin may be normal if iron stores are not significantly increased. HLA typing will identify those most likely to have inherited the disorder (p.**291**).

INVESTIGATION OF SUSPECTED PORPHYRIA

Notify the laboratory and check which type of samples are required. Porphyrins are relatively stable but samples must be protected from light. PBG rapidly polymerizes to uroporphyrins, consequently a random fresh urine sample is more suitable than a 24 hour collection. All samples should be analysed as quickly as possible after collection. Samples should not be sent simply requesting a 'porphyrin screen'. Indicate which type of porphyria is suspected, giving the relevent clinical details, so that the laboratory can select the appropriate tests.

SUSPECTED ACUTE ATTACK

Fresh urine should be tested immediately for porphobilinogen. If PBG is not present it is highly unlikely that the patient is suffering from an acute porphyric attack.

It should be remembered that:

- patients with acute intermittent porphyria who have once had an acute attack may continue to excrete increased amounts of PBG for many years;
- a negative test does not exclude the diagnosis of latent porphyria.

SUSPECTED LATENT PORPHYRIA

A patient with a history of repeated attacks of abdominal pain or neurological symptoms may have acute intermittent porphyria, porphyria variegata or hereditary coproporphyria. Measure:

- *porphyrins in a random sample of faeces.* Raised values suggest porphyria variegata (proto- and coproporphyrin) or hereditary coproporphyria (coproporphyrin);
- *the activity of PBG-deaminase in red blood cells.* Decreased values are found in patients with acute intermittent porphyria. There is often overlap in levels between

affected and normal people but, within a family, carriers can be shown to have levels about half those of unaffected members. This test will also detect affected children. However, the enzyme activity is related to the mean age of the red blood cells; this assay is not suitable for children under about nine months of age or individuals with haemolytic disorders.

SUSPECTED PORPHYRIA WITH SKIN LESIONS

Skin lesions may occur in any, other than acute intermittent, porphyria. Blood, urine and faeces should be sent for testing.

- *Increased erythrocyte porphyrins suggest protoporphyria or congenital erythropoietic porphyria* (very rare). High values may also occur in iron deficiency anaemia and lead poisoning.
- *Increased urinary porphyrins suggest porphyria cutanea tarda or congenital erythropoietic porphyria.* The increased uroporphyrin excretion in these conditions must be distinguished from the coproporphyrinuria of liver disease.
- *Increased faecal porphyrins occur in protoporphyria, porphyria variegata and hereditary coproporphyria.* These may be distinguished by chromatographic separation of porphyrins; this will also demonstrate the abnormal pattern of porphyria cutanea tarda.

Investigation of Family Members

If one of the acute porphyrias is diagnosed it is essential to investigate blood relatives.

Those found to have the condition must be counselled regarding drug usage.

Carriers of porphyria variegata and hereditary coproporphyria can be identified after puberty by demonstration of clearly increased faecal porphyrin excretion. Normal excretion before puberty does not exclude the diagnosis.

Acute intermittent porphyria is detected by measuring red cell porphobilinogen deaminase activity.

Biochemical Effects of Tumours

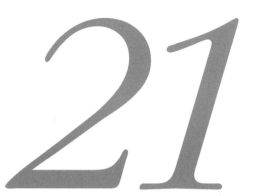

21

Neoplastic cells of differentiated tissues some-times synthesize enough compounds, not normally thought of as coming from that tissue, to be detectable in body fluids. These substances fall into two principal groups; those that:

- *alter metabolism and so usually produce clinical effects,* many of which are hormonal syndromes often indistinguishable from those already described in other chapters;

- *although biologically inactive, may be analytically detectable in plasma or urine.* These are sometimes used as markers for the presence of malignancy.

In this chapter some possible mechanisms involved in the synthesis of these compounds will considered and the limita-tions of their use as tumour markers will be discussed.

*T*HE DIFFUSE ENDOCRINE SYSTEM

Some rare syndromes are associated with neoplasia of cells that have endocrine or neurotransmitter properties, but, because of their scattered nature through tissues of non-ectodermal origin, are not usually thought of as endocrine organs. Many of these cells share common cytological characteristics, originating in the embryonic ectoblast. Staining techniques have shown their ability for *A*mine *P*recursor *U*ptake and *D*ecarboxylation (APUD) with the production of amines. Tumours of these cells have there-fore been called APUDomas. Some secrete physiologically active amines whereas others, such as the pituitary and parathyroid glands, and the calcitonin-producing C-cells of the thyroid, secrete peptide hormones. Many occur in the gastrointestinal tract and pancreas.

Secreting tumours of tissues of the sympa-thetic nervous system, and the amine-secret-ing carcinoid tumour will be discussed in this chapter.

Catecholamines

The sympathetic nervous tissue, comprising the adrenal medulla and sympathetic ganglia, is derived from the embryonic neural crest and is composed of two types of cells, the *chromaffin cells* and the *nerve cells*, both of which can synthesize active catecholamines (dihydroxylated phenolic amines). Adrenaline (epinephrine) is almost exclusively a product of the adrenal medulla whereas noradrenaline (norepinephrine) is predomi-nantly formed at sympathetic nerve endings.

Metabolism of catecholamines. Adrenaline and noradrenaline are formed from the amine precursor, tyrosine, via dihydroxy-phenylalanine (DOPA) and dihydroxy-phenylethylamine (dopamine). DOPA, dopamine, adrenaline and noradrenaline are all catecholamines. Adrenaline and nora-drenaline are both metabolized to the inactive 4-hydroxy-3-methoxymandelate (HMMA), often called vanillyl mandelate (VMA), each by similar pathways on which metadrenaline and normetadrenaline respec-tively are intermediates (Fig. 21.1). Adrenaline, noradrenaline and the metadrenalines, their conjugates, and HMMA, can all be measured in urine.

Action of catecholamines. Both adrenaline and noradrenaline act on the cardiovascular system. Noradrenaline causes generalized vasoconstriction, with hypertension and pallor, whereas adrenaline dilates blood vessels in muscles, with variable effects on blood pressure.

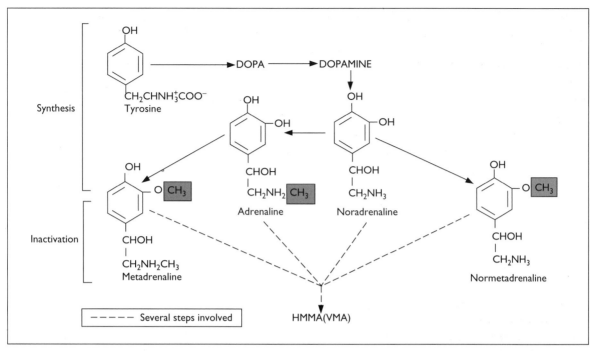

Fig. 21.1 Synthesis and metabolism of catecholamines.

Adrenaline may also cause hyperglycaemia due to stimulation of glycogenolysis and other anti-insulin effects.

A more detailed discussion of the action of these two hormones will be found in textbooks of pharmacology.

CATECHOLAMINE-SECRETING TUMOURS

Although tumours of the sympathetic nervous system, whether adrenal or extra-adrenal, can produce an excess of catecholamines, the two main types have completely different clinical manifestations.

- *Phaeochromocytomas occur in chromaffin tissue*:
    about 90 per cent are in the adrenal medulla;
    about 10 per cent are extra-adrenal.
- *Neuroblastomas are tumours of nerve cells*:
    about 40 per cent are in the adrenal medulla;
    about 60 per cent are extra-adrenal.

Phaeochromocytomas occur mainly· in adults and are usually non-malignant. The symptoms and signs can be related to very high plasma concentrations of catecholamines and include:

- *paroxysmal hypertension accompanied by anxiety, sweating, a throbbing headache and either facial pallor or flushing. Occasionally the hypertension may be persistent, rather than paroxysmal;*
- *hyperglycaemia and, if the plasma glucose concentration is high enough, glycosuria,* which may occur during· the attack.

Phaeochromocytoma is a *rare* cause of hypertension but is potentially curable by surgery; therefore its presence should be excluded if a young adult presents with hypertension for no apparent reason. Table 21.1 summarizes some other relatively rare causes of hypertension, which should also be excluded before 'essential hypertension' is diagnosed.

Neuroblastomas are very malignant tumours of the sympathetic nervous tissue occurring

Table 21.1 Some metabolic causes of hypertension and initial investigations

Cause	Initial investigations	
Renal disease	Plasma urea or creatinine; urine for protein, blood and casts	
Primary hyperaldosteronism	Plasma potassium, bicarbonate, sodium, urea	(p.**51**)
Cushing's syndrome	24 hour urinary free cortisol	(p.**122**)
Primary hyperparathyroidism	Plasma calcium, albumin, phosphate, urea	(p.**179**)
Phaeochromocytoma	24 hour urinary catecholamines or HMMA (VMA)	(p.**395**)

in children. The plasma catecholamine concentrations are often as high as, or higher than, those in patients with phaeochromocytomas, but the clinical syndrome described above is rare. It is not known why this should be. Some neuroblastomas secrete dopamine.

DIAGNOSIS OF CATECHOLAMINE-SECRETING TUMOURS

Chemical diagnosis of these tumours can usually be made by measuring the daily urinary excretion of catecholamines, or HMMA (VMA), the major catabolic product of catecholamines. An excretion of more than twice the upper limit of the reference range is diagnostic of such a tumour, but slightly increased excretion may be found in cases of essential hypertension. Many dietary components and drugs affect some of the analytical methods; *it is important to consult your laboratory before starting a urine collection.*

In some cases, particularly if the tumours are small, hypertension is paroxysmal; consequently metabolite excretion in a 24 hour urine collection may be misleading. If a normal result is obtained the estimation should be repeated, perhaps on a random specimen collected immediately after the onset of symptoms. Estimation of plasma catecholamine concentrations in samples obtained by selective venous catheterization may help to localize the tumour before surgery. It is very important to contact the laboratory *before* taking blood specimens for such estimations.

The Carcinoid Syndrome

Normal metabolism of 5-hydroxytryptamine. Some cells are called argentaffin because they reduce, and therefore stain with, silver salts. They are normally found in tissues derived from the embryonic gut. They are most abundant in the ileum and appendix but are also found in the pancreas, stomach and rectum. They synthesize the biologically active amine, 5-hydroxytryptamine (5-HT; serotonin) from the amine precursor tryptophan, the intermediate product being 5-hydroxytryptophan (5-HTP). 5-HTP is inactivated by deamination and oxidation by monoamine oxidases to 5-hydroxyindole acetic acid (5-HIAA) (Fig. 21.2); the oxidases and aromatic amino acid decarboxylases are present in other tissues, as well as in argentaffin cells. 5-HIAA is usually the main urinary excretion product of argentaffin cells.

Argentaffin cells may also excrete a peptide, substance P, an excess of which causes flushing, tachycardia, increased bowel motility and hypotension.

CAUSES OF THE CARCINOID SYNDROME

Tumours of argentaffin cells, which may be benign or malignant, are commonest in the ileum and appendix; those in the appendix rarely metastasize and may differ histochemically from the other small intestinal argentaffin tumours. More rarely the neoplasm is bronchial, pancreatic or gastric in origin; argentaffin tumours are very rarely found at other sites.

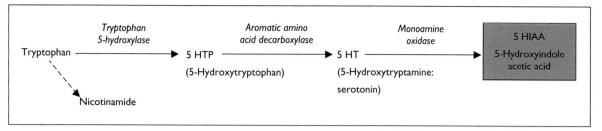

Fig. 21.2 Metabolism of tryptophan.

The carcinoid syndrome is usually associated with abnormally high concentrations of plasma 5-HT. Ileal and appendiceal tumours only produce the typical clinical syndrome when they have metastasized, usually to the liver. Products of intestinal tumours are inactivated in the liver, but those from other sites, such as the bronchus, are released directly into the systemic circulation in an active form and may therefore cause symptoms.

Only one enzyme, tryptophan-5-hydroxylase, is needed to convert tryptophan to 5-HTP (Fig. 21.2) and its derepression in malignant syndromes leads to excessive synthesis of 5-HTP. The decarboxylase and monoamine oxidases are present in normal non-argentaffin tissues so 5-HTP accumulates. In the carcinoid syndrome associated with carcinoma of the bronchus the urinary excretions of 5-HTP and 5-HT, compared with that of true carcinoid tumours, are proportionally higher than that of 5-HIAA.

Clinical features of the carcinoid syndrome. Symptoms and signs of the carcinoid syndrome include:

- *flushing*;
- *diarrhoea*, which may be severe enough to cause the malabsorption syndrome;
- *bronchospasm* and *right-sided fibrotic lesions of the heart*; the heart lesions do not occur if the primary tumour is in the bronchus.

The signs and symptoms are more likely to be due to the presence of substance P than to 5-HT. Histamine has also been suggested as a cause of the flushing. A pellagra-type syndrome may occasionally develop, because tryptophan is diverted from nicotinamide to 5-HT synthesis (Fig. 21.2).

Diagnosis of the carcinoid syndrome. Urinary 5-HIAA secretion is usually very high. A daily excretion of more than 130 µmol (25 mg) is a diagnostic finding if walnuts and bananas, which are high in hydroxyindoles, have been excluded from the diet for about 24 hours before the urinary collection is started. Less elevated levels have been reported in association with small bowel disease and intestinal obstruction.

In very rare cases, usually of bronchial or gastric tumours, the argentaffin cells lack aromatic amino acid decarboxylase. In such cases, despite increased secretion of 5-HTP, urinary 5-HIAA excretion may not be increased to diagnostic levels. If there is a strong clinical suspicion of the carcinoid syndrome despite the finding of a normal 5-HIAA excretion, estimation of total 5-hydroxyindole (5-HTP, 5-HT and 5-HIAA) excretion may be indicated.

Multiple Endocrine Neoplasia (MEN)

In the rare syndromes of multiple endocrine neoplasia (MEN; pluriglandular syndrome), two or more endocrine glands secrete inappropriately high amounts of hormones, usually from adenomas. There are two main groups of syndromes.

MEN I may involve two or more of the following endocrine tissues; the glands involved are listed in order of decreasing incidence of involvement:

- parathyroid gland (hyperplasia or adenoma);
- pancreatic islet cells:
  gastrinomas;
  insulinomas.
- anterior pituitary gland;
- adrenal cortex;
- thyroid.

MEN II includes:

- medullary carcinoma of the thyroid gland;
- phaeochromocytoma;
- adenoma or carcinoma of the parathyroid gland.

Both syndromes are usually familial, inherited as a Mendelian dominant trait with variable penetrance. Other combinations are even more rare. At the time of writing the reason for the grouping is as yet unknown.

HORMONAL EFFECTS OF TUMOURS IN NONENDOCRINE TISSUE

'Ectopic' hormone secretion occurs if a hormone, or hormone-like substance, is secreted from a site other than that normally associated with significant production of that substance; inappropriate secretion may or may not be ectopic (p.**49**), but symptomatic ectopic hormone secretion, because it is not under normal feedback control, is always inappropriate.

Many tumours of nonendocrine tissues secrete hormonal substances very similar to, and sometimes identical with, the natural hormone; some such tumours have been shown to secrete two or more hormones.

'Ectopic' Hormone Production

MECHANISM OF PRODUCTION

Many theories have been proposed as to why 'ectopic' hormone secretion should occur.

Every cell has the potential to produce any peptide coded for in the fertilized ovum. 'Ectopic' hormones or other peptides may be produced by malignant cells if they partly revert to their early embryonic, pluripotential state. This may cause the histological changes

associated with neoplasia, sometimes associated with synthesis of significant amounts of a peptide not normally detectable in the fully differentiated tissue. Two possible theories both include 'derepression':

- *of part of the genome of the tissue cell* that codes for the peptides, which are then synthesized in excess.
- *of specialized neuroendocrine cells*, scattered through many tissues.

Some substances are secreted more often by one type of tumour than others. This may reflect a differing chemical background in different parts of the body. As might be expected some types of tumour secrete more than one 'foreign' substance.

All these explanations are hypotheses.

HORMONAL SYNDROMES

Hormones produced at 'ectopic' sites, like those secreted by pathological overactivity of endocrine glands, are not under normal feedback control, and secretion continues under conditions in which it should be suppressed; such secretion is therefore inappropriate. 'Ectopic' production is most clinically obvious if the peptide has hormone-like effects. Many of the syndromes associated with such hormonal syndromes have been discussed in the relevant chapters. Carcinoid syndrome, due to carcinoma of the bronchus, is possibly caused by overproduction of one peptide enzyme and has been discussed on p.**397**.

The following may be due to hormone secretion by the tumour:

- *hypercalcaemia, due to secretion of PTH-related protein (PTHRP)*, is one of the commonest of these syndromes. It is associated with most types of malignant disease, including squamous cell carcinoma of the bronchus. PTHRP is structurally similar to PTH and may have important actions in mineral metabolism in the fetus (p.**174**). The onset of hypercalcaemia can be very rapid in contrast with that of primary hyperparathyroidism. The presence of hypokalaemia which is commonly associated with hypercalcaemia does not usually indicate simultaneous ACTH production;

- *hyponatraemia due to ADH secretion.* Although *ectopic* ADH production is most commonly associated with the relatively rare oat-cell carcinoma of the bronchus, the syndrome of *inappropriate* ADH secretion has been reported in a wide variety of tumours. The syndrome, which is not confined to malignant disease, has been discussed fully on p.**49**. Because the gradual fall in plasma osmolality allows time for osmotic equilibrium to be established across cell membranes, the patient may not experience clinical symptoms of hypo-osmolality. Therefore, no treatment other than fluid restriction is needed. If the plasma osmolality has fallen rapidly enough to cause symptoms of cerebral oedema more active treatment may be indicated.

   Infusion of a small amount of hyperosmolar fluid with a diuretic will increase plasma osmolality without further volume expansion.

   Demeclocycline, a tetracycline, directly inhibits the action of ADH on the renal tubules. This drug may be given to patients with severe symptoms when simpler methods have failed, or are contraindicated.

- *hypokalaemia due to ACTH secretion.* Ectopic ACTH secretion stimulates the secretion of all adrenocortical hormones except aldosterone (p.**123**); the clinical presentation often resembles that of primary hyperaldosteronism. The condition is most frequently associated with an oat-cell carcinoma of the bronchus but has been described less frequently in association with a variety of other malignant lesions, especially pulmonary carcinoid tumours. The patient presents with severe hypokalaemic alkalosis (p.**124**). Potassium replacement is only effective if administered with spironolactone, amiloride or triamterene (p.**68**), or an inhibitor of steroid synthesis such as metyrapone;

- *polycythaemia due to erythropoietin secretion*, or an erythropoietin-like molecule, is a well-recognized complication of renal carcinoma; erythropoietin stimulates bone marrow erythropoiesis. Because the inappropriate secretion of this is a normal product of the kidney this is not an example of ectopic hormone secretion; however, the syndrome has been reported in association with other tumours, especially hepatocellular carcinoma (primary hepatoma);

- *hypoglycaemia due to insulin or an insulin-like growth factor (IGF)*, although rare, has been reported in association with many tumours. Severe hypoglycaemia, with appropriately low plasma immunoreactive insulin and C-peptide concentrations, has been found in association with very large retroperitoneal or thoracic mesenchymal tumours resembling fibrosarcomas, or with hepatocellular carcinoma (p.**213**);

- *gynaecomastia due to chorionic gonadotrophin secretion* has been reported in association with various tumours, including carcinoma of the bronchus, breast and liver, due to raised circulating concentrations of chorionic gonadotrophin. In children with hepatoblastoma this may also cause precocious puberty. The syndrome is rarely reported, but a mild degree of gynaecomastia may be overlooked;

- *hyperthyroidism due to TSH secretion.* Some tumours of trophoblastic cells, such as choriocarcinoma, hydatidiform mole and testicular teratoma, have been shown to secrete a TSH-like substance. Clinical hyperthyroidism is extremely rare even when plasma hormone concentrations are high.

NON-HORMONAL PEPTIDES AS INDICATORS OF MALIGNANCY

For a measurement of a tumour marker to be clinically useful, the result should clearly separate those patients with, from those without, a tumour. Therefore a tumour marker should be:

- *sensitive*; levels should be raised if the tumour is present;
- *specific*; levels should *not* be raised if the tumour is *not* present.

A tumour marker may be used to:

- *screen for disease. Very few* markers are sufficiently sensitive or specific that they can be use to screen for the presence of a tumour;
- *diagnose a tumour.* If a patient presents with clinical signs or symptoms, the measurement of a marker in plasma or urine may *very occasionally* be used to confirm a diagnosis;
- *determine the prognosis.* In some cases the concentration of a specific marker is related to the mass or to the spread of the tumour;
- *monitor response to treatment.* If a tumour marker is present its rate of fall may be used to assess the response to treatment such as surgery, chemotherapy or radiotherapy;
- *identify recurrence of tumour.* If the concentration of the marker was previously raised intermittent measurement during remission may sometimes be used to identify recurrence. Occasionally tumours may dedifferentiate and fail to express the marker despite continued growth and spread.

Some proteins that can be used as tumour markers are discussed briefly here; others, such as paraproteins are discussed elsewhere in this book.

α-fetoprotein (AFP) is an oncofetal protein, the synthesis of which is suppressed as the fetus matures. Concentrations may be very high in the plasma of patients with germ-cell tumours such as hepatocellular carcinoma (primary hepatomas and hepatoblastomas) and teratoma. Moderately raised concentrations may be due to non-malignant liver disease.

Carcinoembryonic antigen (CEA) may be produced by some malignant tumours, especially colorectal carcinomas. If the initial plasma concentration is raised, serial plasma CEA estimations may sometimes help to monitor the effectiveness of, or recurrence after, treatment. Plasma concentrations correlate poorly with tumour mass but very high ones usually indicate a bad prognosis. Plasma concentrations may also rise due to non-malignant disease of the gastrointestinal tract and therefore results of this assay may be *very misleading* for diagnosis of malignancy.

Human chorionic gonadotrophin (HCG) is normally produced by the placenta. Its measurement can be used to screen for choriocarcinoma in women who have had a hydatidiform mole (p.**145**). Concentrations may be raised in plasma from patients with malignancy of the gonads such as seminomas and measurement may be used to monitor response to treatment and the development of recurrence.

Prostatic specific antigen (PSA) has been discussed on p.**307**. It is a protein present in the prostate and detectable in plasma in men. Plasma concentrations may rise in men with carcinoma of the prostate but also in those with benign prostatic hypertrophy.

Carbohydrate antigens (CA) are a group of tumour markers, raised plasma concentrations of which may be used to monitor the response to treatment and recurrence of certain tumours:

- *CA 125* may be raised in plasma of some patients with ovarian carcinoma;

- *CA 19-9* may be raised in plasma of some patients with pancreatic carcinoma and also with colorectal cancers;
- *CA 15-3* may be raised in plasma of some patients with advanced breast cancer.

At the time of writing tests for these tumour markers are not widely available.

None of the tumour markers discussed above fulfil the criteria of a ideal marker. None is sufficiently sensitive or specific to be used to screen for early disease. Furthermore, some advanced tumours dedifferentiate and fail to produce a marker despite continued growth and spread.

Summary

Some neoplastic cells secrete substances that may be biologically active and produce clinical syndromes or may be inactive but can be detected in body fluids.

Catecholamine-secreting Tumours

1. Tumours of sympathetic nervous tissue are associated with increased urinary excretion of the catecholamines, adrenaline and noradrenaline, and their metabolic products, the metadrenalines and hydroxymethoxymandelate (HMMA; VMA).
2. Phaeochromocytoma is a rare tumour, usually occurring in adults. It originates most commonly in the adrenal medulla, and much more rarely in extra-adrenal sympathetic nervous tissue. It is associated with hypertension and other symptoms of increased catecholamine secretion.

3. Neuroblastoma is a tumour of childhood, occurring either in extra-adrenal sympathetic nervous tissue, or in the adrenal medulla. Catecholamine secretion is increased, but symptoms are rarely referable to this chemical abnormality.

The Carcinoid Syndrome

1. Argentaffin cells synthesize 5-hydroxytryptamine (5-HT) which, after conversion to 5-hydroxyindole acetate (5-HIAA), is excreted in the urine.
2. Tumours of argentaffin tissue are usually found in the intestine, and at this site do not cause typical symptoms of the carcinoid syndrome until they have metastasized to the liver.
3. The carcinoid syndrome is usually associated with increased urinary 5-HIAA excretion.

Multiple Endocrine Neoplasia (MEN)

In these syndromes two or more endocrine glands secrete excessive amounts of hormones.

Hormonal Effects of Tumours of Non-endocrine Tissue

1. Many tumours secrete hormonal substances, usually peptides, normally foreign to them, which are sometimes identical with the hormones produced by normal endocrine glands.

2. Symptomatic hypercalcaemia, probably due to secretion of PTHRP, should be sought and treated in all cases of malignancy.

Non-hormonal Peptides as Indicators of Malignancy

Some non-hormonal peptides may be detected by immunological techniques and used to monitor the response to treatment of some malignancies of specific tissues.

The Cerebrospinal Fluid

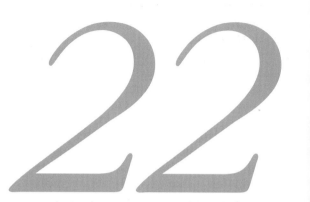

Cerebrospinal fluid (CSF) is mainly formed by ultrafiltration of plasma through the walls of the capillaries of the choroid plexuses in the lateral ventricles of the brain. These plexuses also actively secrete small amounts of substances such as chloride. In the adult the total volume is about 140 ml.

The fluid passes from the lateral, through the third and fourth ventricles, into the subarachnoid space between the pia and subarachnoid mater, from where much is reabsorbed into the circulation by arachnoid villi. The remaining fluid flows through the subarachnoid space, completely surrounding the brain and spinal cord; thus it supports and protects these structures against injury. In addition, like lymph, it removes waste products of metabolism.

CSF circulates very slowly, allowing long contact with cells of the central nervous system (CNS); uptake of glucose by these cells may account for its low concentration relative to plasma. Flow is slowest, and therefore contact longest, in the lower lumbar region where the space comes to an end; therefore the composition of CSF from lumbar is different from cisternal or ventricular puncture.

Concentrations of analytes in the CSF should always be compared with those in plasma because alterations in the latter are reflected in the CSF even when CNS metabolism is normal.

Examination of the Cerebrospinal Fluid

Biochemical investigation of the CSF is usually less important diagnostically than simple inspection and microbiological and cytological examination of the fluid. Textbooks of microbiology should be consulted for further details.

SAMPLE COLLECTION

CSF is usually collected by lumbar puncture. This procedure may be dangerous if the intracranial pressure is raised; the clinician should therefore check that there is no papilloedema before proceeding. If possible a total of about 6 ml of CSF should be collected as 2 ml aliquots into sterile containers and sent first for microbiological examinations; any remaining specimen can then be used, if necessary, for chemical analysis. If the tests are performed in the reverse order bacterial contamination may occur. If measurement of glucose concentration is indicated, a further 0.5 ml should be collected into a tube containing fluoride and sent without delay to the laboratory with a blood sample taken at the same time.

CSF is potentially highly infectious and must be handled and transported with care.

Appearance

Normal CSF is completely clear and colourless; slight turbidity is most easily detected by visual comparison with water.

COLOUR

Bright red colour results from:

- a recent haemorrhage into the subarachnoid space;
- damage to a blood vessel during lumbar puncture.

If CSF is collected as three separate aliquots, all three will be equally blood stained in the first case, but progressively less so in the second.

Xanthochromia is defined as a yellow coloration of the CSF and results from:

- *altered haemoglobin*, the colour appearing several days after a subarachnoid haemorrhage and, depending on the extent of the bleeding, lasting for up to a week or more;
- *excess of white blood cells (pus)* which will often be obvious from the gross turbidity of the sample. The presence of pus cells is detectable by microscopy;

- *a very high protein concentration* due, for example, to cerebral or spinal tumours which impair the circulation of CSF. Specimens from these cases tend to clot spontaneously due to the presence of fibrinogen;
- *jaundice*, which will be clinically obvious and may impart a yellow colour to the CSF.

TURBIDITY

Turbidity is usually due to *pus*. Slight turbidity will, of course, occur after haemorrhage but the cause can be differentiated by microscopical examination of the fluid.

SPONTANEOUS CLOTTING

Clotting occurs when there is an excess of fibrinogen in the specimen, usually associated with a very high protein concentration. This finding occurs classically in association with tuberculous meningitis or with tumours of the CNS.

Biochemical Estimations

The following are the most frequently requested biochemical estimations.

GLUCOSE

The CSF glucose concentration is slightly lower than that in plasma and, under normal circumstances, is rarely less than 50 per cent of the plasma concentration. Provided that CSF for glucose assay has been preserved with fluoride, an abnormally low glucose concentration occurs in:

- *hypoglycaemia*. The CSF glucose concentration parallels that of plasma, although there is a delay before changes in plasma glucose concentrations are reflected in the CSF. Hypoglycaemia may cause coma and low CSF glucose concentrations in the absence of any primary cerebral abnormality. *Both plasma and CSF concentrations must be measured*;

- *infection*. If there is an increased polymorphonuclear leucocyte count or a bacterial infection, the CSF glucose concentration may be very low because of increased metabolism of glucose. If obvious pus is present estimation of CSF glucose yields little additional information. The assay is most useful when the CSF is clear and *tuberculous meningitis* is suspected; CSF glucose may then be low, but not as low as in pyogenic meningitis. In viral meningitis the CSF glucose concentration is often normal. *CSF glucose estimation does not reliably distinguish between different forms of infective meningitis because the result may be normal in any form*;
- *widespread malignant infiltration of the meninges* may be associated with low CSF glucose concentrations; glucose estimation is *not* useful as a diagnostic test for this condition.

PROTEIN

The CSF protein concentration in the lumbar spine is up to three times higher than that in the ventricles; the normal lumbar concentration is below 0.4 g/L. In newborn infants, because of the relatively high vascular permeability, the CSF protein concentration is about three times that of the adult.

As in any ultrafiltrate, concentrations of proteins, including lipoproteins, all of high molecular weight, are very much lower than in plasma. In addition, electrophoresis shows that the proportions of individual proteins are slightly different in CSF compared to serum. For example, the concentration of prealbumin is higher and of γ-globulin lower in CSF relative to other proteins than in plasma. The 'Tau' protein, detectable in the β-γ region in CSF, is a variant of transferrin which cannot be absorbed as the ultrafiltrate passes through the choroid plexus; this modified form cannot be reabsorbed into the circulation and therefore is not found in plasma.

Changes in concentration of, for example, IgG do not necessarily indicate cerebral disease, but may merely reflect changes in plasma. *Results of assays can only be* interpreted if those of the two fluids are compared.

Cerebral disease may change the total concentration of CSF protein and the proportions of its constituents, for two reasons.

- The vascular and meningeal permeabilities can increase, allowing more protein to enter the CSF.
- Proteins (immunoglobulins) may be synthesized within the cerebrospinal canal by inflammatory or other invading cells.

In some conditions both these factors may be present.

MEASUREMENT OF TOTAL PROTEIN CONCENTRATION

Measurement of CSF total protein is a relatively insensitive test for the diagnosis of cerebral disease, because early changes in the concentration of a specific protein do not always cause a detectable rise in the total protein concentration. Serial determinations may be used to monitor treatment.

The CSF total protein concentration may be increased:

- *in the presence of blood*, due to haemoglobin and plasma proteins;
- *in the presence of pus*, due to cell protein, and to exudation from inflamed surfaces.

If either of these is apparent on visual inspection or by microscopical examination of the specimen *no further information is provided by estimating the total protein concentration; the laboratory staff should not be unnecessarily exposed to potentially dangerous infected material.*

- *in non-purulent inflammation of cerebral tissue*, when there may be a definite rise in total protein concentration, despite the absence of detectable cells in the CSF. Cells may also be undetectable in some cases of bacterial meningitis, particularly:
    in children;
    in immunocompromized patients;
    if antibiotics have been given before lumbar puncture.

- *if there is blockage of the spinal canal* which, by impairing the flow of CSF distal to the block, allows longer for equilibrium with the circulation and so brings the composition of CSF slightly nearer to that of plasma. Increased pressure in the CSF may also increase xanthochromia. Such blockage may be caused by:
    spinal tumours;
    vertebral fractures;
    spinal tuberculosis causing adhesions.
- *local synthesis of immunoglobulins* by plasma cells within the CSF.

MEASUREMENT OF INDIVIDUAL CSF PROTEIN CONCENTRATIONS

In the presence of blood or pus tests for individual CSF proteins are not useful and may even be misleading. They may, however, detect abnormalities when the total protein concentration is equivocally raised or normal, and may help to elucidate the cause of a high concentration.

Increased capillary permeability, with a similar increase in the permeability of the blood–brain barrier, may be demonstrated by finding relatively high molecular weight proteins not normally present in CSF. This non-specific pattern is associated with a large number of inflammatory conditions, but may sometimes aid diagnosis. Such a pattern may be due to:

- *cerebral tumours*;
- *acute idiopathic polyneuropathy* (*Guillain-Barré syndrome*), in which acute-phase proteins (p.**319**) and immunoglobulins may also be synthesized locally.

ABNORMAL CSF PROTEIN SYNTHESIS

Identification of *immunoglobulins synthesized within the CSF*, particularly IgG and IgA, may, when interpreted in conjunction with other evidence, help diagnosis of multiple sclerosis or other demyelinating disorders. Abnormal immunoglobulin synthesis may be detected by:

- the finding of a characteristic electrophoretic pattern with multiple (*'oligoclonal'*) bands in the γ-globulin region. *Oligoclonal bands only signify cerebral disease if they are found in the CSF and not in the serum.* Although such bands can be detected in over 90 per cent of patients with multiple sclerosis *the finding is not specific for this condition.* Occasionally intrathecal malignant B-lymphocytes produce a local monoclonal band detectable by electrophoresis;
- *comparison of the IgG and albumin CSF/plasma ratio.* Albumin has a lower molecular weight than IgG and increases disproportionately in CSF if the increased vascular permeability due to inflammation is the cause of the high protein concentration; in this case the CSF/plasma ratio of IgG to albumin will be low or, if permeability is so increased that the two proteins diffuse at almost the same rate, normal. In conditions such as *multiple sclerosis* in which IgG has been synthesized within the

CSF the *ratio is high.* This method is less sensitive than the detection of 'oligoclonal' bands.

Increased CSF immunoglobulin synthesis, with oligoclonal bands, may be found in:

- multiple sclerosis (the most important indication for the test);
- viral infections:
  meningitis;
  encephalitis;
  slow virus infection, for example Jakob–Creutzfeldt disease;
  subacute sclerosing panencephalitis.
- bacterial meningitis;
- neurosyphilis;
- idiopathic polyneuropathy (Guillain-Barré syndrome);
- systemic lupus erythematosus;
- cerebral sarcoidosis;
- cerebral tumours (rarely).

The recommended procedure for examining the CSF is outlined on the next page.

Summary

1. CSF is potentially highly infectious.
2. Biochemical analysis of CSF is less useful than simple inspection and bacteriological examination.
3. Estimation of CSF glucose concentration is rarely useful in acute conditions, but more so in cases of suspected tuberculous meningitis.
4. The CSF total protein concentration may be increased if there is inflammation of the meninges or stasis in the spinal canal above the site from which the CSF was obtained.
5. The finding of multiple ('oligoclonal') bands in the CSF is of diagnostic value in non-purulent cerebral conditions such as multiple sclerosis.

PROCEDURE FOR EXAMINATION OF THE CSF

If the CSF is:

- *very cloudy*, send for microbiological examination. Biochemical estimations are unnecessary;
- *heavily bloodstained* in three consecutive specimens there has probably been a cerebral haemorrhage. Biochemical estimations are useless;
- *clear or only slightly turbid*, send for microbiological examination and for estimation for glucose and protein concentrations. If indicated, intrathecal immunoglobulin synthesis may be confirmed, either using the CSF/plasma ratio of IgG to albumin or by detection of multiple ('oligoclonal') bands in the CSF. *Always send a blood sample at the same time.*
- *xanthochromic*, send the specimen, with blood, for protein estimation. Examine microscopically for erythrocytes and pus cells.

Drug Monitoring

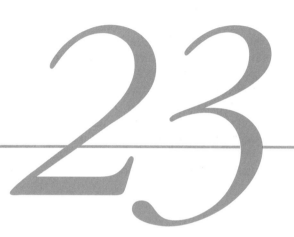

The concentrations of many drugs can be measured in plasma and other body fluids although in only a few situations is this of proven value. Interpretation of results is not straightforward.

Pharmacokinetics is the study of the fate of drugs after administration and is concerned with their absorption, distribution in body compartments, metabolism and excretion. Absorption depends on whether the drug is taken orally, by intravenous or intramuscular injection, sublingually or rectally. Unless stated otherwise, the drugs considered in this chapter are taken orally.

Possible indications for measuring plasma drug concentrations are to:

- monitor their therapeutic use as a aid to:
  checking that the patient is taking the drug as prescribed (*compliance*);
  ensuring that the dose is high enough to produce the required effect but not so high as to be likely to cause toxic effects.
- diagnose obscure conditions;
- elucidate the type of drug or drugs taken in cases of suspected overdose and to assess the need for treatment.

In the last two groups qualitative screening of the urine and/or gastric aspirate for drugs or their metabolites may be helpful.

MONITORING DRUG TREATMENT

The best way of assessing whether the dose of a drug is optimal is to measure, either clinically or by laboratory assays, the desired effect. For example, the effect of antihypertensive drugs is monitored by measuring the blood pressure. Examples of biochemical effects, which are discussed in the relevant chapters, include the monitoring of plasma:

- potassium and bicarbonate concentrations during potassium supplementation;
- thyroxine and TSH concentrations during the treatment of thyroid disease;
- calcium concentration and alkaline phosphatase activity during vitamin D treatment.

The plasma drug concentration may not parallel cellular effects and its measurement is inferior to direct assessment. Measurement of plasma concentrations may be indicated:

- if the desired result cannot be measured precisely; for example, the incidence of epileptic fits is a poor indicator of the optimal dosage of anticonvulsants, both because the frequency of fits may vary even without treatment and because only partial control may be possible, even with the best treatment;

- if the range of plasma levels most effective in producing the desired result without toxic side-effects (the *therapeutic range*) has been defined; this is particularly true if there is a narrow margin between therapeutic and toxic drug concentrations, such as in the case of lithium (p.**415**);
- if the prescribed drug is the principal active compound and is not metabolized significantly to an active metabolite; otherwise the active metabolite may be measured, for example phenobarbitone in primidone treatment.

Pharmacokinetics and how they affect plasma drug concentrations will be discussed so that the limitations of drug monitoring may be understood.

Factors Affecting Plasma Concentrations

The total amount of drug in the extracellular fluid depends on the balance between that entering and that leaving the compartment; the plasma *concentration* depends on the volume of fluid through which the retained drug is distributed.

The following factors may affect the plasma concentration of some drugs.

COMPLIANCE

It has been shown that very few in-patients take a drug exactly as prescribed; compliance with instructions is likely to be even worse outside hospital. The patient may:

- fail to take the drug at all;
- not take, or take more than, the prescribed dose;
- take it irregularly;
- become confused about the timing and dose if more than one drug has been prescribed.

Unless the doctor realizes this he may attribute the poor clinical response, or symptoms of toxicity, to inappropriate dosage. A regular review of therapy and careful explanation to the patient often works wonders and is more rewarding than changing the dosage without further questioning.

Assay of plasma concentrations is a crude method of assessing compliance and only tests the situation at the time when blood was taken if they are very low, and certainly if no drug is detectable; this is strong evidence that the patient is not taking the drug or is taking inadequate amounts. If concentrations are very high he may be regularly taking too high a dose, or, especially if there are no signs of toxicity, he may have taken a large dose just before seeing the doctor, to 'catch up' because of previous undercompliance.

ENTRY OF THE DRUG INTO, AND DISTRIBUTION THROUGH, THE EXTRACELLULAR FLUID

Timing of the sample. Blood samples must be taken at a standard time after ingestion of the drug, the exact time varying with the known differences in rate of absorption, metabolism and excretion of different drugs (Table 23.1).

Table 23.1 Therapeutic drug monitoring in adults. Therapeutic ranges are less reliable for patients taking a number of drugs. Sampling times are only a general guide. In some cases samples taken at other times may be appropriate

Drug	Sampling time	Major route of elimination	Comments
Digoxin	6–8 hours post dose	Liver Renal (60–80%)	Check plasma potassium concentration
Theophylline	*Oral* 2 hours post-dose *Slow release* 4–6 hours *IV:* 6–8 hours into infusion	Liver	
Lithium	12 hours post dose	Renal	May cause hypothyroidism
Phenytoin	Trough	Liver	Undergoes saturable metabolism
Phenobarbitone	Trough	Liver	
Primidone	Trough	Liver	Partially metabolized to phenobarbitone
Valproate	Trough	Liver	Only useful to assess compliance or confirm toxicity
Carbamazepine	Trough	Liver	
Gentamicin	Trough Peak: 30 min post IV 60 min post IM	Renal	
Cyclosporin	Trough	Liver	Monitor renal and liver function

- If blood is taken before absorption of the drug is complete a falsely low concentration may be detected.
- If it is taken after absorption, but before the drug has been completely distributed through the extracellular compartment, the plasma concentration may be high and therefore misinterpreted.

There may also be intersubject, or even intrasubject, variations of these factors, perhaps due to disorders of the organs responsible for absorption; sometimes only serial sampling can determine whether a reasonably steady plasma concentration is being maintained. These factors are discussed below.

Drugs such as phenoxymethyl penicillin (penicillin V) may be degraded within the gastrointestinal lumen and allowance must be made for this when the dose is calculated.

Absorption. *Lipid-soluble* drugs can pass through cell membranes more readily, and are therefore absorbed more rapidly, than water-soluble ones; they reach the highest plasma concentrations at between 30 and 60 minutes after ingestion. The rate of absorption in an individual patient may be affected by:

- the timing of ingestion in relation to meals;
- the rate of gastric emptying. This must be allowed for, for example, during treatment with drugs affecting gut motility or after gastric surgery;
- vomiting, diarrhoea or malabsorption syndromes;
- the administration of compounds, such as the bile acid sequestrants used in the treatment of hypercholesterolaemia (p.287), which may also bind some drugs within the intestinal lumen.

Volume of distribution. The final plasma concentration of a drug reached after a standard amount has been absorbed depends on the volume through which it has been distributed. For example, it may be difficult to predict the appropriate dose in oedematous or obese patients in whom, because they have a larger than normal volume of distri-

bution, may have unexpectedly low plasma concentrations. By contrast, in small children, with a low volume of distribution, there is danger of overdosage. The patient's weight or surface area may need to be allowed for when the dose is calculated.

Binding to plasma albumin. Many drugs, like many endogenous substances, are partly inactivated by protein-, usually albumin-, binding. Most drug assays estimate the total concentration of the free- plus the protein-bound drug. Biological feedback mechanisms do not control free drug concentrations as they do those of plasma calcium and hormones; therefore the method of interpretation to allow for altered protein binding is different. *Measured* plasma concentrations fall little due to a reduction in protein binding; a larger *proportion* of the measured drug will be in the unbound, free active form so that metabolism and excretion will increase. *Unless this is realized, dangerously high plasma free concentrations may be interpreted as being within, or even below, the therapeutic range* if the plasma albumin concentration is very low. The bound proportion varies with differing plasma albumin concentrations and there is no valid correction factor that allows for protein abnormalities (compare calcium, p.172). About 90 per cent of phenytoin, 70 per cent of salicylic acid, 50 per cent of phenobarbitone and 20 per cent of digoxin is protein-bound. However binding may be affected by:

- *abnormalities in plasma albumin concentration*. Blood should be taken without stasis to minimize a possible *rise* in plasma albumin, and albumin-bound drug, concentrations. *Low* concentrations, such as those often found in hepatic cirrhosis or the nephrotic syndrome, may reduce the proportion of protein-bound drugs;
- *competition for binding sites on protein*. Many drugs, unconjugated bilirubin and hydrogen ions, compete with each other for binding sites. If more than one drug is being taken the free concentration of each is likely to be higher than the measured concentrations would suggest. *Plasma*

drug levels in patients taking several differ-ent drugs, or who are jaundiced or acidotic, may be difficult to interpret.

In *renal glomerular dysfunction* the use of drug assays to detect reduced excretion may be partially invalidated by acidosis and by retention of other competing ions. Similarly, in *hepatic disease*, low plasma albumin concentrations or competition for binding sites by unconjugated bilirubin limits the value of monitoring protein-bound drugs.

Interpretation is further complicated because assay methods may vary significantly from laboratory to laboratory.

METABOLISM AND EXCRETION OF DRUGS

The time taken for the plasma drug concen-tration to fall to half its original concentration is called its *effective half-life*. To maintain a reasonably steady plasma concentration drugs with a short half-life should be taken more frequently than those with a long one. After starting treatment a steady state is usually reached after about four half-lives have elapsed; *the first specimen of blood for monitoring should not be taken earlier than this.*

The rate at which the plasma drug concen-tration falls after it has reached peak concen-tration depends on:

- the rate of distribution through the extra-cellular fluid (see above);
- the rate of entry into cells;
- the rate at which it is metabolized and excreted, whether in urine or bile.

The rate of elimination of most drugs depends on their plasma concentration. A small increase in the dose of some, such as phenytoin, may exceed the capacity of the metabolic or excretory pathways and so cause a disproportionate increase in plasma levels; the plasma concentrations of these drugs should be monitored carefully. The rate at which this occurs is known as *saturation kinetics*.

Metabolic conversion to active or inactive metabolites. Some drugs are only active after metabolic conversion; others are inacti-vated, usually by conjugation in the liver. Ideally a drug assay should measure all the active forms, whether the parent compound or its active metabolite, and none of the inactive forms.

Some drugs, given orally and absorbed into the portal system, are partly inactivated by the liver before reaching the systemic circulation. Hepatic dysfunction impairs metabolism, allowing more active drug than usual to enter the systemic circulation; induction of enzymes that inactivate drugs, such as some anticon-vulsants, reduces the amount leaving the liver.

Drug–drug interactions. If a number of different drugs are being prescribed, one may affect the plasma concentration of another by altering its binding to plasma proteins, rate of metabolism or excretion. For example, sodium valproate displaces phenytoin from its protein-binding sites and reduces its rate of metabolism.

Relation Between Plasma Concentrations and Cellular Effects

Plasma concentrations are measured in an attempt to predict biological activity at the cellular level. They only do so if they paral-lel the concentrations at the active sites and if the cells respond predictably to a given concentration at that site. Neither of these conditions is always fulfilled.

Drug concentrations at the active site. In a steady state the plasma concentration may not be the same as that at the active site within the cell, but usually parallels it. This may *not* be true if:.

- *treatment has just begun.* Plasma concen-trations may be relatively high compared with those in cells;

- *treatment has just stopped*. Plasma concentrations may fall more rapidly than those in cells;
- *the drug is taken irregularly or at intervals inappropriate to its half-life*. Plasma concentrations then fluctuate and equilibrium may not be reached with those in cells;
- *there is a change in concentration of hydrogen ions (pH), or other substances that compete for binding to cell membranes or active sites*. This adds to the problem of interpreting plasma concentrations in patients with renal or hepatic dysfunction (p.**413**).

TISSUE SENSITIVITY

Inter-subject variation. Some patients are more sensitive to drugs than others. The rate of metabolism of some drugs depends on the age of the patient.

- *Premature infants*, with immature detoxifying mechanisms, metabolize and excrete some drugs more slowly than adults.
- *Children*, who have a higher metabolic rate than adults, may eliminate some drugs more rapidly than adults.
- *The elderly* may metabolize drugs slowly; they are particularly sensitive to digoxin.

The rate of metabolism of some drugs may be affected by genetic factors. For example, the inactivation of *isoniazid* by acetylation depends on whether the patient is genetically capable of carrying out this process at a normal rate; toxicity is likely at lower plasma concentrations in 'slow acetylators' than in 'fast acetylators'.

Intra-subject variation. The sensitivity of an individual to a drug may vary. Known causes of increased sensitivity to digoxin are hypokalaemia and hypercalcaemia.

Tolerance. Drugs may induce the synthesis of enzymes that inactivate them and consequently higher doses than usual may be needed to produce the desired effect. In other cases reduced receptor sensitivity may require higher doses than normal in order to increase the plasma concentration and to achieve the desired effect.

Additive or antagonistic effects at the active site. Some drugs and endogenous substances, often the same ones as those that compete for plasma albumin-binding sites, compete for binding at the active site within the cell. Some of these have been discussed above. By contrast, some drugs have synergistic effects. These factors further complicate the interpretation of plasma concentrations in patients taking more than one type of drug.

When to measure individual drug concentrations to monitor treatment

Only a few drug assays are of proven clinical value. The clinical picture must be taken into account and all the above factors must be allowed for when interpreting results. The following are some of the drug measurements which have been claimed to be useful for therapeutic monitoring.

Digoxin. Estimation of plasma digoxin concentrations may be useful:

- *to assess compliance*. The elderly, for whom digoxin is frequently prescribed, are *often taking several different drugs* and are liable to be confused about which tablets to take and at what time;
- in patients, such as the elderly who are likely to have a *low threshold for toxicity* and premature infants who have an *increased elimination half-life*;
- if it is difficult to calculate the appropriate dose because of an *abnormal volume of distribution* due to obesity or oedema, or in infants (p.**339**); if excretion is impaired, perhaps due to renal dysfunction;
- if the patient is taking another drug, such as amiodarone that possibly reduces its rate of excretion.

Plasma digoxin concentrations, even within the reference range, are very difficult to interpret in the presence of conditions that may alter receptor sensitivity, such as:

- hypokalaemia, hypercalcaemia or hypomagnesaemia;
- hypoxia or acidosis;
- thyroid disease.

Blood should be taken at least six hours after the last dose, when absorption and distribution are usually complete (Table 23.1; p.**411**).

Anticonvulsants. Once the dose that gives stable plasma concentrations within the therapeutic range has been determined, monitoring is probably only necessary:

- to assess compliance;
- if the frequency of fits increases in a previously well-controlled patient;
- if the clinical picture suggests toxicity;
- if another drug is prescribed that may affect the plasma concentrations.

Plasma concentrations in children and in pregnant women should be monitored more frequently as these groups are more likely to develop toxicity.

Measurement of plasma *phenytoin, phenobarbitone* and *possibly carbamazepine* may be of clinical value. Of these monitoring phenytoin is the most useful because it exhibits *saturation kinetics* (p.**413**). Sodium valproate displaces phenytoin from its binding sites and reduces its rate of metabolism; free plasma phenytoin may then cause toxicity despite apparently appropriate total plasma concentrations.

Plasma concentrations of sodium valproate correlate poorly with the dose prescribed, the clinical response and with toxicity, probably because of the presence of active metabolites. Consequently the only possible justification for measuring plasma concentrations is to assess compliance.

There are several new antiepileptic drugs now available; the need to monitor their plasma concentrations is under evaluation. *Vigabatrin*, an inhibitor of γ-aminobutyric acid (GABA) metabolism, has a very long half-life because it binds avidly to receptors; therefore plasma concentrations are unlikely to predict therapeutic response or toxicity.

Lithium and high-dose salicylate therapy. The margin between therapeutic and toxic concentrations of both lithium and salicylate given at high dosage is narrow and therefore plasma concentrations should be monitored regularly.

Lithium is given to psychiatric patients, who are especially unlikely to comply with instructions. Lithium is not protein-bound and interpretation of results of assays is *not complicated by protein abnormalities*. Plasma concentrations should be measured on a specimen taken 12 hours after the evening dose.

Theophylline assays may be useful, especially in *acute asthmatic attacks that are not responding clinically*; results may help to ensure that the poor response is not due to underdosage, and, if it is not, that increasing the dosage will not lead to toxic plasma levels.

Theophylline and its active metabolite *caffeine* are used in the management of recurrent apnoea in the *newborn*; at this age their clearance is slow and theophylline is partially metabolized to caffeine. *Both* plasma theophylline and caffeine concentrations may need to be assayed if theophylline has been given, in order to assess therapeutic or toxic effects.

Samples for theophylline assays should be taken at between two and four hours after the last dose.

Aminoglycosides, such as gentamicin, are given intramuscularly or intravenously and, in contrast to many other antibiotics, the margin between the therapeutic range and toxic levels is narrow. Toxic levels may cause oto- and nephrotoxicity.

Measurement is indicated if:

- there is *serious infection*, or if the treatment is so prolonged that the risk of toxicity is increased;
- renal function is impaired.

Aminoglycoside concentrations should be measured twice. The *first* specimen should be taken *immediately before injection*, when the 'trough level' is expected, to ensure that concentrations are not already high and that further administration is not likely to cause toxicity, or that they are not so low as to be ineffective. The *second* should be taken *about an hour after injection*, at the time of the anticipated 'peak level', to ensure that an adequate concentration has been achieved for antibacterial action.

Antiarrhythmic drugs, such as procainamide and quinidine, may be measured in special cases. N-acetylprocainamide is a less potent metabolite of procainamide and need not be assayed.

Cyclosporin is an immunosuppressant and is used to prevent rejection of transplanted organs. Dosage may be difficult to assess because there is considerable variation between individuals in the rate of clearance; there is also a relatively narrow margin between therapeutic and toxic drug concentrations. During the first six months, when the risks of rejection are highest, plasma concentrations should be measured regularly.

Monitoring Possible Side-effects of Drug Treatment

Some drugs have harmful side-effects. For example, thyroid function should be monitored during lithium treatment because of the danger of hypothyroidism (p.**164**), and plasma potassium concentrations during diuretic therapy (p.**68**). Assessment of liver damage (measurement of plasma transaminase activities), or of renal function, may be indicated during treatment with potentially hepatotoxic or nephrotoxic drugs respectively.

Diagnosis of Obscure Conditions

Drug overdosage must always be excluded as a cause of coma of obscure origin. This subject will be dealt with in the next section.

Unexplained clinical or laboratory findings may suggest effects due to a drug or alcohol ingestion despite denial by the patient. Hypokalaemia, for example, may be due to purgative abuse (p.**62**) and hypoglycaemia may be a presenting finding associated with alcohol ingestion (p.**213**). Raised plasma transaminase activities, thought to be due to alcoholic liver disease, may be investigated by measuring random plasma alcohol concentrations.

Measurement of plasma drug concentrations may be supplemented by screening the urine for drugs or their metabolites.

_I_NVESTIGATION OF KNOWN OR SUSPECTED OVERDOSAGE

About half the patients attempting suicide take several drugs, sometimes with alcohol. Qualitative screening of plasma, urine or gastric aspirate may be needed to confirm the diagnosis and will often help to identify the drugs.

It is often unnecessary to measure plasma *concentrations* of drugs that the patient is known to have taken in overdose. The need for gastric lavage and measures to increase urinary excretion of the drug and to maintain adequate respiration and circulation are not usually affected by a knowledge of drug concentrations. Only measurements of plasma electrolytes, glucose and blood gases are helpful.

Drugs and other toxins can be considered in three main groups. These are:

- toxins for which there is *a specific antidote*;
- toxins for which there is *no specific antidote* but which are not, or *are only partially, protein-bound*;
- toxins for which there is *no specific antidote and which are strongly protein-bound*.

The case for assay is strongest in the first and weakest in the last group.

Poisons for which there is a Specific Antidote

Paracetamol (acetaminophen). It is *essential* to measure plasma drug concentrations in suspected paracetamol poisoning because:

- a metabolite of paracetamol is hepatotoxic; the patient may die of liver failure despite recovery from the immediate effects;
- a specific antidote to the hepatotoxic effect is available;
- the antidote is only useful if given within a defined period of time and if defined plasma concentrations are reached;
- the likelihood of hepatotoxicity cannot be predicted from the clinical picture at presentation.

N-acetylcysteine, cysteamine and methionine are all relatively effective antidotes, because they enable paracetamol to be converted to non-toxic metabolites. *N*-acetylcysteine is the least toxic and is most often used. Cysteamine may cause nausea, vomiting, abdominal pain and cardiac arrhythmias. Methionine, although less toxic, may cause vomiting. *N*-acetylcysteine is only effective in clearly defined circumstances and should

only be given after the following factors have been taken into account:

- *timing of the specimen.* Plasma concentrations of the drug cannot be interpreted and should not be measured, until absorption and distribution are nearly complete, at about *four hours after ingestion.* If treatment is to be effective it should be started as soon as possible following ingestion and is probably *ineffective after about 20 hours.* Concentrations should be measured on specimens taken *as early as possible between four and 20 hours after ingestion.*
- *plasma paracetamol concentrations.* As a rough guide, treatment is indicated if the plasma paracetamol concentration is 200 mg/L (1300 µmol/L) or more at four hours and 30 mg/L (200 µmol/L) or more at 15 hours after the dose *and falls above the solid line in Fig. 23.1.*

Results of serial measurement of plasma transaminase activities and prothrombin time

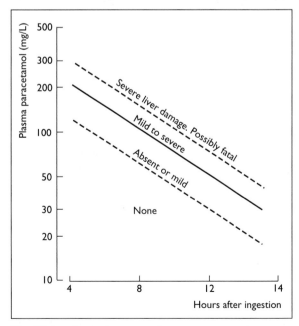

Fig. 23.1 Relation between plasma paracetamol concentration, time after ingestion and potential severity of liver damage. (Paracetamol in mg/L × 6.6 = µmol/L.) Reproduced with kind permission of Prescott LF. In Richens A, Marks V, eds. *Therapeutic drug monitoring.* Edinburgh: Churchill Livingstone, 1983.

may indicate liver involvement, which may become apparent about three days after ingestion.

Iron overdosage is commonest in children who may mistake the tablets for sweets. Desferrioxamine chelates iron and the chelate is excreted in the urine. The concentration of plasma iron at which treatment is indicated have not been clearly defined, but concentrations above 90 μmol/L (500 μg/dl) in young children and above 150 μmol/L (840 μg/dl) in adults are said to be definite indications for treatment. If there is any doubt desferrioxamine should be given.

Poisons for which there is no Specific Antidote

Weakly protein-bound poisons. Forced diuresis may increase the excretion of some free drugs; induction of alkalosis often increases the excretion rate further, but neither forced diuresis nor induction of alkalosis is without risk; in most cases neither is indicated. If an alkaline diuresis is induced plasma potassium concentrations, as well as blood pH, must be monitored because of the danger of acute hypokalaemia (p.**66**). It has been suggested that plasma concentrations of *lithium* (unbound), *phenobarbitone* (about 50 per cent bound) and *salicylate* (about 70 per cent bound) should be measured if overdosage is suspected. Serial measurements

may help the clinician to assess the adequacy of therapy.

Strongly protein-bound poisons. It is agreed that there is no indication to measure concentrations of strongly protein-bound drugs, such as barbiturates other than phenobarbitone, in a suspected case of overdosage (p.**412**); excretion cannot be increased significantly and supportive treatment is based on clinical observation and the results of plasma electrolyte and blood gas estimations.

Monitoring of *methanol* and *paraquat* concentrations may be desirable.

Before blood is taken from any case of suspected overdosage you must contact your laboratory; this is especially important in the case of rare poisons. The local laboratory may not have full facilities and it is then essential to seek specialist advice from a toxicology centre about the value of the assay and the type of specimen needed.

Medicolegal Precautions

Specimens of vomit, gastric washings, urine and plasma from all serious cases of poisoning should be stored in the refrigerator in sealed containers, labelled with the full name of the patient (or, if this is not available, some other form of identification) and the date and time of the specimen. The specimen may be needed later for medicolegal purposes and should be kept for at least three months.

Summary

1. Assay of plasma drug concentrations to monitor therapy is only indicated for a few drugs in defined circumstances.

2. Drug effects are ideally assessed by clinical or laboratory evidence of the response, rather than by the drug concentrations.

3. The specimen must be taken at the correct time after administration if results are to be meaningful.
4. A knowledge of the pharmacokinetics of the drug is necessary in order to interpret results of measurements of plasma concentrations.

5. Screening of plasma or urine to identify toxic substances taken in overdosage may be helpful. It is rarely necessary to measure the concentrations.
6. In most cases of drug overdosage plasma, urine and gastric aspirate should be stored for at least three months in case of medicolegal proceedings.

The Clinician's Contribution to Valid Results

24

Chemical pathology is the study of physiology and biochemistry applied to medical practice and overlaps that of clinical disciplines. An understanding of the basis of chemical pathology is, as we have seen, essential for much diagnosis and treatment.

The medical student and the clinician need only limited knowledge of the technical details of laboratory estimations. However, correct interpretation of results requires some understanding both of achievable analytical accuracy and reproducibility and of physiological variations; these subjects will be discussed in the next chapter. They should also be aware of laboratory organization in so far as it affects the speed at which tests can be completed. Above all they should realize that *the technique of collecting specimens can affect results drastically* and should cooperate with the laboratory in its attempt to produce answers rapidly and accurately and identifiable with the relevant patient. To this end they should understand the importance of:

- accurately completed request forms;
- correctly labelled specimens;
- collection of specimens by the correct technique at the appropriate time;
- speedy delivery to the laboratory.

Treatment based on technically correct results from a wrongly labelled or collected specimen may be as lethal as a faulty surgical technique; moreover, even if the error is recognized, time could have been saved by a little thought and care. *An emergency warrants more, not less, than the usual accuracy in collection and identification of specimens.*

All patient samples are *potentially dangerous,* but those from patients with communicable disorders, such as hepatitis and AIDS, are assayed with special precautions and should be *clearly identified by the clinician. All* blood specimens must be sent in leakproof, sealed plastic bags, with the request form in a different pocket in the bag. Failure to comply with these guidelines may put many people, including porters and laboratory staff, at unnecessary risk and may mean that some assays are not performed, or are, at best, delayed.

If the clinician delegates any part of these tasks to, for example, a nurse or ward clerk he is not absolved from responsibility for their accuracy, any more than senior laboratory staff are absolved from responsibility for the accuracy of analysis and reporting.

*R*EQUEST FORMS

Clinical Information

Most departments take stringent precautions to control the analytical accuracy and precision of results. However, when very large numbers of estimations are being performed under pressure it is impossible to be sure that every result is correct. The clinician must play his part by co-operating with the pathologist to minimize the chance of error, not only by taking suitable specimens, but also by giving *relevant* clinical information. 'Unlikely' results

are checked in most laboratories and if, for example, plasma enzymes had risen from normal to very high activities within a day estimations would be repeated on both specimens to be sure that they had not been transposed with those from another patient. If, however, it were known that the patient had had a myocardial infarction, the result would have been expected and time and money would have been saved. In this example the words 'post MI' would be more informative, and take no longer to write, than any previously stated diagnosis.

Patient Identification

Accurate information about the patient, legibly written, is essential for comparing current with previous results on the same patient. This includes:

- hospital case number;
- the surname and first name(s) correctly and consistently spelt;
- *date of birth*, rather than age.

A surprising number of people have the same names, even when these are apparently uncommon; it is less likely that they will be the same age in years and even less that they will have the same date of birth; they should not have the same hospital number. Any of these may be recorded inaccurately on the form and, unless there is complete agreement with previous details, results may be entered into the wrong patient's record either on a computer or in the patient's case notes, causing confusion and possible danger to the patient. It is equally important to provide accurate information for manual or computerized reporting.

Location of the Patient and Identification of Clinician

It is obvious that if the *ward or department* is not stated it may take time and trouble to determine where the results should be sent. *The requesting doctor must sign the form legibly*. He should also state how he can be notified rapidly, for example by his 'bleep number', in case abnormal results requiring urgent action are found or advice needs to be given about treatment. He must check the completed request form to be sure that the information given is correct; it is also important to include the consultant's name.

Request forms designed by pathology and other departments ask only for information essential to ensure the most efficient possible service to the clinician and therefore to the patient. It is not uncommon to receive a form stating only a common surname and sometimes not even stating the investigations needed. *This is particularly dangerous in an emergency.*

COLLECTION OF SPECIMENS

Collection of Blood

If a clinically improbable result has been checked analytically and the second agrees well with the first, a fresh specimen should be analysed. Before proceeding further it is essential to try to determine why the initial analysis gave a false answer (if it was false). Although contamination at some stage of blood collection is an obvious possibility, this is relatively rare and should not be accepted until other, more common, causes have been excluded.

The errors to be discussed in this chapter arise outside the laboratory and are, in our experience, relatively common. All examples given are genuine.

EFFECT ON RESULTS OF PROCEDURES BEFORE VENEPUNCTURE

Effect of posture. The concentrations of plasma proteins and of substances bound to them are lower if the patient is supine rather than standing up. It is often difficult to standardize this variable and the effect must be taken into account when serial results are interpreted. It will be discussed more fully on p.**435**.

Oral medication. Specimens should not be withdrawn just after a large oral dose of a substance, which may effect the analyte to be measured, has been taken. For example:

- blood should be taken for drug assays at a standard time after the dose; misleadingly high plasma concentrations may occur at the time of peak absorption (p.**411**);
- there may be significant hypokalaemia for a few hours after taking potassium-losing diuretics due to rapid clearance of potassium from the extracellular fluid. The plasma concentration returns to its 'true' level as equilibration occurs between cells and extracellular fluid.

Interfering substances. Previous administration of a substance may affect a plasma analyte concentration for some time. For example, drugs:

- such as salicylates compete with T_4 for binding sites on TBG and may cause a misleadingly low plasma total T_4 concentration, due to reduction in the protein-bound fraction;
- may interfere with chemical reactions used in assays, such as some of those for creatinine.

The effect of interfering substances is probably more common than is recognised and is often difficult to detect.

Intravenous infusion. A spuriously low plasma sodium concentration may be due to gross hyperlipidaemia or hyperproteinaemia (p.**38**). If a lipid solution is being infused it should be replaced by a lipid-free one for at least three hours before sampling. Hyperlipidaemia not only causes spurious results because of the space-occupying effect but may directly interfere with several assays.

Examination of the prostate. Palpation of the prostate, especially by an inexperienced clinician, may release abnormally large amounts of prostatic (tartrate-labile) acid phosphatase and prostatic specific antigen (PSA) into the circulation; the spuriously elevated concentration in blood may persist for several days. Although the effect of this procedure has been questioned, it does, in our experience, sometimes occur. Very high serum activities or levels are unlikely to be due to this cause. If marginally raised, the assay should be repeated on a specimen taken a few days later. The plasma levels of both tartrate-labile acid phosphatase and PSA may rise following a biopsy of the prostate.

EFFECTS ON RESULTS OF THE TECHNIQUE OF VENEPUNCTURE

Venous stasis. It is usual to apply a tourniquet proximal to the site of venepuncture to ensure that, because the vein 'stands out', it is easier to enter with the needle. If occlusion is maintained for more than a short time the combined effect of raised intracapillary pressure and hypoxia of the vessel wall increases the rate of passage of water and small molecules from the lumen into the surrounding interstitial fluid. Large molecules, such as proteins, including immunoglobulins and lipoproteins, and erythrocytes and other blood cells, cannot pass through the capillary wall at the same rate; their plasma concentrations therefore rise. Day-to-day variations in these analytes can often be attributed, at least in part, to the differing amounts of stasis used as well as to changes in posture.

Many plasma constituents are partly bound to protein. Prolonged venous stasis can raise the plasma total calcium concentration, sometimes to equivocal or slightly high levels (Table 24.1). Blood samples for plasma calcium estimation should preferably be taken without stasis, especially if high plasma concentrations have previously been found. Other important protein-bound substances include hormones and drugs.

Prolonged stasis may also cause local hypoxia; consequent leakage of intracellular constituents, such as potassium and phosphate, may cause falsely high plasma concentrations.It is sometimes difficult to

Table 24.1 Some effects of a tourniquet and of its release on plasma concentrations in a normal subject

Time (minutes)	Tourniquet on for						Tourniquet off for	
	0	0.5	1	2	3	4	0.25	0.5
Calcium (mmol/L)	2.38	2.36	2.39	2.39	2.44	2.46	2.42	2.39
Total protein (g/L)	81	81	83	83	88	89	86	84
Albumin (g/L)	44	43	45	46	47	48	47	45
Haemoglobin (g/dl)	13.7	13.8	14.0	14.3	14.6	15.0	14.6	14.0

enter 'bad veins' without applying stasis. A tourniquet may be used and released as soon as the needle is in the vein; a suitable specimen may be obtained after waiting at least a further 15 seconds before withdrawal of blood (Table 24.1).

Site of venepuncture. If the patient is receiving an intravenous infusion the administered fluid in the veins of the same limb, *whether proximal or distal to the infusion site*, has not mixed with the total plasma volume; local concentrations will therefore be unrepresentative of those circulating through the rest of the body. Blood taken from the opposite arm will give valid results. Table 24.2 shows an example of this. All measured constituents except glucose were diluted; the very high plasma glucose concentration supported the suspicion that the sample had been taken from an arm into which dextrose (glucose) was being infused. The house surgeon confirmed. Specimens taken subsequently from the other arm gave normal results and were almost identical with those of the day before. Note that glucose infusion may cause systemic hyperglycaemia and, if the plasma glucose concentration rises above about 11 mmol/L, glycosuria. Only if the hyperglycaemia persists after infusion has stopped should the diagnosis of diabetes mellitus be considered.

Such an extreme example is easy to detect; although time had been wasted and the patient subjected to an unnecessary venepuncture, no serious harm was done. Results might have *appeared* to be correct if isosmolar saline was being infused and only electrolytes had been analysed. The wrong

Table 24.2 Effect of taking a blood sample from an arm into which an infusion of dextrose (glucose) was being administered

		Site of venepuncture	
		'Infusion arm'	Other arm
Bicarbonate	(mmol/L)	14	31
Potassium	(mmol/L)	1.8	3.1
Sodium	(mmol/L)	69	141
Total protein	(g/L)	48	79
Creatinine	(μmol/L)	37	93
Glucose	(mmol/L)	54.2	6.7

interpretation might have been made and inappropriate treatment given.

If it is impossible to obtain blood from another limb the infusion should be temporarily stopped, the tubing disconnected from the needle and 20 to 30 ml of blood aspirated through this needle *and discarded*; only then should the sample for analysis be withdrawn and the infusion restarted.

CONTAINERS FOR BLOOD

Most hospital laboratories issue a list of the types of container suitable for different assays; this list may vary from hospital to hospital. For example, most departments ask that blood for:

- *glucose* estimation be put into a tube containing an inhibitor of erythrocyte glycolysis, such as fluoride;
- *potassium* should be estimated on plasma from *heparinized* blood rather than serum. Potassium is released from cells, especially

platelets, during clotting. Serum potassium concentrations are usually higher than those of plasma by a variable amount; this difference can be clinically misleading. Marked differences may be found in patients with leukaemia in whom the number of white blood cells is usually greatly increased.

Laboratories should only accept blood in the correct containers. Even with this precaution serious errors can arise if blood is decanted from one container to another, although this is less likely to occur if a closed vacuum system for obtaining blood is used. The anticoagulant actions of oxalate and of sequestrene (ethylenediamine tetraacetate; EDTA) depend, respectively, on precipitation or chelation of calcium, so invalidating results of calcium estimation. EDTA is usually in the form of its potassium salt. A typical example of decanting blood from one vial to another is shown in Table 24.3. Blood was received in a vial containing lithium heparin. The house physician confirmed that blood had been put, at the same time, into EDTA for haematological investigations, and that to bring the level in the EDTA vial 'down to the mark', some blood had been tipped into the lithium heparin vial which was sent to the chemical pathology department. Obviously the *more blood that is decanted the greater the potential error.* We have seen a plasma potassium concentration of 6.0 mmol/L in a specimen in which the plasma calcium concentration was later found to be 0.4 mmol/L.

Table 24.3 Effect of decanting some EDTA blood into a lithium heparin vial (the observed effect depends on the amount of EDTA blood added)

		With EDTA aliquot	Without EDTA aliquot
Bicarbonate	(mmol/L)	26	27
Potassium	**(mmol/L)**	**4.9**	**4.1**
Sodium	(mmol/L)	140	140
Total protein	(g/L)	81	80
Urea	(mmol/L)	4.9	4.8
Calcium	**(mmol/L)**	**1.71**	**2.16**
Albumin	(g/L)	41	42

The use of sodium, instead of lithium, heparin may cause a falsely high plasma sodium result. This anticoagulant is often used in specimens taken for 'blood gases'; apparent plasma sodium concentrations of 160 to 170 mmol/L can result from transferring an aliquot of sodium heparinized blood into a lithium heparin vial. *This error is particularly likely to be misinterpreted and the wrong treatment instituted if the patient is unconscious or confused and, therefore, is a likely candidate for hypernatraemia (p.46).* This type of patient is also likely to be having blood gases analysed.

Use of lithium heparin leads to a falsely high plasma lithium concentration in the specimen.

EFFECTS OF HAEMOLYSIS AND DELAYED SEPARATION OF BLOOD

Haemolysis. The concentration of many substances is very different in erythrocytes from that of the surrounding plasma. Haemolysis releases the cell contents into plasma and, consequently, if this occurs *in vitro* some plasma constituents, such as potassium, phosphate and AST, may be falsely increased. The increase is variable and is not related to the intensity of the red colour of plasma due to haemoglobin. This is very uncommon if haemolysis occurs *in vivo* because these constituents are distributed throughout the total extracellular, not just plasma, volume. Haemoglobin may interfere with some chemical reactions, falsely increasing the apparent plasma bilirubin concentration and lowering alkaline phosphatase activity.

The chance of haemolysis is minimized if the blood is treated gently and if a closed vacuum system is used. If a needle and syringe system is used the plunger of the syringe should be drawn back slowly and the blood allowed to flow freely; the needle should be removed from the syringe before the specimen is expelled *gently* into the correct container.

Delayed separation of blood. The differential concentrations of some analytes across cell membranes are maintained by energy, derived from glycolysis. *In vitro*, erythrocytes soon use up the available glucose and therefore the energy source; concentrations of these analytes in plasma will then tend to equalize by passive diffusion across cell membranes with those in erythrocytes. If plasma is not separated from blood cells within a few hours the effect on plasma concentrations will be similar to that resulting from haemolysis. However, there are a few important differences:

- because haemoglobin is not released, the plasma *looks normal*; the error is therefore easily overlooked;
- *the plasma potassium concentration rises* (Table 24.4) as the plasma glucose falls; initially there may be a slight fall in the plasma potassium concentration as it moves into the erythrocytes.

Many plasma constituents, such as bilirubin, deteriorate even if plasma is correctly separated and stored. Whenever possible, blood should reach the laboratory early in the working day, when the bulk of assays is being performed.

Low temperatures *slow* erythrocyte metabolism so that differential concentrations cannot be maintained; *refrigeration of whole blood has the same effect on raising the plasma potassium concentration, but in a shorter time*, as allowing it to stand at room temperature. Blood specimens must be centrifuged and the plasma separated from the cells before storing, for example, overnight.

If the container is not, or is wrongly, dated the error may not be detected.

Table 24.4 Effect of delayed separation of plasma from a lithium heparinized blood specimen, maintained at room temperature

	Blood separated after (hours)				
	0	2	4	8	24
Potassium (mmol/L)	4.1	3.9	4.3	4.8	6.4
Glucose (mmol/L)	4.8	4.6	3.9	3.0	1.9

Reporting of results. If the plasma sample is haemolysed or separation has been delayed, the result of a plasma potassium concentration may still be clinically significant. For example, if the sample is visibly haemolysed and the plasma potassium concentration is only 2.8 mmol/L, this may indicate profound hypokalaemia; the laboratory staff should contact the requesting doctor directly to discuss the significance of the comment 'haemolysed specimen' on the report form.

Collection of Urine

Urine estimations performed on timed collections are expressed as units/time (for example, mmol/24hour); this figure is calculated by multiplying the concentration by the volume collected during the timed period. The accuracy of the final result depends largely on that of the urine collection and this is surprisingly difficult to ensure. Sometimes, if the patient is incontinent, or has prostatic hypertrophy or a neurological lesion which renders him incapable of complete bladder emptying, accurate collection is only possible if a catheter is inserted; because of the risk of urinary tract infection this is undesirable unless indicated for clinical reasons. However, most collection errors are due to a misunderstanding on the part of the nurse, doctor or patient.

For example, a 24-hour specimen may be collected between 08.00 hours on Monday and 08.00 hours on Tuesday. The volume *secreted by the kidneys* during this period is the crucial one. Urine already in the bladder at 08.00 hours on Monday was secreted earlier and should not be included; that in the bladder on 08.00 hours on Tuesday was secreted during the relevant 24 hours and *should* be included in the collection. Therefore, the procedure is as follows:

> *08.00 hours on Monday*. The bladder is emptied completely, whether or not the patient feels the need. *Discard the specimen*.

Collect all urine passed until:

> *08.00 hours on Tuesday.* The bladder is emptied completely, whether or not the patient feels the need. *Add the specimen to the collection.*

The shorter the period of collection, the greater the error if this procedure is not followed.

Before the collection is started a container should be obtained from the laboratory; this may contain a preservative to inhibit growth of bacteria capable of destroying the substance being estimated, but which does not interfere with the relevant assay. The patient must be told that there is preservative in the container which should not be discarded. If the preservative is, for example strong acid, he should be warned of this.

Collection of Faeces

Rectal emptying is usually erratic and, unlike that of the bladder, can rarely be performed to order. Results of faecal estimations of, for example, fat may vary by several hundred per cent in consecutive 24-hour collections. If the collection period lasted for weeks, the *mean* 24-hourly output would be very close to the true daily loss from the body into the intestinal tract. As a compromise most laboratories collect for periods of either three or five days. To render collection more accurate, some departments use orally administered 'markers' (p.**260**).

Faecal collections and estimations are time-consuming and unpleasant for all concerned. Only if *every* specimen passed during the collection period is sent to the laboratory will the timed result be reasonably accurate. Administration of purgatives, enemas or barium before or during the collection period alters conditions and invalidates the result. Before a patient starts a faecal collection for, for example, faecal fat estimation, it is important for the requesting doctor to look at the stool himself; there is little point sending 'sheep droppings' to the laboratory for such an estimation. If the stool is obviously foul-smelling, fatty and bulky there is no need for the test.

Labelling Specimens

Every specimen must be labelled accurately and the information should correspond with that on the accompanying request form in every detail. The date, and sometimes the time, of collecting the specimen should be included, and should be written at the time of collection, either by the doctor or by the phlebotomist. If it is done in advance the doctor may change his mind and the information will then be incorrect; there is also a very real danger of using a container with one patient's name on it for another patient's specimen.

BLOOD SPECIMENS

Specimens in wrongly labelled vials may cause danger to one or more patients. The date of the specimen is important both from the clinical point of view and, as discussed on p.**426**, to assess the suitability of the specimen for the assay requested. The time when the specimen was taken is especially important if, like plasma glucose, the concentration of the analyte varies during the day. If more than one specimen is sent for the same assay on one day, *each must be timed to determine in which order they were taken.*

URINE AND FAECAL SPECIMENS

Timed urine specimens should be labelled with the date and time of starting and completing the collection, so that the volume secreted in unit time can be calculated. Faecal collections are best labelled not only with the date and time, but also with the specimen number in the series; the absence of a specimen is then immediately obvious.

SENDING THE SPECIMEN TO THE LABORATORY

Many estimations can be performed rapidly if the result is needed urgently. However, batching specimens for assay is more economical in staff time and in reagents, as well as being easier to organize. Most laboratories like to receive non-urgent specimens early in the day. A constant 'trickle' may cause delay in reporting the whole batch, and possibly in noticing a result indicating the need for urgent action.

If a patient arrives late in the day it is preferable to delay taking the specimen until the next morning. If this is not possible, and if the result is not needed immediately, the specimen should be sent to the laboratory with a note to that effect. Plasma can then be separated from cells and stored overnight;

this service should not be abused, since it takes a long time to centrifuge and separate plasma from a large number of specimens; the chance of transposition of samples is increased.

In cases of true clinical emergency *the requesting clinician should notify the laboratory, preferably before the specimen is taken, indicating the reason for the urgency*, so that the laboratory may be ready to deal with the specimen as soon as it arrives. Usually a specimen not known to need urgent attention, and certainly one not accompanied by any clinical information, will be assumed to be non-urgent. *It is the clinician's responsibility to indicate the degree of urgency*. The words 'urgent, please phone' should only be

Table 24.5 Some extra-laboratory factors leading to false results

Cause of error	Some possible consequences
Keeping blood overnight before sending to the laboratory	High plasma K^+, total acid phosphatase, LD, HBD, AST, phosphate
Haemolysis of blood	As above, lower plasma ALP
Prolonged venous stasis during venesection	High plasma total and all fractions of protein, total calcium, lipids, total T_4
Taking blood from an arm with an infusion running into it	Electrolyte and glucose concentrations approaching composition of infused fluid. Dilution of everything else
Putting blood into wrong vial or tipping it from this into another vial	For example, EDTA or oxalate cause low plasma Ca^{2+}, with high Na^+ or K^+
Blood for glucose not put into fluoride	Low blood or plasma glucose
Failure to keep sample cool or delay separating and freezing plasma	Low PTH, ACTH, insulin
Palpation of prostate by rectal examination, passage of catheter, enema etc. in last few days	High tartrate-labile acid phosphatase and PSA
Biopsy of prostate	High tartrate-labile acid phosphatase and PSA
Inaccurately timed urine collection	Falsely timed urinary excretion values (for example, per 24 hours). False and erratic renal clearance values
Incorrect or no preservative	Falsely low result, for example, urea or calcium
Loss of stools during faecal fat collection or failure to collect for sufficiently long period between markers	False faecal fat results

used after contacting one of the senior laboratory staff to discuss the indication. Misuse of emergency services delays truly urgent results both by increasing the amount of work and by inducing cynicism in laboratory staff.

Table 24.5 summarizes some of the errors discussed in this chapter.

BEDSIDE INVESTIGATION

Traditionally, urine testing has been performed by medical or nursing staff in ward siderooms; results have varied in accuracy and usefulness. A large range of blood assays can now be performed near the wards or in clinics; examples include 'blood gases', glucose, bilirubin and sodium and potassium estimations. Although the idea is superficially attractive, especially because of the speed of obtaining the result in an emergency, there are many problems to be considered. Some of the more important of these include:

- the difficulty of training staff, particularly if there is a high turnover;
- the possibility of untrained staff performing the analyses and handling potentially infected specimens;
- the difficulty of technical maintainence of equipment and the supply and checking of reagents;
- the difficulty of ensuring correct quality assurance procedures and consequently of obtaining correct results;

- the considerable financial implications associated with duplication of apparatus and its potential misuse by clinical staff.

Whichever bedside investigations are performed, somebody must be ultimately responsible for the selection of the equipment, the choice of reagents, quality assurance programmes, safety and training. Preferably this should be a chemical pathologist or senior biochemist; if not he must be part of the team. Many of these bedside investigations duplicate those performed in the laboratory but, because of the constraints of equipment and reagents, *the results may be numerically different*. The doctor must be aware of the limitations when interpreting the results.

The subject is too complex to be dealt with fully here, but *it should be appreciated that it is safer to have no result than a wrong one*. No type of investigation in wards and clinics should be introduced or continued without full consultation and cooperation with the local laboratory.

Summary

1. The clinician's responsibility for contributing to the accuracy and speed of reporting results includes:

  - taking a suitable specimen of blood:
      at a time when an earlier procedure will not interfere with the result;
      from a suitable vein;
      with as little venous stasis as possible;
      with precautions to avoid haemolysis.
  - putting the specimen in the correct container;
  - labelling the specimen accurately;

- completing the request form accurately, including *relevant* clinical details, drug therapy and potential hazards such as infection;
- ensuring that safety regulations have been complied with;

- ensuring that the specimen reaches the laboratory without delay;
- collecting accurate and complete timed specimens of urine and faeces.

2. Bedside investigations should only be initiated and carried out in collaboration with the local laboratory.

Requesting Tests and Interpreting Results

25

REQUESTING TESTS

Why Investigate?

The clinician has a great many tests at his disposal. If used critically these often provide helpful information; if used without thought the results are at best useless and at worst misleading and dangerous. Writing a request form should not be considered as casting a magic spell which, in itself, will benefit the patient.

Investigations should be used:

- to diagnose disease;
- to assess the complications of the disorder or its treatment;
- to monitor treatment.

They should *not* be used to show how 'clever' the doctor is. Appropriate investigations should only be requested, if after taking a history and examining the patient, a differential diagnosis has been established. Intellectual satisfaction comes from deciding what one hopes to gain from the results of investigation and by achieving this aim as economically as possible in time and money. One test is not necessarily better than another because it is newer, more expensive or more difficult to perform; if it *is* better it should be used instead of, not as well as, the other one.

Over-investigation may actually harm, not help, the patient by causing him unnecessary discomfort or danger, delaying treatment, or more insidiously, by using resources that might be spent more usefully on other aspects of his care. Of course, under- is just as undesirable as over-investigation; the cost to the patient of omitting a necessary test is just as high as carrying out unnecessary ones.

Before requesting an investigation the clinician should ask himself:

- will the result, whether high, low, or normal, *affect my diagnosis?*
- *will the result affect my treatment?*
- *will the result affect* my assessment of the patient's *prognosis?*
- *can the abnormality* I am seeking *exist without clinical evidence of it.* If so, is such an abnormality dangerous and can it be treated?

If, after careful consideration, the answer to any of these questions is 'yes', the test should be performed, If the answer to *all* of them is 'no', there is no need for the test.

Sometimes the test may be necessary even if the clinical diagnosis is obvious. For example, both the clinical and biochemical features of overt hypothyroidism return towards normal once treatment is started, but it is usually necessary to continue such treatment for life. Later another doctor, seeing the patient for the first time, may only be able to confirm the original diagnosis by stopping treatment to see if the symptoms return. This could be avoided if an unequivocally low plasma T_4, with an unequivocally high TSH, concentration provided objective documentation.

Why not Investigate?

The student is warned against the following unqualified statements:

- *'It would be nice to know'.* Will it help the patient?
- *'We must document it fully'.* Will the extra documentation make any difference to the management of the patient, or even to the sum of medical knowledge?
- *'Everyone else does it'.* If they do they may be right, but do you know their reasons? Perhaps they too do it because everyone else does. Do not accept any statement from anyone (not even from this book)

uncritically. Reassess dogma continually. If you lack experience, at least examine the reasoning behind what you read or are taught; use the statements of 'experts' as working hypotheses until you are in a position to make up your own mind.

How Often Should I Investigate?

This depends on:

- *how quickly numerically significant changes are likely to occur.* For example, concentrations of the main serum protein fractions are most unlikely to change significantly in less than a week, and the plasma urea concentration will not change significantly during the first 12 hours of oliguria;
- *whether a change, even if numerically significant, will alter treatment.* For example, plasma transaminase activities may alter within 24 hours in the course of acute hepatitis. Once the diagnosis has been made this is unlikely to affect treatment. By contrast, the plasma potassium concentrations may alter rapidly in patients given large doses of diuretics and these

may indicate the need to instigate or to change treatment.

Investigations are very rarely needed more than once in 24 hours, except in some patients receiving intensive therapy. If they are, repeat only those that are essential. Being more selective helps to reduce laboratory costs and speed up the 'turn around' for results.

When is an Investigation 'Urgent'?

The only valid reason for asking for an investigation to be performed 'urgently' is that an earlier answer will alter the patient's management. This is very rare. More often an investigation is called 'urgent' because the doctor has:

- forgotten to request the test electively on a patient who arrived earlier and the result of which may be asked for during the ward round;
- failed to reach a firm diagnosis on emergency admission and is using unselective investigations in the hope that 'something will turn up'.

*I*NTERPRETING RESULTS

Before considering the diagnosis or treatment based on the analytical results the clinician should ask himself three questions.

- If it is the first time the test has been performed on this patient, *is it normal when the appropriate reference range is taken into account or abnormal with*

respect to the appropriate reference range?
- If it is abnormal, *is the abnormality of diagnostic significance* or is it a nonspecific finding?
- If it is one of a series of results, *has there been a change and, if so, is this change clinically significant?*

Is the Result Normal?

REFERENCE RANGES

By convention, a reference ('normal') range usually includes 95 per cent of the test results obtained from a healthy and frequently age- and sex-defined population. For the majority of tests the individual's results for any constituent are distributed around this mean in a 'normal' or Gaussian distribution, the 95 per cent limits being about two standard deviations from the mean. For other tests the reference distribution may be skewed, either to the right or to the left about the population median. Remember that 2.5 per cent of the results at either end will be outside the reference range; such results are not necessarily abnormal for that individual. All that can be said with certainty is that the *probability* that a result is abnormal increases the further it is from the mean or median until, eventually, this probability approaches 100 per cent. Furthermore, a normal result does not necessarily exclude the disease being sought; a test result within the population reference range may be abnormal for that individual.

Very few biochemical tests clearly separate a 'normal' healthy population from an 'abnormal' population. For most there is a range of values in which 'normal' and 'abnormal' overlap (Fig. 25.1), the extent of the overlap differing for individual tests. For each individual test, the percentage of patients correctly diagnosed with 'positive' test results (*diagnostic sensitivity*), the percentage of patients correctly diagnosed with 'normal' results (*diagnostic specificity*), and predictive value, if the prevalence of the disorder within the population is known, can be calculated.

The numerical value of a biochemical test, and consequently the reference range, is affected by various non-pathological factors including:

- physiological differences, such as sex and age;
- physiological variations, such as diurnal or circadian rhythms;

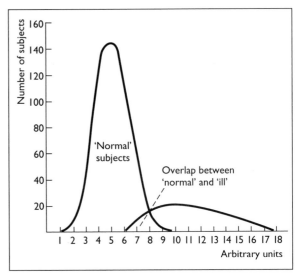

Fig. 25.1 Theoretical distribution of values for 'normal' and 'abnormal' subjects, showing overlap at the upper end of the reference range.

- methodological differences between laboratories.

No result of any investigation should be interpreted without consulting the reference range issued by the laboratory carrying out the assay. For this reason we have decided not to include a table of our reference ranges.

PHYSIOLOGICAL DIFFERENCES

Physiological factors affect the interpretation of results. For example there are:

- *sex differences* in the reference ranges of tests, such as plasma urate and iron (p.**370** and p.**378**) and, of course, of sex-hormone concentrations;
- *age related differences* in children, which have already been discussed (Chapter 17); other biochemical variables, such as plasma urea concentration, tend to rise with age especially in men;
- *geographical differences*, which may occur, either because of racial or environmental factors.

It is therefore clear that *we are not so much expressing 'normal' ranges, rather than the most usual ones for a given population.* A plasma urea concentration of 7.5 mmol/L (45 mg/dl) at the age of 20 suggests mild renal glomerular impairment, which may progress to clinically severe renal damage in later life; the same numerical result at the age of 70 suggests the same degree of renal impairment but, if it is not rising, the individual will usually die of some other disease before renal impairment becomes severe. In other words, this rising *mean* population concentration with age is not strictly normal and probably does reflect disease. However, in an individual there may be no change with advancing years. By contrast, many of those values found in children and at puberty, which differ from those in adults, are associated with growth and are therefore true physiological differences.

METHODOLOGICAL DIFFERENCES BETWEEN LABORATORIES

It has been pointed out that, even if the same method is used in the same laboratory, it is difficult clearly to define normality. Interpretation may sometimes be even more difficult if results obtained in different laboratories, using different analytical methods, are compared. Agreement between laboratories is close for most constituents. However, for others, such as plasma enzymes, different methods give different results. We have also seen that the definition of 'international units', in which the results of enzyme assays are usually expressed, does not, for example, include the temperature at which the assay is performed. Different laboratories, for various technical reasons, use temperatures varying from 25°C to 37°C; results on the same specimen at these two temperatures will differ significantly, although apparently expressed in the same units. Even if temperatures were standardized, results would still vary unless the substrate, pH and all the other variables were the same. If precision is acceptable one method is often no better than another *if the results are compared with the reference ranges for the laboratory in which the estimation was performed and if serial estimations are carried out by the same method.*

Is the Abnormality of Diagnostic Value?

Results of assays on plasma or serum only express extracellular concentrations. Moreover, some abnormalities are so non-specific as to be of no diagnostic or therapeutic significance.

RELATION BETWEEN PLASMA AND CELLULAR CONCENTRATIONS

Intracellular constituents are not easily sampled, and plasma concentrations do not always reflect the situation in the cells; this is particularly true for those constituents, such as potassium, which are at much higher intracellular than extracellular concentrations. A normal, or even high, plasma potassium concentration may be associated with cellular depletion if equilibrium across cell membranes is abnormal, such as in diabetic ketoacidosis. In the short term the aim should be to correct the plasma potassium concentration whatever the cell content, but the possibility of a rapid change associated with treatment of the underlying abnormality should be anticipated (p.**65**).

Plasma phosphate concentrations, like those of potassium, may fall as phosphate moves into cells when, for example, glucose and insulin are being infused. Hypophosphataemia does not necessarily indicate phosphate depletion.

RELATION BETWEEN EXTRACELLULAR CONCENTRATIONS AND TOTAL BODY CONTENT

The numerical value for a concentration depends not only on the total amount of the constituent measured, but also on the amount of water through which it is distributed. Hyponatraemia is rarely due to sodium depletion, but more often to an excess of water; total body sodium is usually increased, as in severe congestive cardiac failure (p.**48**). Conversely, hypernatraemia is much more often due to a water deficit than to sodium excess. It is very important to recognize these facts and to adapt treatment accordingly.

NON-SPECIFIC ABNORMALITIES

Plasma concentrations of, for example, albumin, calcium and iron, vary considerably in disorders unrelated to a primary defect in their metabolism.

The concentrations of all protein fractions including immunoglobulins, and of protein-bound substances, may fall by as much as 15 per cent after as little as 30 minutes recumbency, possibly due to fluid redistribution in the body. This may account, at least in part, for the low plasma albumin concentrations found in even quite minor illnesses. In-patients usually have blood taken early in the morning, while recumbent and tend to have lower plasma concentrations for these parameters than out-patients.

Most plasma calcium methods measure the total concentration, which includes the protein-bound and free-ionized fractions. Changes in albumin concentrations cause changes in those of the calcium bound to it, without alteration of the physiologically active free-ionized fraction; this can occur either artefactually, as discussed on p.**424**, or because of true changes in albumin. It is dangerous to try to raise the plasma total calcium concentration to within the reference range if there is significant hypoalbuminaemia since this may cause a high free-ionized concentration.

Plasma iron concentrations are very variable and fall in most types of anaemia, whether due to iron deficiency or not; it is dangerous to give iron to patients with anaemia, especially by the parenteral route, unless there is other, more reliable evidence of iron deficiency (p.**381**).

Has There Been a Clinically Significant Change?

Before one can interpret day-to-day changes in results and decide whether the patient's biochemical state has altered, one must know the degree of variation to be expected in results derived from a normal population.

REPRODUCIBILITY OF LABORATORY ESTIMATIONS

Most estimations should give results reproducible to well within five per cent; some, such as sodium and calcium, should be even more precise but the variability of, for example, some hormone assays is much greater. Changes of less than the precision of the method are not likely to be clinically significant.

PHYSIOLOGICAL VARIATIONS

There are physiological variations of both plasma concentrations and urinary excretion rates of many constituents; results may be incorrectly interpreted if this is not taken into consideration. Physiological variations may be:

- *regular*. Such changes occur throughout the 24 hour period (circadian or diurnal rhythms, like those of body temperature), or throughout the month.

 The time of meals affects plasma *glucose* concentrations; correct interpretation is often only possible if the blood is taken when the patient is fasting, or at a set time after a standard dose of glucose (p.**217**).

 The daily (circadian) variation of plasma cortisol is of diagnostic value (p.**106**), but superimposed on this regular variation, 'stress' will cause an acute rise. Plasma *iron* concentrations may fall by 50 per cent between morning and evening. To eliminate the unwanted effect of circadian variations blood should, ideally, always be taken at the same time of day, preferably in the early morning with the patient fasting. This is not usually possible, and these variations should be taken into account when serial results are interpreted.

 Some constituents vary monthly, especially in women (again, compare body temperature). These can be very marked, as in the results of *sex hormone* assays, which can only be interpreted if the stage of the menstrual cycle is known; plasma iron may fall to very low concentrations just before the onset of menstruation (p.**379**). Some constituents may also vary seasonally. Some of these changes, such as the relation between plasma glucose and meals, have obvious causes, but many appear to be regulated by the so-called 'biological clock', which is often predominantly affected by the alternation of light and dark.

- *random.* Day-to-day variations in, for example, plasma iron concentrations are very large and may swamp regular cycles (p.**379**). The causes of these are not clear, but they should be allowed for when serial results are interpreted. The effect of stress on plasma cortisol and other hormone concentrations, and the many factors affecting those of serum proteins, have already been mentioned.

CONSULTATION WITH LABORATORY STAFF

The object of citing the examples given in this and in the preceding chapter is to stress the pitfalls of interpreting laboratory results in isolation without relevent clinical information. Clinical findings are the lynch-pin of diagnosis and management, and usually, if the specimen has been taken with care, a diagnosis can be made and treatment instituted *by relating the result to the clinical condition of the patient.* If there is any doubt about the interpretation of a result, consultation between the clinician and chemical pathologist or biochemist can be mutually helpful.

Inevitably laboratory errors do occur, even in the best departments, but a discrepant result should not be assumed to be due to this cause before consultation. It may have already been checked in the laboratory. The staff will, in any case, repeat the test on that specimen if there is doubt, provided that it has been stored appropriately. Usually the first result agrees with the second. A fresh specimen should then be sent to the laboratory, after consultation to determine if and why the first was unsuitable. If the result is still the same, every effort must be made to find a clinical cause for the apparent discrepancy.

Laboratory staff of all grades take an active interest in the patients from whom they receive specimens and take trouble to keep the clinician informed of changes that may need urgent action; they may suggest further useful tests. The clinician should reciprocate by giving the chemical pathologist or biochemist information relevant to the interpretation of the results and of the clinical outcome of an interesting problem. Such exchange of ideas and information is in the best interest of the patient.

Summary

The clinician should use the laboratory intelligently and selectively. When interpreting test results the following facts should be remembered.

1. The relation of results to the reference range only indicates the *probability* that it is 'normal' or 'abnormal'.
2. There are physiological differences in

reference ranges, due, for example to sex and age; there are also day-to-day physiological variations.

3. There are small day-to-day variations in results due to technical factors; reference ranges may vary with the assay method used.

4. Plasma concentrations reflect those in the extracellular compartment, but do not always reflect intracellular ones. Plasma concentrations may depend more on the amount of extracellular water than on the body content of the analyte.

5. Changes in the concentration of a given constituent may be unrelated to a defect in the metabolism of that constituent.

Finally, when in doubt, two heads are better than one. Pathologists and clinicians bring different expertise to a problem and full consultation between the two is of great importance.

Appendix

1

UNITS IN CLINICAL CHEMISTRY

Results in clinical chemistry have been expressed in a variety of units. For example, concentration of electrolytes were formerly usually quoted in mEq/L, those of protein in g/100 ml and of cholesterol in mg/100 ml. The units used might vary for laboratory to laboratory: calcium concentrations might be expressed as mg/100 ml or mEq/L; in Britain plasma urea concentrations were expressed as mg/100 ml of urea, whereas the United States it is usual to report mg/100 ml of urea nitrogen. This situation can be confusing and with patients moving, not only from one hospital to another, but from one country to another, dangerous misunderstandings have arisen.

Système International D'Unités (SI Units)

International standardization is obviously desirable; such standardization has long existed in many branches of science and technology.

The main recommendations for clinical chemistry are as follows:

- if the molecular weight (MW) of the substance being measured is known, the unit of quantity should be the mole or a subunit of a mole.

$$\text{Number of moles (mol)} = \frac{\text{weight in g}}{\text{MW}}$$

In clinical chemistry millimoles (mmol), micromoles (μmol) and nanomoles (nmol) are the most common units.

- the unit of volume should be the litre. Units of concentration are therefore mmol/L, μmol/L or nmol/L.

EXAMPLES

Results previously expressed as mEq/L

$$\text{Number of equivalents (Eq)} = \frac{\text{weight in g}}{\text{Equivalent weight}}$$

$$= \frac{\text{weight in g} \times \text{valency}}{\text{MW}}$$

- In the case of univalent ions, such as sodium and potassium, the units will be numerically the same. A sodium concentration of 140 mEq/L becomes 140 mmol/L.
- For polyvalent ions, such as calcium and magnesium (both divalent), the old units are divided by the valency. For example, a magnesium of 2.0 mEq/L becomes 1.0 mmol/L.

Results previously expressed as mg/100 ml.
If results were previously expressed in mg/100 ml the method of conversion to mmol/L is to divide by the molecular weight (to convert from mg to mmol) and to multiply by 10 (to convert from 100 ml to L). Thus effectively the previous units are divided by a tenth of the molecular weight. For example, the molecular weight of urea is 60, and of glucose 180. A urea concentration of 60 mg/100 ml and a glucose concentration of 180 mg/100 ml are both equivalent to 10 mmol/L. The factor of 10 is, of course, only used for concentrations. The *total amount* of urea excreted in 24 hours in mg is numerically 60 times that in mmol.

EXCEPTIONS

- *Units of pressure* (for example mmHg) are expressed as pascals (or kilopascals – kPa). 1 kPa = 7.5 mmHg, so that a Po_2 of 75 mmHg is 10 kPa. Pascals are SI units.
- *Proteins.* Body fluids contain a complex mixture of proteins of varying molecular

weights. It is therefore recommended that the gram (g) be retained, but that the unit of volume be the litre (L). Thus a total protein of 7.0 g/100 ml becomes 70 g/L.
- 100 ml should be expressed as decilitre (dl).
- *Enzyme units* are not yet changed. Note that *the definition of international units for enzymes does not state the conditions of the reaction* (p.**437**).
- Some constituents, such as some hormones, are still expressed in 'international' or other special units.

Different countries are still at different stages of implementation. We have adopted the following policy.

- If old and new units are numerically the same, we have given only the SI units (for example, sodium and potassium).
- We express protein concentrations only as g/L.
- If it is generally accepted that SI units be adopted we have used these, with the equivalent old units in brackets.

A conversion table for some of the commoner results is listed in Table A.1. Note that:

1 mol	=	1000 mmol (millimoles)
1 mmol $(10^{-3}$ mol)	=	1000 µmol (micromoles)
1 µmol $(10^{-6}$ mol)	=	1000 nmol (nanomoles)
1 nmol $(10^{-9}$ mol)	=	1000 pmol (picomoles)

Table A.1 Some approximate conversion factors for SI units

	From SI units		**To SI units**	
Bilirubin	µmol/L × 0.058	= mg/dl	mg/dl ÷ 0.058	= µmol/L
Calcium				
Plasma	mmol/L × 4	= mg/dl	mg/dl ÷ 4	= mmol/L
Urine	mmol/24hours × 40	= mg/24 hours	mg/24hours ÷ 40	= mmol/24hours
Cholesterol	mmol/L × 39	= mg/dl	mg/dl ÷ 39	= mmol/L
Cortisol				
Plasma	nmol/L × 0.036	= µg/dl	µg/dl ÷ 0.036	= nmol/L
Urine	nmol/24hours × 0.36	= µg/24hours	µg/24hours ÷ 0.36	= nmol/24hours
Creatinine				
Plasma	µmol/L × 0.011	= mg/dl	mg/dl ÷ 0.011	= µmol/L
Urine	µmol/24hours × 0.11	= mg/24hours	mg/24hours ÷ 0.11	= µmol/24hours
PO_2	kPa × 7.5	= mmHg	mmHg ÷ 7.5	= kPa
PCO_2	kPa × 7.5	= mmHg	mmHg ÷ 7.5	= kPa
Glucose	mmol/L × 18	= mg/dl	mg/dl ÷ 18	= mmol/L
Iron	µmol/L × 5.6	= µg/dl	µg/dl ÷ 5.6	= µmol/L
TIBC	µmol/L × 5.6	= µg/dl	µg/dl ÷ 5.6	= µmol/L
Phosphate	mmol/L × 3	= mg/dl	mg/dl ÷ 3	= mmol/L
Proteins				
All serum	g/L ÷ 10	= g/dl	g/dl × 10	= g/L
Urine	g/L × 100	= mg/dl	mg/dl ÷ 100	= g/L
	g/24hours		No change	
Urate	mmol/L × 17	= mg/dl	mg/dl ÷ 17	= mmol/L
Urea				
Plasma	mmol/L × 6	= mg/dl	mg/dl ÷ 6	= mmol/L
Urine	mmol/24hours × 60	= mg/24hours	mg/24hours ÷ 60	= mmol/24hours
5-HIAA	µmol/24hours × 0.2	= mg/24hours	mg/24hours ÷ 0.2	= µmol/24hours
HMMA	µmol/24hours × 0.2	= mg/24hours	mg/24hours ÷ 0.2	= mmol/24hours
Faecal 'fat'	mmol/24hours × 0.3	= g/24hours	g/24hours ÷ 0.3	= mmol/24hours

Appendix

2

COMMON ABBREVIATIONS

ACE	Angiotensin converting enzyme
ACP	Acid phosphatase
ACTH	Adrenocorticotrophic hormone (corticotrophin)
ADH	Antidiuretic hormone (Pitressin; arginine vasopressin; AVP)
AIDS	Acquired immune deficiency syndrome
ALA	5-aminolaevulinate
ALP	Alkaline phosphatase
ALT	Alanine transaminase (GPT)
AMS	α-amylase
Anti-HB$_c$	Antibody to hepatitis B viral core
Anti-HB$_s$	Antibody to HB$_s$Ag
APRT	Adenine phosphoribosyl transferase
APUD	Amine-precursor uptake and decarboxylation
AST	Aspartate transaminase (GOT)
AVP	Arginine vasopressin (antidiuretic hormone; ADH)
BJP	Bence-Jones protein
BUN	Blood urea nitrogen (in mg/dl)
	= 28/60 $\times$ plasma urea in mg/dl
	(*or* 2.8 $\times$ plasma urea in mmol/L)
CAH	Congenital adrenal hyperplasia
CBG	Cortisol-binding globulin (transcortin)
CK	Creatine kinase
CoA	Coenzyme A
CRH	Corticotrophin releasing hormone
CSF	Cerebrospinal fluid
DDAVP	1-Deamino-8-D-arginine vasopressin (desmopressin acetate)
DNA	Deoxyribonucleic acid
DOC	Deoxycorticosterone
DOPA	Dihydroxyphenylalanine
Dopamine	Dihydroxyphenylethylamine

ECF	Extracellular fluid
EDTA	Ethylene diamine tetracetate (sequestrene)
EM Pathway	Embden-Meyerhof pathway (glycolytic pathway)
ESR	Erythrocyte sedimentation rate
FAD	Flavine mononucleotide
FFA	Free fatty acids (NEFA)
FMN	Flavine mononucleotide
FSH	Follicle-stimulating hormone (follitropin)
GDH	Glutamate dehydrogenase
GFR	Glomerular filtration rate
GGT	γ-glutamyltransferase (γ-glutamyltranspeptidase; γ-GT)
GH	Growth hormone (somatotrophin)
GnRH	Gonadotrophin-releasing hormone
GOT	Glutamate oxaloacetate transaminase (AST)
G-6-P	Glucose-6-phosphate
G-6-PD	Glucose-6-phosphate dehydrogenase
GPT	Glutamate pyruvate transaminase (AST)
GTT	Glucose tolerance test
HAV	Hepatitis A virus
HBD	Hydroxybutyrate dehydrogenase
HB$_s$Ag	Hepatitis B surface antigen
HCG	Human choriogonadotrophin
HDL	High-density lipoprotein
hGH	Human growth hormone
HGPRT	Hypoxanthine guanine phosphoribosyl transferase
5-HIAA	5-hydroxyindole acetate
HIV	Human immunodeficiency virus
HMMA	4-hydroxy-3-methoxy-mandelate (VMA)
HPL	Human placental lactogen
5-HT	5-hydroxytryptamine (serotonin)

5-HTP	5-hydroxytryptophan
ICD	Isocitrate dehydrogenase
ICF	Intracellular fluid
ICSH	Interstitial cell-stimulating hormone (LH)
IDDM	Insulin-dependent diabetes mellitus
Ig	Immunoglobulin
IGF	Insulin-like growth factor
LCAT	Lecithin cholesterol acyl transferase
LD	Lactate dehydrogenase (LDH)
LDH	Lactate dehydrogenase (LD)
LDL	Low-density lipoprotein
LH	Luteinizing hormone
MEN	Multiple endocrine neoplasia (pluriglandular syndrome)
MPS	Mucopolysaccharidosis
NAD	Nicotinamide adenine dinucleotide
NADP	Nicotinamide adenine dinucleotide phosphate
NEFA	Non-esterified fatty acids (FFA)
NIDDM	Non-insulin dependent diabetes mellitus
5′-NT	5′-nucleotidase (NTP)
NTP	5′-nucleotidase (5′-NT)
17-OGS	17-oxogenic steroids
11-OHCS	11-hydroxycorticosteroids ('cortisol')
17-OHCS	17-hydroxycorticosteroids (17-oxogenic steroids)
PBG	Porphobilinogen
PIF	Prolactin-release inhibitory factor
PP factor	Pellagra preventive factor
PRPP	Phosphoribosyl pyrophosphate
PSA	Prostatic specific antigen
PTH	Parathyroid hormone
PTHRP	Parathyroid hormone related protein
RF	Releasing factor (RH; liberin)

RH	Releasing hormone (RF; liberin)
RNA	Ribonucleic acid
RTA	Renal tubular acidosis
SG	Specific gravity
SGOT	Serum glutamate oxaloacetate transaminase (AST)
SGPT	Serum glutamate pyruvate transaminase (ALT)
SHBD	Serum hydroxybutyrate dehydrogenase (HBD)
SHBG	Sex-hormone binding globulin
T$_3$	Triiodothyronine
T$_4$	Thyroxine (tetraiodothyronine)
TBG	Thyroxine-binding globulin
TBPA	Thyroxine-binding prealbumin
TBW	Total body water
TCA cycle	Tricarboxylic acid cycle (Krebs' cycle; citric acid cycle)
TIBC	Total iron-binding capacity (usually measure of transferrin)
TP	Total protein
TPP	Thiamine pyrophosphate
TRF	Thyrotrophin-releasing factor (TRH)
TRH	Thyrotrophin-releasing hormone (TRF)
TSH	Thyroid-stimulating hormone (thyrotrophin)
UDP	Uridine diphosphate
UTP	Uridine triphosphate
VLDL	Very-low-density lipoprotein
VMA	Vanillyl mandelate (HMMA)
WDHA	Watery diarrhoea, hypokalaemia and achlorhydria (Verner-Morrison syndrome)
Z-E syndrome	Zollinger-Ellison syndrome

Index

The main page references are in **bold** type.